MW00782753

PSYCHOLOGICAL ASSESSMENT

EVIDENCE-BASED PRACTICE IN NEUROPSYCHOLOGY

Kyle Brauer Boone, Series Editor

Clinical Practice of Forensic Neuropsychology:
An Evidence-Based Approach
Kyle Brauer Boone

Psychological Assessment:
A Problem-Solving Approach
Julie A. Suhr

Psychological Assessment

A Problem-Solving Approach

Julie A. Suhr

THE GUILFORD PRESS

New York   London

© 2015 The Guilford Press
A Division of Guilford Publications, Inc.
370 Seventh Avenue, Suite 1200, New York, NY 10001
www.guilford.com

Printed in the United States of America

This book is printed on acid-free paper.

Last digit is print number: 9 8 7 6 5 4 3 2 1

The author has checked with sources believed to be reliable in her efforts to
provide information that is complete and generally in accord with the standards
of practice that are accepted at the time of publication. However, in view of the
possibility of human error or changes in behavioral, mental health, or medical
sciences, neither the author, nor the publisher, nor any other party who has
been involved in the preparation or publication of this work warrants that the
information contained herein is in every respect accurate or complete, and they
are not responsible for any errors or omissions or the results obtained from the
use of such information. Readers are encouraged to confirm the information
contained in this book with other sources.

Library of Congress Cataloging-in-Publication Data

Suhr, Julie A.
  Psychological assessment : a problem-solving approach / Julie A. Suhr.
    Includes bibliographical references and index.
  ISBN 978-1-4625-1958-3 (hardback : alk. paper)
  1. Psychodiagnostics.   2. Psychological tests.   I. Title.
  RC469.S88 2015
  616.89′075—dc23

                                                              2014030630

*To the many clients I have evaluated over my years
of training, teaching, and supervision*

*And to my students, from whom I have learned
more than they likely learned from me*

About the Author

Julie A. Suhr, PhD, is Professor of Psychology at Ohio University. Her current research interests include the effects of psychological (non-neurological) variables on neuropsychological performance and aspects of executive functioning in individuals with various neurological conditions. Dr. Suhr has taught graduate courses in personality assessment, intellectual assessment, and clinical neuropsychology, and supervises clinical assessments in the training clinic as part of the doctoral training program in clinical psychology.

Contents

PSYCHOLOGICAL ASSESSMENT

1

Introduction

"You see," he explained, "I consider that a man's brain originally is like a little empty attic, and you have to stock it with such furniture as you choose. A fool takes in all the lumber of every sort that he comes across, so that the knowledge which might be useful to him gets crowded out, or at best is jumbled up with a lot of other things so that he has a difficulty in laying his hands upon it. Now the skillful workman is very careful indeed as to what he takes into his brain-attic. He will have nothing but the tools which may help him in doing his work, but of these he has a large assortment, and all in the most perfect order. It is a mistake to think that that little room has elastic walls and can distend to any extent. Depend upon it there comes a time when for every addition of knowledge you forget something that you knew before. It is of the highest importance, therefore, not to have useless facts elbowing out the useful ones."

—SHERLOCK HOLMES, *A Study in Scarlet*

HOW THIS TEXT DIFFERS FROM MOST "ASSESSMENT" TEXTS

Although there are many assessment texts available to assist in the training of the next generation of assessors, they tend to be focused on training in testing rather than in assessment. Similarly, although there has been an important movement toward the practice of empirically based assessment in clinical work, thus far the empirical evidence for such has focused primarily on psychometric properties of specific tests or test batteries to answer very specific diagnostic questions. The goal of the present text is to present an empirically informed approach to the entire process of psychological assessment.

1

A Focus on Assessment, Not Testing

Assessment is a conceptual, problem-solving process of gathering dependable, relevant information about an individual in order to make an informed decision (American Psychological Association, 2000). At its heart, assessment is a decision-making process in which the assessor iteratively formulates and tests hypotheses by integrating data in a dynamic fashion (Hunsley & Mash, 2007). Like a good detective, a good assessor needs to know what information is relevant to gather, what tools are the most reliable and valid for gathering the relevant information, and the best methods for putting that information together in a way that allows for good decision making. In addition, the assessor needs to use that information in a way that benefits the person being assessed, and thus must effectively communicate both the assessment process and the decision or decisions resulting from that process to relevant individuals.

One vital "tool" essential for assessors to have in their toolbox is a comprehensive understanding of the processes involved in the administration, scoring, and interpretation of psychological tests. A competent assessor needs a competent understanding of psychometrics in order to critically consider the psychometric strengths and weaknesses of different assessment methods, including tests, for use with a particular client for a particular clinical purpose. However, testing and assessment are not the same thing, as assessment requires the integration of information collected from a number of sources, only one of which is formal test data (American Educational Research Association, American Psychological Association, & National Council on Measurement in Education, 1999). Although tests can be used to improve assessment decision making, they are not always used well. Furthermore, as with other tools, when tests are used by those who are not trained to use them well, they can actually detract from good decision making.

Whereas a competent assessor needs knowledge about tests and their psychometric properties, he or she also needs a comprehensive understanding of the science underlying human behavior (both normal and abnormal). Thus, a competent assessor must understand psychopathology, neuroscience and neuropsychology, health psychology, developmental psychology, and diversity issues, to name a few, in order to guide decisions about the appropriate questions to ask and the appropriate (test and nontest) data to gather for a particular client and a particular assessment goal. Furthermore, a competent assessor needs well-developed clinical skills for gathering data, interpreting and integrating data, and presenting the interpretation of evaluation results, as well as their implications, to clients and other referral sources.

Where does one begin learning the assessment process? Training programs (and beginning "assessment" textbooks) often start with (1) teaching students basic interpersonal skills relevant to clinical interviewing and (2) training students in psychometrics, administration, scoring, and interpretation of specific psychological tests in isolation. Although this approach is a good start and a critical foundation to assessment, there is so much more to assessment that an assessor must learn through continued training and experience. For example, even though an assessor may possess good clinical skills, such as being comfortable asking strangers difficult questions in what can be a stressful interaction, that assessor will not conduct a good intake interview until he or she has in his or her "brain-attic" the relevant biopsychosocial and developmental information needed to guide decisions about important questions to ask and data to gather. In addition, even though an assessor may have memorized all the diagnostic criteria for disorders based on a particular diagnostic system, and has learned to ask about them reliably in a structured diagnostic interview, the assessor will not use that tool accurately if he or she doesn't understand the underlying science of the disorders that he or she is simply asking about descriptively. Furthermore, although an assessor may know the psychometrics of any one psychological test, the assessment task at hand requires the assessor to integrate knowledge about results from that test with other assessment data, including the results of other tests and assessment data gathered using other methodology—a process that involves much larger and more integrative psychometric and statistical considerations. Those data, in turn, need to be integrated into a scientific understanding of the potential disorders or diagnoses (as well as normal human conditions) under consideration in order to interpret the findings accurately. In addition, the assessor needs to be aware of potential biases in decision making that affect every stage of the decision-making process, from the first hypotheses formed, the questions selected, the choice of data to gather, and the way in which those data are integrated together. Thus, it is not surprising that Acklin (2002, p. 15) stated that "competency in the field of assessment psychology is probably best viewed as an advanced postdoctoral specialization."

In 2002, the Board of Educational Affairs and Education Directorate of the American Psychological Association sponsored a Competencies Conference that outlined a model of training identifying specific foundational or functional competencies for psychological practice and described the development of these competencies in an additive fashion across various levels of training (Rodolfa et al., 2005). In 2009, the Competency Benchmarks workgroup articulated clearly defined competencies within these foundational and functional areas to guide programs in using the competency-based model in their training of students (Fouad et al., 2009). In the functional competency area of assessment, the student at the beginning level of training should be focused on developing basic knowledge of the scientific, theoretical, and contextual basis of assessment, including initial knowledge of the constructs being assessed, the psychometric properties of measures of those constructs, and how to administer and score traditional psychological measures as well as both standardized and nonstandardized clinical interviews. As noted above, these are the topics covered in most current assessment texts and in core assessment training at the predoctoral level. In addition, however, the beginning student should be developing (1) an appreciation of the decision-making complexities of reaching a diagnosis, (2) an awareness of the need for multiple sources of information to make a diagnosis or to conduct a case conceptualization, and (3) an understanding of the presentation of normal and abnormal behavior in the context of diverse individuals and contexts. These competencies develop as part of more advanced assessment courses and practica, as well as in crucial psychological breadth courses, and are core topics in the current text.

As students become more advanced in their training and are nearing readiness for internship, they are expected to apply their scientific knowledge in the accurate and consistent selection, administration, scoring, and interpretation of measures with attention to their psychometric properties and the population and context at hand; to adapt, as necessary, to environmental and client needs; and to integrate knowledge across diverse sources of data, with consideration of the strengths and limitations of those data, to inform clinical decision making. In addition, the more advanced students should be able to communicate assessment results in both written reports and in verbal report (e.g., a case presentation or feedback to the client). These are competencies that are expected to be developed prior to the internship year, and thus should also be the focus of formal assessment training during the predoctoral training years. Unfortunately, managed care has led to both underutilization of assessment in clinical practice and to a deemphasis on assessment training in graduate school, with most programs focusing on testing rather than on the problem-solving skills necessary to good assessment (Handler & Smith, 2012; Naglieri & Graham, 2012).

The current text takes the reader beyond a focus on the initial learning of basic assessment skills to using the scientific literature to address these other aspects of the entire assessment process. Using the competency training model, this text focuses on the level between that of the beginning graduate student who has not yet entered practical training and that of the student who is immersed in practical training at either the advanced practicum or beginning internship level. Thus, the present text includes a more integrative coverage of assessment competencies for beginning graduate students, so that they can gain an appreciation for "what comes next" after they have begun to tackle fundamental assessment tasks in isolation, but also for more experienced trainees who have mastered the foundational assessment competencies and are now conducting assessments during their more advanced training or internship. In addition, the text may serve as a "refresher course" for practitioners seeking to enhance their assessment competencies.

A Scientific Approach to the Detective Work of Assessment

The overall assessment approach advocated in this text is one in which the assessor considers him- or herself to be a "scientific detective." The decision-making processes essential to good assessment are, in fact, similar to those utilized by that most famous (if fictional) of detectives, Sherlock Holmes. Those not familiar with Sherlock Holmes and his creator, Sir Arthur Conan Doyle, may find it interesting that Doyle, who was a physician, chose to model the character of Sherlock Holmes after one of his own medical professors (Dr. Joseph Bell, a surgeon with expertise in diagnostic assessment). As is seen in Chapter 2, although Sherlock Holmes was assumed to be a master of deductive reasoning, he also provides models for the appropriate use of inductive reasoning in the decision-making process.

Like the detective viewing "evidence" through the lens of the magnifying glass, an assessor must view the data at hand through various lenses, knowing when to focus in and take a closer look, and knowing when the information has no clinical value. To be a good scientific detective, an assessor needs to know the science of many subfields in psychology, as mentioned above, and must use scientific knowledge from those fields to examine available assessment data through multiple lenses (i.e., multiple hypotheses that have been informed by that scientific literature). The assessor also needs to become aware of when his or her lenses have become "biased" in some way and take appropriate steps to address that bias. Furthermore, just as detective work is dynamic, so too is the assessment process. A scientifically minded detective knows that, as evidence flows in, evidence in support of or against the working hypothesis/hypotheses may change. So too an assessor must realize that the dynamic process of assessment may lead to changes in the weight of evidence leaning toward or away from various diagnostic considerations—depending on what is learned from the interview, from collaterals, from behavioral observations, from prior records, and from test scores—and that such a dynamic process may even affect what additional data need to be gathered beyond that initially conceptualized as relevant to the specific case.

There is no question that a scientifically minded assessor must, first and foremost, respect the validity of the data at hand, both that gathered directly by the assessor and that available from other sources. Thus, Chapter 6 focuses on the importance of understanding the psychometrics of assessment tools, including formal psychological tests; understanding the importance of standardized administration/data gathering; considering assessment factors that may affect the reliability and validity of any test or other assessment data in an individual setting; and considering decision-making issues related to interpreting any given test (and its subtests) in isolation. Because the focus of this text is assessment, not testing, the text does not include a comprehensive review of individual tests, but instead presents selected, well-validated psychological tests (Chapters 9–12) to illustrate key decision-making points about their use in assessment. It is hoped that these examples model (1) how assessors can use empirical methods for the selection and use of the most empirically validated tests for the specific assessment purpose under consideration; and (2) the need for assessors to update their knowledge of instruments they are accustomed to using, as new versions or updated psychometric and normative information become available.

As the most learned proponents of evidence-based assessment point out, an empirically based assessment approach is not just about the psychometric validity of any given psychological test in isolation, but also emphasizes the use of research and theory to (1) identify which constructs are most important to assess in any given case, (2) select the appropriate methods and measures used to assess those critical constructs, and (3) select the assessment process to undergo (Barlow, 2005; Hunsley & Mash, 2005, 2007). That assessment process requires integration of not only assessment data for multiple constructs across multiple methods of measurement, but integration with what is known about normal and abnormal development in relation to the particular constructs that are part of the presenting problems.

Assessment is inherently a decision-making task in which the assessor iteratively formulates and tests hypotheses by integrating data in a dynamic fashion. Indeed, examination of the evidence base for assessment should include evaluation of the accuracy and usefulness of this decision-making process, but at this point most of the existing literature on evidence-based assessment has focused on evidence for the value of specific tests or groups of tests for particular conditions (Barlow, 2005; Hunsley & Mash, 2005, 2007). Such "evidence" presumes that the first stages of the assessment process were already valid (determining which specific hypotheses—that is, diagnoses—to consider for the individual being assessed); yet, the decisions made in this first stage of assessment are critical to an ability to interpret the validity of the tests under consideration, and require scientific knowledge well beyond that of test psychometrics. A major competency for students to master prior to independent practice is that of empirically informed clinical decision making (Fouad et al., 2009), and there is an identified need for more of this training during the predoctoral years (Belar, 2009; Gambrill, 2005; Harding, 2007) Thus, in several chapters, the scientific literature pertaining to other critical aspects of the assessment process are discussed. Because good assessment requires integration and decision-making processes at every step of the assessment, Chapter 2 discusses the decision-making biases that can affect every stage of the assessment process. In addition, research-informed guidelines for obtaining and using important assessment data from sources beyond formal tests are presented in Chapter 8. Furthermore, although little evidence currently bears on the last stage of the assessment process (integration of multiple sources of assessment data to reach informed decisions), Chapter 13 focuses on this vital aspect of the assessment process. Overall, the goal of this text is to demonstrate that inductive and deductive decision making by a scientifically minded assessor can lead to more accurate decisions and better care.

Emphasis on the Use of a Developmentally Informed Biopsychosocial Lens

As previously mentioned, knowledge of psychopathology from developmental, neurobiological, psychological, and sociocultural perspectives is important to every stage of a scientifically supported assessment, from the initial hypotheses developed to selection of the relevant test and extratest data to gather all the way to how to integrate the available information to make clinical decisions. Thus, a developmentally informed biopsychosocial perspective (see Chapter 3) is a crucial "lens" for a scientifically minded detective to wear when conducting an assessment. Furthermore, knowledge of neurobiological, developmental, psychological, sociological, and cultural contributions to test behaviors and test performance is crucial not only to interpreting performance on individual tests, but also to integration of material across tests and nontest data and may be highly important to the formulation of recommendations following the evaluation.

To illustrate this point with a nonpsychological example, consider a fever. A person can self-report symptoms of a fever ("feeling hot"), an examiner can observe signs of the fever (flushed face, shivering), and the fever can even be measured with a standardized instrument (thermometer). However, none of that information explains *why* the person has the fever, which is essential to its correct treatment. Now consider the example of depressed mood. A person can self-report symptoms of depressed mood ("feeling sad"), an examiner can observe signs of the depressed mood (psychomotor retardation, restricted affective expression), and the depressed mood can even be measured with standardized (self-report) instruments. However, none of that provides information that explains potential contributory factors to the depressed mood, which could include neuroendocrine problems, brain damage, family history of depression, stressful life events, difficulty coping with other more serious psychological disorders, etc., and this information is essential to its correct treatment (and even to whether the person's depressed mood is consistent with any particular psychological diagnosis). Thus, a scientifically minded assessor is one who has adequate knowledge of developmental, psychological, cultural, sociological, and medical contributions to psychological complaints and concerns and examines the client's presenting, observed, and measured history and current symptoms through each of these informed lenses.

It is important to note that, in proposing the use of a biopsychosocial lens in assessment, the present text does not advocate any particular therapeutic orientation or etiological lens, but rather a consideration of all potentially relevant causal factors to the client's presenting concerns, based on existing scientific knowledge of both normal and abnormal human behavior. Just as psychologists who wear only a biological or only a sociological lens when assessing a client will miss relevant information, psychologists who wear the lens of only one specific psychotherapeutic orientation, regardless of the nature of the individual client's presentation, will view whatever the client brings to the very first session in a biased fashion, by focusing assessment attention only on issues consistent with that theoretical lens. It is also important to note that, even if there appear to be medical contributions to a presenting concern (which may as yet be undiagnosed), this does not entirely preclude a psychological approach to treatment (though it may certainly indicate a need for medical assessment/treatment in addition to psychotherapy, and in some cases, may suggest that psychotherapy is not indicated). What this text advocates for is the careful definition of the problems or concerns presented by a client and the gathering of information on all potential developmental, biological/medical, psychological, and sociocultural contributions to that client's presentation (i.e., a problem-focused assessment).

It is important for the reader to note that, because the focus of this book is on assessment for the purpose of understanding a client's presenting condition and the etiological factors that contribute to that presentation, there is little focus on psychological measures that have been specifically validated for the purposes of case conceptualization in treatment planning. Certainly, once an assessor has conducted a valid assessment for understanding the etiological factors relevant to the presenting concern (and has potentially reached a diagnosis), and who has determined that psychotherapy might be indicated for the client, the assessor might administer additional psychological measures specifically developed and validated for the purposes of case conceptualization/treatment planning. Those measures typically place the client's symptom complex into a particular therapeutic orientation and/or are used for following a client's progress through therapy. However, measures of case conceptualization and treatment outcome are not necessarily valid measures for the purposes of initial assessment and thus are beyond the purposes of the present text. For further information on empirically validated measures specific to these clinical purposes, readers are referred to recently published materials that provide excellent summaries of such measures (e.g., Antony & Barlow, 2010; Hunsley & Mash, 2008b).

A Focus on Assessment That Does Not Always Lead to Diagnosis

When one wears the lens that sees the only goal of assessment as one of confirming (or disconfirming) a particular diagnosis, that lens may be biased in that it can lead the assessor to the wrong conclusion, due to faulty information seeking and decision making. For example, consider the following case: A female in her early 30s was referred for treatment of her anxiety disorders. She had been diagnosed with social anxiety and generalized anxiety disorder by another psychologist, who administered several self-report questionnaires focused on DSM-IV symptoms of both disorders, as well as a structured diagnostic interview. However, upon meeting the client, it was clear that the other psychologist had merely asked the client whether she had any medical disorders (with the limited "exclusionary" questions in the structured interview), rather than fully considering the possible contribution of medical or physical conditions to her presentation. The client's appearance (bulging eyes) and other symptoms that she reported upon questioning (changes in menstrual cycle, issues with her skin) led the second psychologist to refer the client to a physician for further evaluation, and the client was eventually diagnosed with Graves' disease, which is known to include symptoms of anxiety, irritability, sleep problems, rapid heart rate, tremor and sweating, all of which at first glance (and with shallow focus only on descriptive symptomatology) would have been consistent with a number of anxiety disorder diagnoses. Had the second assessor focused only on the referral question, only asked questions about symptoms, and given only cursory attention to possible medical conditions by merely asking about previous medical diagnoses, the client would have been harmed: The etiological factor that was the primary cause of her "anxiety" symptoms would not have been identified, and she would have received unnecessary psychotherapy for symptoms that were entirely related to her medical condition.

Unfortunately, in a world in which "informed" clients present for evaluation insisting that they "know" what their diagnosis is, and where there are potential biases (e.g., compensation for services) for an assessor to "find" a diagnosis, this may be the most common biased lens that psychologists (and other mental health professionals) wear. The overfocus on a need to identify a specific diagnosis can bias the assessment from the moment it begins, including the referral question (e.g., "Please assess for depression") or the first comment the client makes in the first session (e.g., "I think I have ADHD"). Again, one main goal of this text is to emphasize that assessment should be problem-focused and not diagnosis-focused, should go beyond psychological diagnosis, and in fact may not lead to a psychological diagnosis. As Exner and Erdberg (2002) emphasized, "psychodiagnosis" is much more than simply placing a diagnostic label on a person. It is a multitest procedure to examine and assess the person as a unique entity, including all of his or her strengths and weaknesses as well as the person's awareness and insight into his or her presenting problems, the developmental nature of the presentation, and the potential etiological contributions to all of the above—all of which may influence treatment goals or approach. Two people with same psychological diagnosis are still two unique people in many other respects and actually are often still quite unique in their overall symptom pattern (and thus in their treatment needs).

Unfortunately, many factors lead to a restricted focus on assessment for diagnosis only, including a bias toward the assumption that quick screening and immediate decisions are equivalent to a comprehensive assessment. Assessment occurs in diverse contexts, and a scientifically minded assessor recognizes the differences between screening evaluations and more comprehensive assessment approaches that allow for integration across disparate sources of assessment data and use of instruments that are more accurate and less likely to result in false-positive diagnoses. Such differences are considered further in Chapters 6, 9, 11, and 12. A bias toward assessment as a diagnostic-only tool also arises from biases in our culture and in reimbursement systems for diagnosing conditions to reinforce "finding" a reimbursable label for clients. This issue is discussed further in

Chapter 2. However, a bias toward assessment as serving only a diagnostic function can also occur because early training in assessment often focuses only on specific tests for specific diagnoses and specific methods to reach a diagnosis.

The goal of this text is to provide some correction for this overall bias by providing additional information on the scientific foundation for the entire assessment process beyond just diagnosis. On the other hand, sometimes diagnosis is highly appropriate; the goal of this text is not to bias assessors against using what can be an important communication tool (if done correctly). Instead this text presents a balanced viewpoint on the relationship of diagnosis to the process of assessment. To minimize a diagnostic bias, assessors should remember that assessment should focus on the person and his or her problems in their full developmental and biopsychosocial context.

AN EMPHASIS ON ASSESSMENT AS A THERAPEUTIC PROCESS

There are some psychologists (and other mental health professionals) who believe that doing any sort of assessment prior to beginning therapy will "bias" them in some way in their treatment of the client. However, such sentiments seem to be mostly aimed against the idea of using standardized testing instruments that are focused on reaching a diagnosis. Although I share those concerns about the overfocus on diagnoses only in assessment, I also caution clinicians against "throwing the baby out with the bathwater" and assuming there is no value to assessment prior to treatment. Such a viewpoint does not acknowledge that (1) in order to correctly treat a person, you have to know "what is wrong"; and (2) talking with a person and making behavioral observations about him or her during the course of therapy *is* assessment (albeit limited). Individuals with this belief also do not recognize the biased lens of their therapeutic orientation, which can lead to bad decision making, because it will focus their attention on only certain aspects of a client's presentation and cause them to ignore other aspects that may be important to fully understanding the client's situation (see Chapters 2 and 3).

As Exner and Erdberg (2002) pointed out, assuming that relevant assessment information will "emerge" during therapy means a much slower and less validated approach to data gathering. "No one would go into surgery or begin some other form of medical intervention without first being assured that the relevant tests had been completed and that the attending physician had a good understanding of all the issues and treatment alternatives" (Exner & Erdberg, 2002, pp. 11–12). Clinicians who fail to conduct adequate assessments prior to beginning therapy are potentially practicing in an unethical manner, by not basing their decision making on adequate evidentiary data to support their conclusion (American Psychological Association, 2010; Butcher, 2002). Furthermore, because results of assessment often lead to consequences for the individual being assessed, assessment in itself can be viewed as an intervention.

Assessment is necessary to treatment, regardless of diagnosis. Although diagnosis will certainly influence treatment decisions, an assessor needs to consider assessment data beyond any diagnosis to make effective treatment decisions. Even within medicine, the idea that specific symptoms dictate specific treatment is oversimplified and leads to poor assessment. For example, whether a pattern of sinus symptoms is due to viral or bacterial infection is vital information toward determining the treatment for the same symptom complex. Similarly, in the case of the person with "anxiety," above, her symptom picture met DSM-IV symptom criteria for two different anxiety disorders, yet neither would be addressed successfully by psychotherapy, even if empirically supported treatments for anxiety had been provided, because the major etiological contribution to her symptom pattern was neuroendocrine in nature. Even when a psychological disorder *is* present, data such as past and present contributing biopsychosocial factors, levels of current impairment/dysfunction, and presence/absence of inter- or intrapersonal supports and strengths may influence treatment decisions. Assessors should remember that assessment should focus on the person in his or her context and should ultimately be therapeutic, even if the final "diagnosis" (or lack thereof) is not the answer the person seeks. Literature on therapeutic assessment is presented in Chapter 14 to support the contention that an assessor should wear the lens of therapeutic assessment from the moment the case begins, not just at the point of feedback.

The Use of Case Examples

Although the text presents case examples from my (or my colleagues') clinical experience as a way to illustrate key issues in an empirically based approach to assessment, they have often been changed in ways not germane to the main clinical issue but to de-identify the individuals described. In some instances, the cases are prototypical examples merged across several similar clients to represent the critical issue at hand. Furthermore, although quotes from clients are included, they have been slightly paraphrased in ways that remain true to what was said but to further protect against identification.

2

Assessment as a Decision-Making Process

Like all other arts, the Science of Deduction and Analysis is one which can only be acquired by long and patient study, nor is life long enough to allow any mortal to attain the highest possible perfection in it.
—From "The Book of Life," an article by Sherlock Holmes quoted in *A Study in Scarlet*

Because assessment is a dynamic decision-making process, it is vulnerable to decision-making errors at any point in an evaluation, beginning with the referral question/statement itself. Errors can be made in the types of questions that are asked, the hypotheses that are considered, the data that are gathered (or not gathered), and the way in which data are integrated to reach a conclusion. Often these errors are the result of decision-making biases. Such biases can cause an assessor to collect the wrong data, fail to collect the relevant data, and/or to examine the worth of data collected through the wrong interpretive "lens." The purpose of this chapter is to review research on the decision-making process and to discuss the decision-making errors and biases that have been identified as important when health care professionals are making diagnostic decisions. Examples of these decision-making errors and biases are presented throughout the text to illustrate how important it is to be aware of their pervasive nature and to take proactive steps to minimize their effects on assessment decisions.

Diagnostic decision making has been described in the medical literature as a "wicked problem" (Rittel & Webber, 1973). This blunt description is not surprising, given that 75% of diagnostic failures in medical settings are due to failed decision-making processes (Graber, Franklin, & Gordon,

2005). Diagnostic decision making may be even more "wicked" in the realm of psychological diagnosis, where there are no gold standards for judging accuracy of the diagnostic decision. This absence of gold standards renders potential diagnoses only better or worse than other alternatives, rather than unambiguously true or false. Psychological assessors should note that this dilemma is present in some medical decision making as well, particularly in areas of medicine that rely more heavily on self-report for diagnosis, rather than on objective laboratory findings.

Another issue adding further complexity to the decision-making process in psychological assessment is that psychological disorders are often comorbid. Much of the research on accuracy of decision making is focused on narrowing to one decision; within the realm of real-world assessment, the typical decision is arriving at the correct diagnosis. Yet, given the high co-occurrence of mental health disorders (American Psychiatric Association, 2013), narrowing the possibilities to one diagnosis is not necessarily the correct decision to make. Thus, existing research on diagnostic decision making actually oversimplifies this "wicked problem" because there is no consideration of the fact that sometimes there is more than one diagnosis and sometimes there is no diagnosis. Furthermore, decision-making research minimizes the reality that real-world assessment decisions must often be made under incredible time and resource pressures (Crupi, Tentori, & Lombardi, 2009). Regardless of these limitations, existing decision-making research can still be useful as a guide to understanding the decision-making processes that occur within an assessment context and help assessors to identify where those processes can go wrong.

INDUCTIVE AND DEDUCTIVE REASONING

Generally, decisions are made using both inductive and deductive reasoning. In inductive reasoning, a decision maker starts with specific observations and moves to broader generalizations about the likely implications of those observations. Thus, inductive reasoning is a "bottom-up" approach that begins with specific observations (which, in assessment, may include reported symptoms or complaints, observed behavior/mental status of a client, test scores, etc.), detection of potential patterns within those initial observations, and formulation of potential explanations for those patterns (which may include potential diagnoses to consider). Generally, inductive reasoning is viewed as a more open-ended and exploratory process and certainly should not be the isolated process used to reach a decision.

Conversely, in deductive reasoning, an assessor starts with a general concept, idea, and/or hypothesis and works down to specific conclusions or observations that would be expected if the concept, idea, or hypothesis were correct. In this more "top-down" approach to reasoning in assessment, an assessor might start with a hypothesized diagnosis, consider what he or she would expect to observe if the diagnosis were to be confirmed (and, ideally, what should be observed or not observed to *disconfirm* the diagnosis), and then gather the relevant data to confirm or disconfirm the hypothesized diagnosis. As a result, deductive reasoning tends to be much more structured and confirmatory, rather than exploratory.

Real-world decision making is a dynamic process that often alternates between deductive and inductive reasoning, and both methods of reasoning have their strengths and weaknesses. As noted in the quote at the beginning of this chapter, the character Sherlock Holmes is best known as an expert in deductive reasoning, but there are many hints throughout his stories that he was a master of inductive reasoning and that he recognized the potential for error that can result from using deductive reasoning too soon in an assessment of a situation. For example, in *The Adventure of the Speckled Band*, when Holmes discusses with the good Dr. Watson his initial errors in reasoning about the case, he says, "I had come to an entirely erroneous conclusion, which shows, my dear Watson, how dangerous it always is to reason from insufficient data" (Doyle, 1892/2011, VIII. The Adventure of the Speckled Band, para 248). He acknowledges his assessment error of jumping from specific observation to a conclusion too early in the data-gathering process, and then using deductive reasoning to further "confirm" observations based upon that faulty deduction—an error that was almost fatal to him in this case. Similarly, in both *A Study in Scarlet* and *A Scandal in Bohemia*, Holmes comments specifically on the "capital mistake" it is to theorize before you have evidence or data, because when a person does so, "Insensibly one begins to twist facts to suit theories, instead of theories to suit facts" (Doyle, 1892/2011, I. A Scandal in Bohemia, para 24).

Traditional models of reasoning and decision making, as applied to diagnostic decision making, emphasized the distinction and the dynamic relationship between inductive and deductive reasoning. For example, the Michigan State medical inquiry project led to the development of the "hypothetical-deductive" model of medical reasoning, based on review of the diagnostic process in medical data (Elstein, Shulman, & Sprafka, 1978). The researchers showed that clinicians typically formulate a limited number (three to five) of initial hypotheses from specific observations, using inductive reasoning, and then consider these hypotheses when obtaining additional clinical evidence, using deductive reasoning to narrow the hypotheses until a final diagnosis is made. More recent models of decision making have considered the cognitive processes that most likely underlie these different stages of the diagnostic reasoning process.

THE DUAL-PROCESS MODEL OF DECISION MAKING

Recent decision-making models describe two systems, or processes, that underlie decision making as applied to a diagnostic context. The first system is nondiscursive and intuitive in nature and the second is discursive and analytical in nature. The intuitive system tends to be fast, automatic, and reflexive, requiring minimal cognitive effort (in fact, it often occurs at an unconscious level), and the principal mode of operation is often assumed to be pattern recognition/matching—an inductive process. The analytical system, in contrast, is slow, deductive, deliberate, rule-based, and linear in its reasoning. This system requires a great deal of cognitive effort and time (Croskerry, 2009; Glockner & Witteman, 2010; Norman & Eva, 2010).

Generally, it is assumed that clinicians begin their reasoning with the intuitive system because humans are "cognitive misers" and default to a state of using the fewest cognitive resources (Croskerry, 2009). Thus, it is likely that the first initial hunches or hypotheses in the beginning of a clinical assessment arise from the inductive system in a relatively automatic and mostly unconscious fashion (Marcum, 2012; Norman, 2009). If clinicians are able to obtain a "diagnostic match" using this less cognitively effortful system, they quickly move to deductive confirmation of the diagnosis. However, in circumstances where there is a less than clear automatic match so that the pattern is not recognized through the intuitive system, or where there are conflicting data, clinicians use the second, more cognitively effortful analytical system to "deliberately deliberate" about the data.

Developers of versions of this decision-making model argue that, although it is assumed that decision makers usually start with the intuitive system, they typically oscillate back and forth between the two systems. In addition, most dual decision-making models also include cognitive processes that provide feedback to the two systems, particularly when their conclusions are in conflict with one another (Arango-Munoz, 2011; Croskerry 2009; Marcum, 2012; Proust, 2010; Stanovich, 2011). Marcum (2012) argued that a feedback system (which serves as a metacognitive monitor in his model) not only provides corrective feedback during a specific decision-making situation, but also serves to reinforce or alter the cognitive processes a decision maker engages in, allowing for more efficient and accurate decision making over time, as a result of experience.

Some researchers argue that the intuitive system is more vulnerable to error than the analytical system because the analytical system has better reliability (because it typically follows standard rules) (Croskerry, 2009). However, there is potential for error in both systems. It is also important to note that, whereas reliability is necessary for validity, it does not guarantee validity; the decision-making rules and algorithms will only work to the extent that (1) they are well spelled out and well validated; and (2) the user gathered the correct information, using valid techniques, to apply the rules. In addition, the intuitive system is a normal, evolutionarily adaptive, and efficient system used in many cognitive processes, including visual perception, social perception, and learning/memory retrieval (Glockner & Witteman, 2010; Norman, 2009), and can lead to accurate decisions as long as the information it is fed is unbiased, representative, and sufficient. There are some data to suggest that there might be different contexts/situations in which it is best to rely on the two different systems (Elstein, 2009), and that using a combination of both processes reduces the likelihood of diagnostic errors (Norman & Eva, 2010).

SPECIFIC SOURCES OF ERROR IN CLINICAL JUDGMENTS

Research has identified diverse sources of error in clinical judgment and decision making, many of which are well characterized in a quote from Kamphuis and Finn (2002): "We expect to see what we are used to seeing, we see what we expect to see, and we inquire about what we expect to see, rather than about what we don't expect to see" (p. 262). Below is a brief review of some of the major sources of error that an assessor should watch for when conducting an assessment. As noted above, although researchers and decision-making theorists have suggested that the intuitive system is more vulnerable to these sources of error, thinking about these heuristics only as cognitive errors or biases belies their long-standing role as generally efficient mental strategies for guiding much decision making in real life. In addition, the deductive/analytical system is also vulnerable to decision-making errors. Furthermore, because much deductive reasoning starts with the output of the inductive/intuitive system, these errors are important to understand; use of a deductive process to confirm (and not disconfirm) already faulty reasoning may only further convince the assessor that he or she has reached the correct decision when that is not the case.

Representativeness Bias

A well-studied phenomenon in reasoning and decision-making processes, and one that is likely more of a vulnerability for the inductive/intuitive system, is the representativeness bias. As mentioned above, using the term "bias" always implies an error; perhaps it is more appropriate to call this a representativeness *heuristic* because in both everyday and diagnostic decision making, representativeness heuristics often work. Representativeness heuristics are typically based on actual data: some observations, signs, symptoms, and characteristics are more strongly related to certain diagnoses. Thus, using a representativeness heuristic can frequently yield efficient and accurate results. However, whether or not those results are efficient and accurate depends on the accuracy of the representativeness heuristic.

Although there are many examples of specific symptoms or observations being correlated with specific diagnoses, a correlative relationship is not enough to take an inductive leap from specific behavioral observation or symptom to one diagnostic hypothesis. The ability to make such an inductive leap is also dependent upon the *specificity* of the correlative relationship between symptom and hypothesized diagnosis, as well as the prior probabilities (base rates) of the diagnosis being considered. For example, memory complaints certainly correlate with head injury. However, memory complaints are also commonly seen in many other neurological as well as non-neurological disorders. In fact, memory complaints occur with high base rates in nonclinical samples. Thus, starting with a presenting symptom of "memory complaints" and automatically "matching" the symptom to a diagnosis of head injury is potentially a representativeness error. Similarly, a client's report of "attacks of anxiety" should call to an assessor's mind a possible diagnosis of an anxiety disorder, but should also call to mind many other psychological, as well as medical, disorders as potentially representative of this complaint (consider the person with anxiety presented in Chapter 1). In each of these examples, other potential diagnoses and conditions also correlate with the presenting symptoms, and some of those potential diagnoses (including no diagnosis) may occur with much higher base rates than the first disorder considered a match to the symptom. Unfortunately, in the real world, clinicians often make a leap from a specific symptom or symptoms to a "representative" disorder without consideration of the specificity of the symptom or symptoms—and then, in a time-pressured situation, prematurely "close" the diagnostic decision-making process, or, in an erroneous deductive reasoning process, gather select assessment information that will confirm the faulty initial reasoning without consideration of disconfirming evidence or alternative hypotheses.

The representativeness heuristic likely interacts with other biases (e.g., the availability bias) and likely contributes to others (e.g., the confirmatory bias). Thus, although the representativeness heuristic can be accurate to the degree that symptoms correlate with the likelihood of a certain disorder, it can place too much decisional "weight" on highly representative evidence and too little decisional weight on relevant prior probabilities for a particular diagnosis and/or discrepant evidence. For example, based on an assessor's own experience, certain symptoms may seem more representative of certain diagnoses than others, or a potential disorder may seem more common than it actually is. In fact, there are data to suggest that when a clinician has experience with only one specific disorder, such as occurs in a specialty clinic, the disorder that is the focus in that clinic takes on a higher mental probability in the clinician's head and may thereby make what is a low base-rate disorder seem more common (Norman & Eva, 2010). The representativeness heuristic can also be influenced by the prior setting in which a clinician worked. So, for example, if the clinician worked in an inpatient setting and often saw people with this complaint, but then worked in an outpatient setting where the overall base rate of severe psychopathology is much lower, the clinician is likely to give too much cre- dence to that complaint because his or her concept of representativeness has been formed with the wrong population in mind.

Availability Bias

The availability bias occurs when information that is most readily acces- sible or most easily recalled unduly influences the decision at hand. This could be the first information presented by the person (primacy bias), such as the presenting concern or referral question, but it could also be the most recent information (recency bias) obtained during the testing, such as the results of a personality measure. Primacy and recency biases have been well documented in the decision-making literature (Tverskey & Kahne- man, 1973, 1974).

The most available information may also be the most vivid and detailed information given by the individual during the assessment. Consider the following case: A family physician referred a 70-year-old individual for eval- uation for "late-onset schizophrenia." The physician noted that the patient was experiencing visual hallucinations, and this unusual and highly salient symptom overrode other diagnostic considerations during the physician's workup. However, given the extremely low base rate of the onset of a first episode of schizophrenia in a 70-year-old individual with no family history of schizophrenia, the physician should have considered other higher base-rate disorders that may also be associated with hallucinations. In this case, the neuropsychological evaluation, together with neurological workup, eventu- ally led to diagnosis of Alzheimer's disease with Lewy bodies. Unfortunately, the physician had already begun treatment with antipsychotic medications based on the diagnosis of schizophrenia; fortunately, this error was quickly addressed after the more thorough assessment was completed. Because the physician was unused to such unusual symptoms being reported by his patients, the presence of hallucinations easily overwhelmed the physician's attention to and recall of any other information (e.g., any reports of memory problems, or perhaps evidence of an inability to complete independent acts of daily living) that would have led to a consideration of other diagnostic hypotheses; for that physician, the most available diagnosis to go with the salient symptom (hallucinations) was schizophrenia.

The presence of availability biases can play a role in the information-gathering process. For example, the initial referral request ("Assess for X") may lead the assessor to think only of follow-up questions pertaining to that bit of information that was most readily recalled. Similarly, as the assessor decides upon other information to obtain (including what tests to adminis-ter or records to send for), whatever information is available at first thought may bias those choices. The presence of an availability bias may also play a role in the interpretation of the assessment data. When so much informa-tion is available about a client, the assessor may more easily recall both the information that was first presented (perhaps the initial "diagnostic" presentation) and/or information that was most recently reviewed (perhaps a test score or scores from something given last in a test battery), and such information will tend to hold more weight in the overall decision, simply due to its being more readily accessible to the assessor.

Similarly, if the client presented a piece of data that was particularly unusual or described in vivid detail, that information is more likely to come into conscious access when the assessor is trying to put together all the available information. Unfortunately, this is a bias frequently encountered in cases of individuals who are convinced that they have incurred severe and impairing cognitive deficits from a mild head injury from some time in their past. A clinician subject to availability biases will give great weight to the first thing learned from such individuals (the presenting concern of severe memory problems—a primacy bias) and great weight to the test results indicating impaired memory (recency bias), while ignoring the hours (and sometimes days) of observations and testing in between, during which the client was able to give detailed and accurate accounts of past and present behavior, able to remember the examiner, and able to find and drive to the clinic. The availability bias may also influence the clinician to ignore records and other extratest evidence indicating that the injury itself was not severe and that the person is continuing to function independently in the home or (in many cases) still working or attending school successfully, in contradiction to the obtained test scores.

The examples above document availability bias that occurs because of information, due to its primacy, recency, or vividness/saliency, presented by the client. Other information that may be more readily accessible in an assessment, and thus create bias, may originate in the assessor, not the client. For example, as noted above in the discussion of the representative bias, the assessor's own personal experience with particular disorders may make certain diagnoses and their presentations more accessible to his or her mind, leading the assessor to call them up more readily as hypotheses to consider and overriding their base rate.

Hindsight Bias

Hindsight bias occurs when an assessor overestimates the probability of a particular diagnosis when the diagnosis is already known. This could happen in an assessment situation if an individual mentions already receiving a certain diagnosis, or if medical records show the diagnosis was already given. However, an assessor should always consider the validity of the procedure that was undergone by the prior evaluator to reach that diagnosis. For example, it is not uncommon in some community mental health settings for an individual to be seen in a crisis, and for a very brief intake evaluation to result in several provisional diagnoses (or, unfortunately, diagnoses that are not listed as provisional but rather as confirmed). Starting a later evaluation with diagnostic hypotheses based solely on conclusions drawn from that limited and potentially faulty initial assessment invites the hindsight bias. The same sort of bias can occur with the results of a screening evaluation, which may suggest the presence of a particular diagnosis. If a clinician using a screening tool doesn't remember that the screening tool likely has a high rate of false positives, given that its purpose is to screen individuals for further assessment or evaluation and not to confirm or establish diagnoses, then that clinician may well experience hindsight bias.

Consider the following case in which hindsight bias carried through to multiple evaluations. A woman in her 60s was referred for a dementia evaluation. Before she arrived, a glance at her medical chart showed that she had been seen by several physicians and medical residents in the prior 3 months. Each time the diagnosis of dementia was raised, and each time it was mentioned in the chart, the dementia diagnosis became less provisional and stated as more certain, with further procedures being considered while she awaited her scheduled neuropsychological evaluation. Yet each time, the only evidence clearly described as indicative of dementia was "disorientation to personal information." A copy of a mental state exam from her most recent visit documented that the only questions she missed were her birthday (she was off by a year, according to the stamped ID card in the corner of each medical page) and her age (she was off by a year, but in a way consistent with her stated birthday). When she arrived for her appointment, the first thing the neuropsychologist asked were orientation questions, and she provided the same answers she had been giving doctors for 3 months—which, while although completely consistent across multiple mental status evaluations, did not match the stamped ID card. The neuropsychologist then asked the client for her driver's license, which confirmed that she had been right all along; the stamped medical card had a typographical error on it. After passing all aspects of the neuropsychological evaluation with flying colors, the other expensive medical workups were cancelled; the client was encouraged to return to the records area to have her hospital ID fixed. In this case, each physician or medical student who saw the woman was biased by the information already in the chart, which suggested (ever more strongly over time) that the woman had dementia; thus, her "disorientation" on a mental status exam "confirmed" their hindsight bias, and the faulty diagnoses was passed along to the next professional.

Regret Bias

Regret bias occurs when an evaluator overestimates the base rate of a potential diagnosis that has a possibly severe outcome because of anticipated regret should the evaluator miss the diagnosis (Dawson & Arkes, 1987). In medicine, such a bias has led to a "Let's go ahead and treat it as if it's X" approach, which also has potential for harm—in some cases more harm than that caused by not making the correct diagnosis and failing to treat the disorder correctly. Probably the best examples of this kind of bias come from the prediction of very low base-rate but dangerous behaviors, such as suicidal or homicidal intent, where the costs of being wrong can be fatal. However, assessors need to remember that there are costs associated with incorrect diagnosis as well. Consider the case of the 70-year-old with an atypical presentation of dementia presented above. The use of antipsychotic medications is actually contraindicated in a dementia with Lewy bodies (McKeith et al., 2005), and thus the physician's faulty diagnostic reasoning may have led to harm for this patient had the antipsychotics not been discontinued in a timely fashion.

The aforementioned biases tend to be considered automatic, intuitive, and thus related to failures in inductive reasoning. The next bias, however, is one to which both inductive/intuitive and deductive/analytic decision-making systems are vulnerable.

Confirmatory Bias

Confirmatory bias is the general tendency to give greater attention to confirmatory evidence and/or actively seek confirmatory evidence, while undervaluing disconfirming evidence and/or not actively seeking to disconfirm a hypothesis. Although the initial working hypotheses might have arisen due to representative bias, availability bias, hindsight bias, regret bias, or even other inductive processes, this next stage of the decision-making process should be active and deliberate and not focused solely on confirmatory evidence.

The presence of a confirmatory bias is likely to lead to inaccurate information gathering during the assessment process. For example, an assessor (1) may ask questions during the interview that seek only to confirm the working hypothesis, (2) may ask only for other relevant data that are confirmatory, or (3) may choose to administer only instruments that have known sensitivity (but not specificity) to that working hypothesis. The patient with Graves' disease (described in Chapter 1) is an excellent example of this kind of confirmatory bias: The assessor focused on the initial report of "anxiety" and administered instruments and interviews solely to confirm anxiety disorder diagnoses, with little attention to exclusionary criteria. Thus, even though the assessor used testing methods empirically supported by the literature for use in cases involving anxiety, the assessor's quick intuitive focus on only anxiety and lack of attention to disconfirmatory evidence and differential diagnosis led to an inaccurate diagnosis.

The confirmatory bias can also contribute to errors in interpretation by causing an examiner to put more evidentiary weight on the confirmatory evidence and to discount any collected evidence that is in contradiction to that hypothesis. In this context, it is important to point out that absent findings can be equally informative in making correct diagnosis. For example, there is evidence of an overdiagnosis of attention-deficit/hyperactivity disorder (ADHD) in both children and young adults (Bruchmuller, Margraf, & Schneider, 2012; Harrison, Alexander, & Armstrong, 2013). The most common pattern that appears to lead to misdiagnosis (aside from malingering; see Chapter 4) is that the assessor put weights on the client's self-reported "impairment" of academic functioning (primacy availability bias) and his or her very low scores on cognitive and achievement tests administered at the time of the evaluation (recency or saliency availability bias), with no consideration of the actual academic records or evidence of current functioning. In many such cases, the academic record reveals that the individual showed no evidence of impairment (and in fact was often functioning above peers) in course grades and on standardized tests, with no accommodations, and that the scores on current testing were highly inconsistent with scores obtained by the client during those school years. The assessor in these cases may not have considered the base rate of these conditions in young adults who have heretofore been functional; the absence of actual evidence of academic impairment in the client's history was either discounted (or perhaps never even considered) as relevant to the diagnosis that was ultimately given.

Confirmatory bias errors are likely to lead to premature closure, which Graber and colleagues (2005) described as the tendency to stop the diagnostic decision-making process (i.e., stop considering other possibilities) before a correct diagnosis is reached. Jumping to a wrong tentative initial diagnosis has been shown to occur frequently in medical decision making, particularly when it occurs under time pressure (Bornstein & Emler, 2000). Managed care has likely contributed to this bias, especially in the case of complex differentials such as those that occur in the mental health field. The current health care environment leads to reinforcement of quick answers despite insufficient data obtained at a first visit and with reliance on self-report and what others have concluded before, or perhaps on results from quick-to-administer screening measures with high false-positive rates (Singh & Weingart, 2009).

Diagnostic Bias

As pointed out in Chapter 1, the most common biased lens a psychologist may wear is the one through which a diagnosis of *some kind* is always seen (Garb, 1998). Overperceiving pathology may be built in by clinical training and experiences (Gambrill, 1990; Lopez, 1989; Shemberg & Doherty, 1999) and reinforced in a world where overpathologizing many common life ailments is common (Frances, 2010). At the very least, a clinician must maintain constant awareness of the possibility of "no diagnosis" in each and every case as part of the differential, and remember that many of the "symptoms" of psychological disorders are extremely common, nonspecific, and thus not necessarily indicative of a disorder. In addition, the clinician must constantly be reminded that evidence of impairment and dysfunction is part of the diagnostic criteria for many, if not most, diagnoses.

As noted above, it is hard for an assessor to resist starting with a diagnostic bias when the referral question or request from a health care provider lists a specific potential diagnosis that the referent wishes the evaluator to consider (e.g., "Evaluate for depression," "Test for dementia"). Diagnostic bias may be even more powerful if, instead of being presented as a referral question or request, the potential diagnosis is one that has been given by some other clinician in the past. Awareness that someone else has made that diagnosis for that particular client is biasing information (see section on hindsight bias, above); a scientifically minded assessor would want to examine the data that were used in the prior evaluation in order to confirm or disconfirm the diagnosis that was given (see Chapter 8).

Even when a client is self-referred, he or she often presents with a specific diagnosis in mind (e.g., "I think I have ADHD"). An assessor with diagnostic bias will then observe, attend to, collect, record, remember, and highlight only a narrow range of information concerning pathological, clinically identifiable features and evidence consistent with the hypothesis at hand. Deductive reasoning, after all, is only as effective as the initial premise is correct. Of course, the same sort of bias could occur even when an assessor starts with inductive reasoning. For example, a self-reported symptom "I have trouble paying attention" leads the assessor, via representativeness bias, to a diagnostic hypothesis of ADHD; then, rather than viewing this generalization as only one of many hypotheses, moves too quickly to deductive reasoning and tries to confirm that one hypothesis. As pointed out above, holding a stereotypical view of specific symptoms and how they fit with specific disorders can contribute greatly to this sort of bias.

WAYS TO MINIMIZE DECISION-MAKING ERRORS

Researchers have shown that, in general, experts are not better than new clinicians in making psychological diagnoses (Witteman, Harries, Bekker, & Van Aarle, 2007). However, both groups are subject to diagnostic errors. Other researchers have suggested specific types of experience and/ or training that might help to minimize errors in this "wicked problem."

Experience

With regard to the effects of experience on the use of decision-making processes, Graber (2009) suggested that, whereas beginning assessors tend to use the deductive/analytical system, assessors intermediate in their experience are more likely to use inductive/intuitive heuristics, and assessment experts take a more conscious reflective approach that uses both processes in a dynamic and interactive way. Marcum (2012) argued that what separates beginning assessors from experienced assessors is the *accuracy* of their intuitive system.

What type of experience is necessary to improve decision making? Interestingly, Graber (2009) argued that, to become an expert, an assessor needs subspecialization training to become an expert in one particular type of condition. Given the potential for this kind of limited and focused condition-specific experience to contribute to decision-making biases (as discussed above), this seems a dangerous suggestion. In fact, researchers have shown that subspecialists tend to overdiagnose pathology in the particular organ system in which they specialize (Hashem, Chi, & Friedman, 2003), consistent with the representativeness bias. Even Graber pointed out that his argument assumed that the individual would be referred to the *correct* specialist. Given the decision-making literature, a more strongly supported argument could be made that, to become an expert, an assessor needs exposure to a wide variety of cases in order to understand differential diagnosis and to resist the decision-making biases that are reinforced by narrow training and experience.

Another potential limitation of experience is its potentially inflating effects on confidence. Decision-making researchers have expressed the opinion that overconfidence may be a major contributor to diagnostic errors (Berner & Graber, 2008; Croskerry, 2009). Jumping too soon to only one hypothesis, about which one feels quite confident, will lead to bias at every level of decision making, from the questions that are asked, to the data that are collected, and to integration of that data. A deductive reasoner who does not temper his or her self-confidence by using good scientific procedures and specifically attempting to consider and confirm or disconfirm multiple hypotheses is particularly vulnerable to error. For example, if the assessor has confidence in his or her initial hypothesis ("My client likely has disorder X"), then the assessor may ask questions only relevant to data that would confirm the presence of disorder X, notice only client behaviors that are supportive of disorder X, give tests known to be sensitive to disorder X (but perhaps not specific to disorder X), and so on. An overconfident assessor expects to see what he or she is used to seeing (Kamphuis & Finn, 2002), and as a result observes, inquires about, and assesses for only what he or she expects to see.

Some assessor overconfidence may arise from lack of specific feedback on the accuracy of prior clinical judgments. Marcum (2012) suggests that, in addition to experience over time, assessors need reflective feedback to improve their intuitive decision making. However, fairly often clinicians do not receive feedback about the accuracy of their diagnoses. In fact, most of the feedback any assessor receives is the personal validation from the client after the assessment is completed, particularly when the client hears what he or she wanted to hear or responds to the generic and nonspecific feedback that is often present (à la the P. T. Barnum effect). Thus, the feedback, although reinforcing, may be inaccurate. For these reasons, broad-based experience under mentorship and with mentor/supervisor feedback is a strong recommendation for training in assessment; for those out in the field, consultation and continuing education, as well as seeking feedback, are also recommended.

Decision-Making Training

It has been suggested that decision-making training should focus on educating the assessor about the decision-making errors that are described above, with the assumption that awareness of these decision-making biases would minimize their influence (Arnoult & Anderson, 1988). However, it is unclear whether mere awareness of these errors is sufficient to counter them in the actual clinical setting, especially given that they typically occur in an automatic and nonconscious manner (Norman & Eva, 2010).

Graber (2009) described the approach to teaching diagnostic decision making in most medical school settings as analytical and deductive in nature. Using case review, medical students are taught to deliberately consider all possible diagnoses, estimate the likelihood of each possible diagnosis, consider the consequences of making or missing each diagnosis, and administer tests to further examine those diagnoses with the highest probability in that deductive process. However, Graber also points out that using cases with already known diagnostic outcomes in the abstract setting of training works well, but that such an approach is not how decision making works in actual practice. For example, in clinical practice, assessors typically don't have a full symptom picture at the outset of a case, but instead must ask the right questions—which requires that the correct diagnosis already be under consideration among a list of potential diagnoses, based on initial partial information. Thus, from the outset, the accuracy of a deliberative and deductive process depends upon the output of the automatic and less conscious intuitive system.

Several researchers offer advice about specific training for both inductive and deductive reasoning and the need for each of these systems to cross-check the other. For example, Graber (2009) suggests that training to develop decision-making expertise should emphasize invoking conscious and deliberative "stop and think" approaches in order to check on the accuracy of the intuitive system. Norman, Brooks, Colle, and Hatala (2000) found that previously untrained individuals benefited from training in both intuitive and analytical decision making. Norman (2009) cites evidence that training should be based on level of experience, in that less experienced assessors may be advised to use experience/intuition in their decision making, whereas experts (who may be overconfident in their intuitive system) should be reminded to use their analytical system. Overall, however, there is little empirical information available that speaks to the efficacy of training in either inductive or deductive reasoning methods.

Training in Base-Rate Analysis

As noted above, consideration of base rates is often a part of deductive decision-making training. It has been argued that training individuals in the use of statistical decision rules will lead to better decision making (Bell & Mellor, 2009; Grove, Zald, Lebow, Snitz, & Nelson, 2000). Although statistical decision rules can help an assessor attend to important information and assign it proper weight in the decision-making process, there are no well-validated decision formulas for most psychological disorders. Generally, such rules and procedures require knowledge of the base rate(s) of the conditions(s) under consideration, the specific relationship of symptom(s) to conditions(s), and the specific relationship of test finding(s) to condition(s).

BASE RATES OF DISORDERS

At the very least, knowing the base rate(s) of the disorder(s) under consideration in a particular assessment provides an assessor with a priori odds for whether certain hypotheses ("Does this person have schizophrenia or dementia?"; "Does this person have anxiety or Graves' disease?") can be weighted as likely or unlikely before the evaluation even begins. However, it is clear that clinicians still do not use this information (Bell & Mellor, 2009), and studies show that consciously considering base rates does not aid diagnostic decision making (Kamphuis & Finn, 2002). One of the difficulties in using such information correctly is that the assessor needs to know the base rates for the disorder relative to contextual factors. Base rates are defined for specific populations and are restricted to them. Thus, the base rate of schizophrenia in the general population is far less than 1% (American Psychiatric Association, 2013), but in an inpatient psychiatric ward is much higher, and at certain ages it is lower, but if there is a family history, it is higher. In short, base-rate knowledge needs to be specific to the context, the person being assessed, and other individual factors unique to the case at hand.

SPECIFIC RELATIONSHIP OF SYMPTOMS TO DISORDERS

The starting point for most assessors' decision making is the client's presenting symptoms. Some disorders are clearly identifiable by their combination of symptoms; rarely, a disorder may be identifiable by a single pathognomic symptom. However, as noted above, a presenting symptom is often not specific to one disorder, but can be seen in many disorders. Thus, it is critical for assessors to be aware of the true relationship between any specific symptom and a specific diagnosis. The assessor needs to know the likelihood not only of seeing that symptom within a diagnosis under consideration, but also the likelihood of seeing that symptom in any of the differential diagnoses under consideration, or even in the general population. Obviously, then, to be useful to statistical decision making, a symptom must be sensitive to the disorder, but also specific to it (see Chapter 6 for more on these concepts). When an assessor uses symptoms of very poor validity (i.e., usually sensitive to, but not specific to, a favored diagnosis), diagnostic error is increased via a representativeness bias. Unfortunately, many of the symptoms, complaints, and concerns presented by individuals seeking psychological assessment or treatment are not specific to any one disorder; in fact, many of those symptoms are commonly reported by members of the non-treatment-seeking general population and thus not even indicative of any disorder. McCaffrey, Palav, O'Bryant, and Labarge (2003) provide useful examples of the base rates of common psychological and cognitive complaints across a wide variety of psychological and medical populations. Such information can be very helpful to assessors when considering whether the presenting concern is one that is associated not only with the disorder under consideration, but also with other potential differential diagnoses and/or is common in the general population.

SPECIFIC RELATIONSHIP OF TEST RESULTS TO DISORDERS

In a similar vein, information is needed not only on whether test results are sensitive to a disorder under consideration, but whether they are specific to that disorder. Chapter 6 discusses the need to know the psychometric properties of the clinical tests an assessor uses on a regular basis, in order to make a scientifically informed decision about the value of any test results to the decision-making process. For example, many mental health professionals assume that continuous performance tests are diagnostic of ADHD; however, there are so many different conditions (e.g., medication use, level of fatigue/arousal, anxiety, even time of day) that can affect performance on such tasks that they are not considered appropriate for the assessment of ADHD (American Academy of Pediatrics, 2000; Pelham, Fabiano, & Massetti, 2005).

USE OF BASE RATES IN DECISION MAKING

As noted above, it is still uncommon to see the use of statistical decision-making processes in clinical practice because of the complexity of the real-world decision-making realities. First, base rates are defined for very specific populations, meaning that such statistical formulas would have to account for many factors prior to determining a priori odds for any particular disorder. Second, the sensitivity and specificity of reported symptoms and/or test scores would have to be known and utilized in the statistical formula in order to make it accurate. As Bell and Mellor (2009) emphasized, suitable statistical formulae or actuarial tables do not exist or are not sufficiently developed in many fields of psychological judgment. Third, Newman and Kohn (2009) point out that testing is not conducted in sequence, but occurs in parallel, and test scores are usually not independent from one another. Thus, when multiple types of information are combined together to move to posterior probabilities, the formula needs to consider whether the data points are conditionally independent (i.e., that the data points are not correlated with one another once disease status is taken into account). Only conditionally independent data add to the calculation of accurate likelihood ratios. It is highly unlikely, given the lack of specificity of many symptoms and complaints (as well as test scores) in psychological assessment, that such conditional independence could occur.

As Bell and Mellor (2009) noted, clinical and statistical approaches do *not* differ in the types of data gathered, the setting in which clinical decisions are made, or the methods by which data are collected (i.e., interview, tests). They argue that clinical approaches may be more appropriate when the explicit prediction rules are not available, or when relevant data in a particular case are not part of the statistical model. They argue further that a clinical approach may be most appropriate in the earliest phases of an assessment, while initial hypotheses are being formed. The main distinction between a clinical and statistical decision-making approach is in how the data are integrated: either through informal, subjective methods or with a statistical formula. Although some argue against the use of both approaches simultaneously because they may lead to contradictory conclusions (Grove et al., 2000), the use of both (when available) may help clarify uncertainty. We return to this discussion in Chapter 13.

SUGGESTIONS FOR ASSESSORS

Given the data reviewed above, the following recommendations are made to help assessors prepare to conduct an empirically validated assessment, including suggestions for developing appropriate knowledge and experience and for every stage of an ongoing assessment.

Knowledge and Experience

1. An assessor needs *exposure to a wide variety of cases* in order to understand the differential diagnoses and to resist the decision-making biases that are reinforced by narrow training and experience.

2. An assessor also needs *broad training*, as suggested in Chapter 1 and as emphasized in Chapter 3. In order to ensure accurate inductive heuristics (thus minimizing a representative bias), an assessor needs broad-based knowledge across a wide variety of domains, including biological, sociological, cultural, developmental, and psychological contributions to the potential concerns and symptoms with which clients might present.

3. An assessor should obtain experience *under mentorship and with feedback*; for those out in the field, consultation and continuing education, as well as seeking feedback, are also recommended.

In the Assessment Setting

1. An assessor should *obtain a complete history* (guided by the biopsychosocial model; see Chapter 3) in order to generate initial hypotheses about factors that contribute to the client's concerns and symptoms. These factors may include potential diagnostic "matches" (and, if some come to mind, the assessor should deliberately consider other potential matches as well, including that there is no diagnosis), but may also include contributory "matches" that lie outside consideration of any specific diagnosis.

2. In order to minimize a diagnostic bias (while also taking a therapeutic approach to assessment), an assessor should consider the purpose of the initial interview as one of *developing hypotheses about the causes of the problems and symptoms presented by the client*, rather than only to reach a diagnosis (Witteman et al., 2007). Such a focus is a "situation assessment" rather than a diagnostic decision-making approach to assessment, and emphasizes the importance of explaining why symptoms or behaviors are occurring rather than focusing merely on diagnosis. Using a biopsychosocial framework when listening to the client's "story" allows for development of hypotheses regarding causes or contributions to the presenting complaints, some of which may lead to a consideration of specific diagnoses. See Chapter 7 for more on viewing the initial interview within that framework.

3. As the history is obtained, the assessor should *consider base rates specific to the context* for any diagnoses that arise for consideration. As the evaluation commences, *listing all possible diagnoses* (and their base rates)

will give the assessor a priori weights with which to consider any further observations and data points as the assessment progresses (Millis, 2009).

4. In the interview and through the entire assessment, the assessor should *consider base rates of symptoms and symptom sets* and how their presence (or absence) affects the weighting of any of the various diagnoses under consideration. The assessor should be careful to *consider both confirmatory and disconfirmatory data for each hypothesis.*

5. The assessor should use a systemic approach to *obtain additional data* (tests [Chapters 9–11] and nontest data [Chapter 8]) beyond that obtained in interview and behavioral observation (Chapter 7) to both *confirm and disconfirm* various diagnostic possibilities under consideration.

6. When the assessor chooses to administer tests, he or she should *use empirically supported instruments with known sensitivity and specificity* to the disorder(s) under consideration (see Chapters 9–12). Use of well-validated and well-standardized instruments can help to minimize diagnostic errors, whereas poorly constructed and validated tests can serve to enhance errors. For example, as noted above, although continuous performance tests are often administered as part of evaluations for ADHD, their extremely poor specificity makes it clear that it is inappropriate to utilize data on such tasks to diagnosis this condition (American Academy of Pediatrics, 2000; Pelham et al., 2005).

7. An assessor needs to *consider statistical and base-rate information when using test scores* in the evaluation process. For example, an assessor may be drawn into an availability bias by the salience of one very extreme score in a test battery, ignoring the fact that this could be a statistical artifact (Bornstein & Emler, 2000; Millis, 2009). It is also important for the assessor to consider the number of data points that arise through a test battery and the impact that number has on using any set of "abnormal" scores for making decisions (see Chapters 10–12).

8. In integrating the assessment data, the assessor should *deliberately consider all evidence (both confirmatory and disconfirmatory) and how it should be weighted, when considering each potential hypothesis.* In so doing, the assessor should carefully review all notes and data and not base this integration on recall, in order to minimize the decision-making biases noted above. If possible, the assessor can use base-rate information or statistically based formulas to further examine the likelihood of any of the differential diagnoses under consideration (Bornstein & Emler, 2000; Millis, 2009). This point is discussed in more detail in Chapter 14.

3

Use of a Developmentally Informed Biopsychosocial Lens in Assessment

One's ideas must be as broad as Nature if they are to interpret Nature.
—SHERLOCK HOLMES, in *A Study in Scarlet*

As mentioned in Chapters 1 and 2, there is a bias in both medical and psychological assessment toward reaching a diagnosis and reaching that diagnosis quickly, which has lead to a focus on self-reported symptom sets to see if they match with consensus diagnoses, rather than giving attention to the client's whole "story." This diagnostic bias leads to only cursory consideration of differential diagnoses, some of which might be suggested by consideration of various factors in the client's story beyond his or her report of a current pattern of symptoms. Furthermore, there is often little to no consideration of the multitude of factors that might contribute to the client's presenting concerns or areas of dysfunction—factors that might not only rule out a diagnosis completely and/or lead to other nonpsychological diagnoses, but might also have important treatment implications.

Interestingly, one stated advantage of diagnoses is that, when done correctly, they "tell the story"; that is, they quickly communicate information about potential etiological factors, contributing concerns, and treatment recommendations. With some medical conditions a diagnosis can explain not only what is causing the person's symptoms, but also predict the prognosis for that person and determine the appropriate treatment options to consider. For example, a clinician working with someone who has the diagnosis of Huntington's disease knows from that diagnosis alone that the individual is suffering from an autosomal-dominant genetic condition in which a mutant huntingtin protein causes neural destruction, that the individual is likely to experience both motor and psychological symptoms that will grow progressively worse over time, and that treatment is likely to include use of medications that address the motor symptoms as well as use of antidepressant and/or antipsychotic medication and potentially psycho-therapy to address the psychological symptoms (Paulsen & Mikos, 2008).

However, even for many medical conditions, there may be genetic, biologi-cal, environmental, psychological, and sociocultural contributing factors that could lead to highly variable prognoses and to any number of treatment approaches. For example, headaches have many potential etiologies, all of which may lead to different prognoses and different recommendations for appropriate treatment. By focusing primarily on symptoms and giving only cursory consideration to "the rest of the story," an assessor can reach an incorrect diagnostic conclusion, leading to inappropriate treatment.

Similarly, in psychological conditions, merely considering the symp-tom set and conducting a diagnostic pattern analysis leave out highly rel-evant information that is crucial not just to a correct diagnosis, but also to considering predictions for outcome and treatment recommendations. Fur-thermore, because psychological disorders are not discrete entities, a sole focus on symptom subsets and whether they can distinguish or differentiate disorders is even less appropriate in this context than for many medical conditions. Because most psychological disorders are on a spectrum, and many psychological disorders are closely related in that they share not only symptoms but also environmental and biological risk factors as well as neu-ral substrates, they do not necessarily have clear and well-defined bound-aries that can be identified with a focus merely on symptom presentation (American Psychiatric Association, 2013). As a result, for any given client, an assessor must take a careful clinical history and consider all the factors that may have contributed to the symptom presentation. "It is not sufficient to simply check off the symptoms in the diagnostic criteria to make a men-tal disorder diagnosis" (American Psychiatric Association, 2013, p. 19).

Taking a careful clinical history and considering other factors that might contribute to the presenting complaints is more complicated than simply asking the client whether he or she has any other diagnoses (or symptoms of such) that were listed in the diagnostic rule-out criteria for any given disorder. For example, someone complaining of poor attention/concentration could have an as-yet-undiagnosed sleep disorder leading to those complaints, rather than ADHD. By asking only "Do you have any medical conditions?", the assessor may miss relevant information that might suggest sleep issues and lead to an appropriate referral for a sleep evalu-ation. In contrast, an assessor attuned to the need to ask for the client's whole story, who recognizes the potential importance of sleep to daytime complaints of attention/concentration, would be careful to ask about time to bed, time to rise, perceived quality of sleep, presence/absence of apnea symptoms, whether the client feels rested in the morning upon awakening, and whether the client is sleepy during the day. Specific attention to this potential etiological factor during the intake interview might lead to appropriate treatment for the true cause of the client's attention difficulties, thereby preventing misdiagnosis.

Even in the case where a mental disorder diagnosis is clearly appropriate, knowing the person's story has important implications beyond diagnosis, because, as with many medical disorders, contributions from other potential factors can have implications for prognosis and for treatment. No two people with major depressive disorder have the same "story": They may have different patterns of symptoms, experience symptoms with different levels of severity, have additional strengths/weaknesses that impact their functioning, and/or experience their disorder in unique sociocultural contexts that may have implications for their daily functioning and their treatment or intervention needs.

STRUCTURE FOR EVALUATING A CLIENT'S STORY

As mentioned in Chapter 2, finding out the client's story is one way to reduce decision- making bias, as a "story" focus may help an assessor focus his or her attention beyond just one salient symptom (availability bias) or beyond only characteristic symptoms of the referral question that mentions a specific diagnosis (representativeness bias). By examining the client's story, the focus of the assessment becomes one of explanation for the presenting concerns, symptoms, and behaviors rather than a focus purely on diagnosis. However, in order to obtain a client's story in a more reliable manner (see Chapter 7), it is useful to have a general structure or framework for elements of the story the assessor should consider relevant. A developmentally informed biopsychosocial "lens" is one structure that is well supported by empirical research in psychopathology and is the framework recommended, not only for the initial interview of a client, but also for gathering relevant assessment data and for conceptualizing the case when integrating all of the information obtained.

The purpose of this chapter is to present a brief summary of a developmental biopsychosocial approach to understanding psychological symptoms and disorders to guide an assessor in the use of this lens during all stages of an assessment. An assessor wearing a biopsychosocial lens will consider and assess for biological, psychological, and sociocultural contributions to a client's presenting concerns; a developmental focus reminds the assessor that obtaining the history of the individual and of his or her concerns is needed to understand the dynamic contributions of any of these elements (and their interaction with one another), in order to place the client's current complaints in an appropriate historical context.

Use of a developmentally oriented biopsychosocial model for understanding psychopathology is supported by decades of research, but can only be presented briefly in this text. Obviously, a more complete coverage of developmental, biological, psychological, sociological, and cultural factors relevant to specific psychological conditions should be part of the training of anyone planning to conduct assessments for psychological disorders. This should include coursework across the breadth of the field (experimental psychopathology, neurochemistry, neuropsychology, behavioral genetics, developmental psychology, social psychology, diversity issues, among others), as well as experiential training in applying these concepts in a clinical context. (See Chapter 1 for more discussion regarding the training implications of this recommendation.)

There has been some criticism raised about the biopsychosocial model in that, incorrectly applied, it can lead to use of whichever "lens" the clinician most favors, thereby allowing clinicians to justify their conclusions about the etiology of and treatment recommendations for any given psychological disorder (Ghaemi, 2009). An assessor who favors a biological lens might examine only those symptom subsets and then consider medication as the first-line treatment for any symptom subset consistent with a specific psychological disorder, whereas an assessor who focuses on sociological contributions to pathology would consider only family and relationship dynamics when assessing and considering treatment for the same individual. However, these approaches constitute an incorrect application of the model, not a criticism of the model per se. Assessors who view a client through only one aspect of a biopsychosocial lens will definitely miss important information about the person's story and make biased decisions. In order to use the model correctly in assessment, an assessor would consider every one of the model's elements, in a dynamic and interactive way, to develop hypotheses that then require further examination and empirical support before any diagnostic or other conclusions could be drawn.

Correct use of a developmentally informed biopsychosocial lens requires the assessor to focus, *at the symptom and behavior level*, on any and all possible contributions to the behavior under investigation, and to assess the client using validated methods (beyond mere self-report) to determine the most likely etiologies and contributing factors for those behaviors and symptoms (which may or may not include a diagnosis of a particular condition) in order to guide treatment recommendations. For example, in the case of the sleep-disordered client with attention/concentration complaints, mentioned above, an assessor who prematurely settled on an ADHD diagnosis, leading to follow-up questions focused only on ADHD symptoms and outcomes, is not applying the biopsychosocial model correctly. On the other hand, an assessor who started with the attention/concentration complaints of the client and hypothesized about all the biological, medical, familial, genetic, lifestyle, cognitive, and cultural factors that could be related, and then explored all of those contributing factors before reaching any diagnostic decision, would be more likely to correctly identify sleep and daytime fatigue factors as potentially contributing to the presenting complaints—which would then lead to appropriate referral for a sleep evaluation and prevent inappropriate and potentially harmful effects of misdiagnosis and mistreatment.

In the next section, components of a biopsychosocial model are briefly discussed as a way to orient an assessor to the importance of all these factors to the typical presenting concerns of individuals seeking psychological assessment. Case illustrations demonstrate the importance of different elements of the model to understanding the case. Presentation of the components of the biopsychosocial model as separate elements inappropriately simplifies the model, however; the final section presents a case example in which elements of the model are considered together in an integrative and dynamic fashion.

THE BIOPSYCHOSOCIAL MODEL

Engel (1977) developed the biopsychosocial model as a way to understand functional medical conditions, although he believed that the model applied equally well to psychological conditions. Most, if not all, psychological disorders are the result of complex interactions of an array of biological vulnerabilities and dispositions (that may or may not be familial or genetic), with many significant environmental and psychosocial events that can exert their effects over time. Psychological symptoms and predisposing psychological characteristics are responsive to a wide variety of neurobiological, interpersonal, cognitive, and other mediator and moderator variables that lead to the development of any individual's overall psychological health and/or psychopathology.

The biopsychosocial lens is useful not just at the beginning of an assessment, when first trying to understand the client's story, but through every step of the assessment. During the interview, when assessing the client who is presenting with specific symptoms, concerns, or complaints, using a developmentally oriented biopsychosocial lens will help in formulating hypotheses about contributing factors, both past and present, to the current concerns of the client. During other data gathering, using the biopsychosocial lens is helpful in deciding the nature of the additional data (both past and present) that might be needed to test the hypotheses generated as a result of the initial interview. Finally, use of a developmentally oriented biopsychosocial lens in the final interpretation and conceptualization of the client's concerns will assist the assessor in making decisions about whether any particular psychological diagnosis (or diagnoses) is appropriate, whether the client should be referred for other workups to rule out other contributing factors suggested by the biopsychosocial history and data, and to make treatment recommendations based on the biopsychosocial context in which the symptoms are presented.

An important aspect of applying this model to the assessment context is focusing attention on the *specific symptoms and behaviors* presented by the client, rather than focusing on diagnosis at the start. This suggestion is paralleled by a recent paradigm shift in experimental psychopathology research. Traditionally, experimental psychopathology studies were designed to examine biopsychosocial etiologies for particular disorders or diagnoses and to understand how they may interrelate over time. The level of understanding, then, was typically limited to a specific disorder or diagnosis, rather than an underlying symptom/complaint or construct. As noted in more recent research in psychopathology, however, this kind of work has limited our understanding of the underlying causes for psychological dysfunction (Insel et al., 2010). Thus, paradigm shifts are occurring within the field, with a focus on understanding the many potential etiologies of specific symptoms and behaviors, rather than symptom sets and diagnoses, in order to truly understand what leads to psychopathology and ultimately how to treat it (Insel et al., 2010). The most empirically attuned assessor should also start at the level of specific symptoms or presenting problems and concerns, rather than at the level of diagnoses, and should use research findings about contributing factors for specific symptoms when generating hypotheses about causes of a client's concerns. In other words, if an assessor makes the decision-making error of jumping to a diagnostic conclusion too soon, based merely on the symptom pattern, and then considers only what research tells us about biopsychosocial contributors to that specific disorder, the assessor would still have erred in his or her application of the biopsychosocial model to the presenting concerns and symptoms of the person being assessed.

The Biological Lens

There is well-documented evidence of brain dysfunction as a correlate to, or predisposing factor for, many psychological symptoms, presentations, and disorders. In addition, there is strong evidence for the contribution of many chronic medical conditions and many temporary physical conditions to the function of the brain, thus causing them to be related to the predisposition for, onset of, or presentation with a wide range of psychological symptoms and disorders. Table 3.1 is a brief list of some common psychological symptoms and complaints and potential biological and medical contributions to them; keep in mind that this list is in no way complete but is meant to illustrate the need to carefully consider the biological lens when evaluating psychological complaints. What is important to note is how many different contributions to common psychological symptoms there are; when coupled with the fact that many of these psychological symptoms appear across many different psychological disorders, it is clear that consideration of all of these factors is crucial both to correct diagnosis (or no diagnosis) and to appropriate intervention. It is also important to note that transient health factors, not just medical diagnoses, can contribute to psychological symptoms and complaints.

How does an assessor conducting an initial assessment take these biological factors into account? Some assessment guidebooks suggest that a obtaining a brief medical history is usually sufficient to determine whether symptoms can be explained by an underlying medical condition, whereas others offer the opinion that a complete physical is necessary for all psychological diagnoses. There needs to be a balance between comprehensiveness and time/efficiency in managing the biological lens in the context of psychological assessment. Clients may or may not know that they have some of the medical conditions listed in the table, because they have not as yet been evaluated for or diagnosed with them, and some biological factors are not medical diagnoses per se. Therefore, taking a brief medical history that simply asks what diagnoses a client currently has received is clearly not sufficient for addressing biological contributions to the presenting concerns. An assessor must remember to ask about the *symptoms* of medical disorders that are known to be related to the complaints of the client, as well as interviewing for evidence of other biological contributors, including the client's general health, last known physical exam, use of medications (including over-the-counter medications), lifestyle factors (including eating, exercising, and sleeping patterns), substance use, and family history for medical conditions that could contribute to the presenting symptoms (especially those that are known to be genetic in nature). Obviously to do

TABLE 3.1. Common Psychological Symptoms and Complaints and Potential Medical and Biological Contributors to the Complaints

Symptom	Medical disorders that might contribute to the complaint	Other potential physical contributors to the complaint
Panic symptoms	Hyperthyroidism, hypoglycemia, allergies/asthma, pain disorders, various cardiovascular diseases and abnormalities, seizures	Caffeine/amphetamine/nicotine misuse, drug withdrawal, chemotherapy, pregnancy, side effects of medications, nutritional deficiency
Worry, rumination	Many chronic illnesses	Pregnancy
Feeling agitated or irritable, having mood swings, feeling "stressed"	Pain disorders, HIV/AIDS, chronic fatigue syndrome, diabetes, hyperthyroidism, seizures	Chemotherapy, substance misuse/withdrawal, sleep deprivation, pregnancy, nutritional deficiency, medication side effects
Lack of energy, fatigue	Hypothyroidism, anemia, hypotension, pain disorders, chemotherapy, chronic fatigue syndrome, allergies, cancer, cardiovascular diseases and disorders, diabetes, HIV/AIDS, kidney disease	Sleep deprivation, pregnancy, nutritional deficiency, dehydration, fever/infection, medication side effects
Feeling depressed	Pain disorders, HIV/AIDS, pain disorders, diabetes, hypothyroidism, chronic fatigue syndrome	Chemotherapy, pregnancy, nutritional deficiencies, sleep deprivation
Hallucinations, delusions	Delirium, dementia, seizures, sleep disorders, liver failure, kidney failure, HIV/AIDS, brain tumor, stroke	Sleep deprivation, substance misuse/withdrawal, fever/infection, sensory deprivation
Attention, concentration, memory complaints	HIV/AIDS, many cardiac conditions, pain disorders, head injury, brain diseases (stroke, seizure)	Chemotherapy, substance misuse/withdrawal, sleep deprivation, nutritional deficiencies, dehydration, side effects of medications

this well, an assessor needs a good understanding of the potential medical and biological contributions to the specific symptoms being presented. Table 3.1 provides a brief summary that is by no means comprehensive; thorough training in psychobiology and medical psychology and experience applying that knowledge is needed. In addition, if a potential biological or medical contribution is expected or revealed during the initial interview, the assessor should make an appropriate referral to an expert in the area for further evaluation.

It is also important for the assessor to consider the accuracy of the client's report of prior/current medical problems, illnesses, injuries, or health concerns. When possible, confirmation of the client's report may be needed. In my clinical experience, some clients overpathologize their past medical histories and others minimize or even omit these histories, relative to data available in medical records and/or through collateral report. As is noted below, there can be psychological and contextual reasons for this type of inaccurate report, which may, in and of themselves, be diagnostic.

As noted in Chapter 1, identifying a clear-cut biological explanation for the presenting concerns might preclude further psychological treatment, but the biopsychosocial assessment was nonetheless successful in that the client was ultimately directed toward the correct treatment for his or her presenting concerns. However, even in the case of a clearly biologically mediated condition, there may still be contributions from other factors that suggest that psychological interventions could assist in the client's care.

The Psychological Lens

Examining the symptoms the client reports can help the assessor identify cognitive processing biases that can occur in many psychological disorders: for example, the tendency for individuals with depression to view past, present, and future in a more negative or pessimistic light (Alloy et al., 2000, 2005), or the tendency of someone with a somatization disorder to be hyperfocused on somatic symptoms and dysfunction despite objective evidence to the contrary (Ursin, 2005; Vervoort, Goubert, Eccleston, Bijttebier, & Crombez, 2006). Furthermore, clients who are currently in a state of high distress may report more extreme symptoms or distorted views of their current symptom severity, their current level of impairment/dysfunction, or their past symptoms/functioning, due to their current distress (De Figueiredo, 2013; Thompson, Bogner, Coyne, Gallo, & Eaton, 2004; Watson & Pennebaker, 1989). Thus, an assessor attuned to the psychological lens is listening not only for symptom sets and developmental patterns that might be consistent with a psychological disorder diagnosis, but is also paying attention to the mental status of the individual who is being interviewed and to the collateral evidence that is either consistent or inconsistent with the client's report of his or her current situation and past history.

Consistent with the psychological lens, the psychologist must also consider how much of the current presentation reflects long-standing characterological issues or is something new, acute, and responsive to stressors, supports, or treatments. This distinction can be important because long-standing behavioral or personality characteristics might interact with other causative factors (e.g., be a vulnerability factor) or may themselves have led to the client's experience of a stressful situation, which then led to other symptoms and concerns (Watson & Pennebaker, 1989). Again, this can be difficult to judge from only the current presentation of the client, pointing to the importance of both gathering data beyond self-report and the need to have a developmental context for the current presentation. In some cases these long-standing behavioral characteristics are in themselves diagnostic (e.g., in personality disorders), but in other cases are merely normal individual difference variables that, in the context of the client's current situation, are perhaps less than adaptive, which may have implications for recommendations but do not lead to a diagnosis per se.

Furthermore, the psychological lens requires that the assessor consider the full psychological profile of the individual, including cognitive, affective, and/or motivational factors that may exacerbate the presenting concerns, weaknesses, or impairments or actually serve as buffers or strengths that mitigate the presenting problem. These factors have bearing on prognosis and treatment recommendations and are what can take an assessment beyond diagnostic to therapeutic. Obviously, thorough knowledge of psychological disorders, their developmental trajectories, and their typical presentations, as well as knowledge of "normal" diversity in psychological characteristics and symptoms, is necessary to wear the psychological lens well. As noted in Chapter 2, extensive knowledge in only one type of psychological disorder, to the neglect of broad-based knowledge in psychopathology, is likely to introduce biases in the assessor that lead to poor assessment and differential diagnosis.

Another aspect of the psychological lens might be the etiological contributions specific to given therapeutic orientations. However, a psychologist who tries to use a particular therapeutic orientation to provide a top-down psychological explanation of a client's presentation before a full biopsychosocial examination of that presentation has occurred is likely to make decision-making errors. Starting assessment of a client using only a particular theoretical orientation that would guide treatment planning results in interpretations based on limited data, and is not much different than using the client's personal explanation for why certain behaviors have emerged; both reflect a belief that explanations for a client's presenting concerns can be found merely through attention to the client's perceptions of his or her symptoms (Pennington, 2002). The assessor who uses a particular therapeutic framework to interpret the presenting symptoms with the client prior to gathering the client's full story from multiple data sources is making many of the decision-making errors outlined in Chapter 2.

The Sociocultural Lens

Exploration of potential sociocultural contributions to a client's presenting problem includes an examination of current and historical environmental stressors and supports within all interactional circles the client could experience: family of origin, current family structure, friend networks, broader social and cultural networks, and broader environmental contexts. Understanding the context of the clinical case places all aspects of the assessment into their appropriate framework, including what the initial referral question truly is, the likelihood that the client will be willing/able to participate in the assessment, adaptations to assessment procedures that may need to occur given the context, and potential etiological factors underlying the client's concerns.

With regard to the initial referral question, the context of the evaluation may reveal that the stated reason for referral is only the surface of more complex issues and questions. For example, it is possible that a client who appears to have self-referred for a psychological concern is actually attempting to seek an evaluation in order to send the report to his or her attorney as part of ongoing litigation or for workman's compensation or disability application (the "lurking lawyer" cases). If the assessor assumes that the context of the evaluation is merely one in which the client is seeking help for a problem, the assessor will not understand the true context of the evaluation. Chapter 4 provides more discussion relevant to the effects of a compensatory context on psychological assessment. However, other contexts may provide clarity to the stated referral question, and it is the job of the assessor to seek these out; in order to best help the person referred, the assessor must know the actual questions that need to be answered.

For example, consider the case of an 18-year-old high school senior who was referred by her parents for evaluation for a math or other learning disability. She was a second-generation Indian, and her parents were concerned about her "poor" scores on the ACT and SAT, which they felt would preclude her from entering any prestigious colleges for a premedicine major. Her academic history was one of perfectly normal functioning in all academic and cognitive arenas, and her scores on the ACT and SAT were average relative to her grade peers, consistent with her academic history. She was reluctant to speak with the examiner, repeating over and over that she was willing to undergo the evaluation but also stating that she was only there because "my parents wanted me to have the evaluation." Eventually, after testing for answers to the stated referral question, during which she performed well below expectations given her academic history and possibly suggestive of diminished effort, the examiner probed more into the student's thoughts about the likely outcome of the evaluation. She reported that she "hoped" she did so poorly that her parents would see that a premed major was "not for her," but she was concerned that they would actually just "fight for accommodations" and "force" her to complete this major. It became apparent that she had no desire to be a premed student but was struggling to communicate this to her parents; her motivation for purposely failing her assessment clearly affected the validity of the results and led to a very different kind of feedback session than what was anticipated, given the initial referral question and the test results.

The assessor should also consider whether contextual factors affect the accuracy of the client's report of symptoms, the reason for referral, and the contextual factors themselves. For example, sociocultural differences may lead the client to over- or underemphasize symptoms, behaviors, or evidence of impaired functioning, or to define constructs differently than the dominant society might. Sociocultural differences could also create barriers to communication, such as through language fluency, or perhaps through the client's perception of the assessor as different or as lacking understanding of the client's sociocultural context. Cultural context is discussed further in Chapter 5, but is also something to consider in regard to the sociocultural lens, because it is important for an assessor to remember that clients' identifications with any particular culture or subculture might influence their understanding of symptoms, how they express the symptoms, whether they view the symptoms as dysfunctional or impairing, how they respond to test materials, etc.

In addition to their effect on self-report, sociocultural variables may also have direct etiological significance for the presenting concerns of a client, necessitating their evaluation in order to make appropriate treatment recommendations. For example, the presence of environmental stressors and supports might be related to the onset, exacerbation, relapse, or recovery from symptoms over time (Butzlaff & Hooley, 1998; Cromer, Schmidt, & Murphy, 2007; Hammen, Kim, Eberhart, & Brennan, 2009; Kendler & Gardner, 2010). Thus an assessor should consider the client's experience of any recent stressors that might be temporally related to the onset of his or her presenting concerns, as well as considering whether there is a developmental pattern to stressors and to the experience of symptoms in their overall history. Interestingly, research suggests that stressful life events are particularly predisposing when the client's own behavior led to the stressful life event (Hammen, 2006; Liu & Alloy, 2010), which might suggest an interaction between premorbid psychological vulnerability factors and current environmental stressors in the etiology of the presenting concerns. For example, a severely depressed individual may stop performing well in the work setting, leading to getting fired, which may worsen the client's depression and overall functioning. Thus an assessor should not automatically assume that the "causal arrow" points in the direction of the stressor (getting fired) leading to the symptoms or disorder, as the presence of a disorder and its symptoms or a psychological vulnerability factor may have led to the stressor, which may have exacerbated the symptoms. Following the developmental story over time can help the assessor examine these directional relationships.

It is also important for an assessor to remember that it is the client's *perception* of the event as stressful that is most likely to be associated with the presenting concerns (Francis-Rainier, Alloy, & Abramson, 2006; Kapci & Cramer, 2000), and this perception might represent the client's own cognitive distortions or biases (the psychological lens) rather than an accurate report about the event itself. For example, a client reporting significant anxiety and depression may attribute the symptoms to a recent stressful event, which is described as extremely distressing and catastrophic in nature, whereas additional data from others present at the event, including those who were with the client and gauged the client's reaction at the time, may paint a very different picture of the event itself, the client's reaction, and his or her mental status at the time of the event. The wearing of a distorted lens in the present, due to client's present level of distress, may have caused the individual to view the past event as more stressful than it really was.

As an example of a family stress for which there is a wealth of research support, expressed emotion is a construct characterized by the presence of hostile, critical family members that are both overly emotionally involved in the client's situation and critical of that person. Initially implicated as a factor in the onset and relapse of schizophrenic episodes, it has since been related to prognosis in several psychological conditions (Butzlaff & Hooley, 1998). However, a clinician examining for the presence of this kind of family stressor needs to bear in mind that a client currently in distress may inaccurately report information about his or her past and current family environment. The assessor would need to interview family members, as well make observations of the family dynamics during a group conversation, in order to truly understand whether expressed emotion is contributing to the client's ongoing problems. In addition, the assessor should consider that the client's psychological condition may have contributed to unusual family dynamics by creating parenting difficulties, for example, or increasing caregiver burden, suggesting that the client's disorder has led to impairment in the interpersonal domain. Furthermore, the relationship between a client's presenting symptoms and family relationships may reflect a shared genetic vulnerability (e.g., as in conduct problems; Bornovalova, Blazei,

Malone, McGue, & Iacono, 2012). Thus, more information would be needed to determine the etiological significance of family conflict and interactional style in the context of an individual's presenting concerns.

Similarly, although research evidence suggests that social support from family or peers can buffer against the effects of stressful life events (Alloy et al., 2000; Cacioppo, Hawkley, & Thisted, 2010; Cacioppo, Hughes, Waite, Hawkley, & Thisted, 2006), when the only evidence for presence or absence of supportive others is the client's report, the assessor must recognize that, as with many aspects of client self-report, this information may be inaccurate. Although it is important to understand the client's perception of his or her social network, it may be important to also gather data from that social network to put that perception into perspective.

Historical Context

Just as the current sociocultural context of symptoms may be affected by biases in report, so may a client's recall of his or her past. So, just as medical history should be validated by records, variables such as educational background or socioeconomic status (SES) should be validated by collateral information. Consider, for example, the case of a college senior who referred himself for evaluation for a learning disability after he did not receive a score that he liked on the GMAT; he was planning to attend graduate school in business. He described himself as having come from an "impoverished" family background, being a "first-generation student" and having received a "minimal" education in a high school in a "poor urban area." He also described himself as having to earn his own way through college, working close to full time while also attending classes. The astute graduate student clinician conducting the evaluation noted the watch that was peeking out from under the client's shirtsleeve, which was several hundred dollars in value, in seeming contrast to his report of extreme economic stress. A review of academic records confirmed that his high school was actually in an extremely affluent area and that he took virtually all the advanced placement (AP) courses offered, passing the AP exams at a very high level, suggesting that he had received a very good public school education. In addition, interview with one parent confirmed that his report of his family background was inaccurate, with both parents (and one set of grandparents) having advanced degrees beyond college, both parents being employed in high-income positions, and with three older siblings who had at least college educations or beyond.

Another example of the incomplete picture that can be taken from only self-reported academic histories is the example of a college freshman who was failing out of her first semester of university. She reported that she did not understand why she was failing, given that she received all A's and B's in high school and was the class valedictorian. She reported that she was feeling depressed and suicidal about her failure in school. A clinician who "stopped there" might have developed only one hypothesis: that the student's depression was leading to her current academic impairment. However, a clinician who asked for school records would have noticed that the student was class valedictorian out of a class of only about 12 students in an urban "magnet" school. Looking up records on the school would have revealed that it did not have a good academic reputation, and further evaluation of the client's school records would have revealed that the student took the state graduation test five times before passing it, which was set at about a ninth-grade achievement level, and that she received ACT and SAT scores that were definitely indicative of a lack of readiness for college-level work (with scores falling less than the fifth percentile relative to others planning to attend college). When cognitive testing was conducted, the client's borderline intellect and achievement scores were consistent with this more detailed knowledge about her academic history, and she was successfully counseled to seek career services, to apply to two-year training programs in career areas of interest to her, and to participate in psychotherapy for her depression—which was clearly a reaction to her academic failure, rather than the cause of it.

Family History

It is important to place clients' symptoms in the perspective of others in their immediate family (both genetic and nongenetic) who may or may not have similar psychological histories or may have experienced similar symptoms or life problems. Thus, an assessor should ask whether others in the client's family have experienced similar symptoms, similar life problems, or have a history of psychological treatment. Certainly one reason for examining family history is to determine the potential biological contribution, including the heritability of some psychological disorders. However, family history can also place the client's presenting concerns in a sociocultural context. For example, asking about family history is more likely to "pull for" some of the cultural definitions and understandings of whether "symptoms" are considered pathological or impairing in the cultural background of the person being assessed. It is also important to examine family history of similar problems because of the social model of illness and diagnosis. In the common-sense model of health and illness, for example, it is hypothesized that individuals create illness representations of their symptoms along the lines of factors such as having a particular illness, what the causes of the symptoms or illness might be, the likely chronicity of the symptoms or illness, and the likely effect of the symptoms or illness on functioning. Individuals develop these illness representations based on information from their social environment, including family members/friends, layperson accounts of the illness, public access to information about the illness (e.g., through the Internet, television, and other media) and authoritative resources such as health care providers. The illness representations that arise from this sort of information influence how people view their past history and present symptoms, what they communicate in assessment, and are predictive of outcomes in a wide variety of illnesses (Hagger & Orbell, 2003; Leventhal, Brissette, & Leventhal, 2003).

For example, consider the case of a young adult female referred for evaluation for a learning disability. The self-report of the client and the client's mother was one of significant physical and cognitive dysfunction and impairment. An assessor focused on this information (and coupled with the severely impaired performance across all areas of academic achievement during the testing) would have incorrectly reached conclusions about the presence of a learning disability. However, an assessor attuned to sociocultural factors would have attended to the client's mention of applying for disability on the basis of the learning disability and found the rest of the story by examining the client's actual educational history, history of functioning, activities and hobbies, and by interviewing the mother about the client's developmental history and family history. Such examination would have revealed that the client's maternal grandmother and mother were both recipients of Social Security Disability payments from their early adulthood, for unclear reasons, and that the client's mother had applied for full disability for the client in her early adolescence on the basis of mild scoliosis, even though the client was actively involved in dance classes and other physical activities at the time. In addition, further examination would have revealed that the reason for the learning disability evaluation was due to continued denial of disability for the scoliosis claim and her mother's insistence that her daughter would be unable to work due to a learning disability—whereas actual school records revealed normal functioning without any need for accommodations throughout elementary, middle, and high school years. The attuned assessor would have also taken note that the self-report (significant physical and cognitive dysfunction and impairment) and behavioral performance (test scores in the impaired range) of the client were in contrast to her ability to participate in a lengthy interview and evaluation. Models of disability/impairment seeking were an important part of the assessment picture that would have been missed if the conclusion were based on the client's self-report during a simple interview, coupled with her current achievement test results.

The Broader Sociological Context

An assessor also has to consider the broader sociocultural lens in which the client is presenting. This broader lens requires examining the systems in which the client is operating on a day-to-day basis to determine whether they provide barriers to functioning or whether they provide resources that might be helpful to consider when making recommendations to the client. Consideration of this broader lens also means considering who, in addition to the client, may need to receive the assessment report, and thus how the results should be communicated (see Chapter 14).

In addition, however, as noted in the common-sense model, clients' illness identities can be informed and reinforced by the broader sociocultural context in which they experience their problems. Certainly in the case above, the client's familial experience with disability may have reinforced her own belief in having a disability, but so too might her school have reinforced her and her family's belief that she was impaired. In fact, my clinical experience has revealed many cases in which schools provided academic accommodations and services to students based on strong familial advocacy rather than documented evidence of their need, thus reinforcing a belief in an impairment that carries through to adulthood. At an even broader level, psychologists and sociologists have documented the larger cultural "push" for pathologizing all common problems of everyday living as psychological disorders and disabilities (Conrad & Potter, 2000; Frances, 2010), in part driven by pharmaceutical companies, support and advocacy groups that are motivated to make "their" disorder stand out for receipt of services, clinicians who are motivated to get reimbursed for services, and even researchers motivated to receive grant funding for their research—but also by our culture's lowering threshold for normal variation in behavior and a tendency to believe that any mistake, error, weakness, or "just average" performance is not acceptable and even indicative of a problem.

The Developmental Lens

Even when an assessor's work is primarily with adults, he or she needs to remember that most psychopathology has origins in development. These origins could be found (1) in the distant past, such as continuing consequences of a developmental disorder or the experience of early life stressors that may increase likelihood of later psychopathology; or (2) in the more recent past, such as a recent life stressor, lifestyle change, or medical problem. In addition, there may be multiple developmental paths contributing to the current presentation, and those contributions are themselves changing and have a circular causality, with feedback loops that can sustain, diminish, or exacerbate any specific behavioral pattern over time (Borrell-Carrio, Suchman, & Epstein, 2004). Many of the cases described above illustrate the importance of considering present symptoms in a developmental context. An assessor who stays attuned to the developmental nature of psychopathology will remember to explore the client's history, not just from the client's phenomenological perspective of "when things started," but by asking about early life history and how the present symptoms might have manifested themselves in the past, etc.

The client's full psychological picture can look like a circle with complex bidirectional interactions, making a determination of "which came first" impossible, but the developmental context must be considered to accurately interpret the current presentation. For example, consider the case of a student in his first year of college who was failing a basic math class. He and his parents were convinced he had a math disability. He was given an achievement test and performed at the fifth percentile, relative to his same-age peers, in math skills. However, a careful look at the client's developmental history, via his mother's report and a review of all of his school records, revealed that he had no problems with math achievement through the ninth grade. Although both the client and his mother reported that he had always "hated" math, he was never behind in math, never referred for services, never scored below proficient in yearly math achievement tests, never received formal interventions or accommodations based on math difficulties, and passed the math section of the state graduation test on his first attempt during 10th grade. However, because he "hated" math, the student took only the required classes to graduate high school and did not complete college-level math courses while in high school; his lowest scores on high-stakes testing (ACT, SAT) were in the math domain, although his scores still fell near the 35th percentile relative to other high school students planning to attend college (the comparison population for such tests). What was most notable, then, was the sharp contrast in his fifth percentile performance, relative to his same-age peers, on a math achievement test administered at the time of the evaluation as compared to his academic history, which documented much higher levels of math achievement. From a developmentally oriented perspective, this client was able to develop and use mathematical skills without any evidence of impairment throughout his precollege academic experience, although he did not enjoy it and was not motivated to continue to develop those skills past what he needed to graduate from high school. Now, when faced with a college-level math course, he expected to do poorly, was not motivated to do well, did not utilize the supplemental instruction and peer tutors available to him because he felt they would not be helpful, and believed his failure in the course was due to a disability rather than to these developmental factors.

Now consider the case of a young man being evaluated in the context of an inpatient neurological rehabilitation setting. He had an accident while riding his motorcycle (without a helmet), resulting in a head injury with about 1 day loss of consciousness and about 3 days of posttraumatic amnesia; he was now awake, alert, and oriented consistently, but was referred for neuropsychological evaluation due to "inappropriate behavior." The nursing staff noted that he often pinched or grabbed them inappropriately when they were treating him and that he often made comments about them that were sexual in nature. The referring physician wrote in the patient's chart that this behavior was consistent with frontal lobe dysfunction due to the head injury and made several predictions about his low likelihood of returning to "normal" functioning based on this information; he also made recommendations for neurorehabilitation focused on the patient's disinhibition. However, the neuropsychologist who came to the patient's room to conduct the evaluation found a pile of *Playboy* and other similar magazines sticking out from the patient's mattress; the patient reported that his father had brought them in for him at his request, as they were part of the patient's "collection." His neuropsychological profile revealed perfectly normal functioning in all areas of cognition assessed. An interview with his father and mother, as well as rating forms about their son's behavior before and after the injury, revealed not only that they saw no differences in his premorbid and postaccident personality or behavior, but that the father engaged in the same behavior as his son, actually pinching the neuropsychologist and making whistling noises behind a nurse who was taking his son's blood pressure, appearing to indicate with gestures something about the nurse's body to his son. Further information from his school revealed a premorbid history of normal academic functioning but a long list of behavioral and conduct problems clearly indicative of disinhibition. Although the neurologist's prediction about this patient's long-term outcome may have been accurate, the hypothesized etiology for his current behavior was not, and it would be unlikely that such long-standing characterological problems in a family system that appeared to reinforce them would respond well to neurorehabilitation for his brain injury.

PUTTING IT TOGETHER

Biopsychosocial models seek to understand human health and illness in their fullest contexts. Both natural and social sciences are basic to the model, and both are needed to understand human behavior. Different clinical presentations must be understood scientifically at several levels of the natural systems continuum, from the individual symptom or predisposition to the final symptom set or diagnosis. Whereas genetics or neurochemistry may explain the dysfunction of a brain system and contribute to behavior, the sociocultural context in which a client develops and in which that client lives can influence how this behavior presents and what it means for his or her overall presentation. Viewing a client's presenting problems through a developmentally oriented biopsychosocial lens means that the assessor will acknowledge the existence of multiple developmental pathways and contributions to behavioral dysfunction, and that these multiple risk and protective factors influence the likelihood of certain outcomes in a probabilistic fashion. A clinician attuned to and experienced in identifying which factors are most supported by research for any given symptom or symptom set will remember to ask the right questions to lend weight or diminish belief in any particular hypothesis raised by these broad lenses.

Case Example

Although several cases above illustrate important aspects of the biopsychosocial model in psychological assessment, this chapter ends with one more case to further illustrate the principles above and for discussion in a group setting.

A psychologist was referred a young woman with a diagnosis of bipolar disorder for psychotherapy, following a brief inpatient stay after emergency admission during a "manic episode." The client had been placed on lithium and was described as "not responding well to medication."

What is known based on this referral information? What else might an assessor want to know prior to the first appointment with this client? What hypotheses are raised by this limited information? What sets of questions might the assessor/psychologist be ready to ask? What additional data might the assessor need other than interviewing the client?

In the intake interview, the client was relatively nonresponsive, with limited eye contact, blunted affect, minimal movement or gestures, and little facial expression. She was dressed sloppily in sweats and her hair was uncombed. She indicated that she had recently gained a lot of weight due to the lithium and that none of her clothes fit her. When asked to describe the symptoms and experiences that brought her to psychotherapy, she grew extremely agitated, wringing her hands and shaking her legs. She began to hyperventilate and then indicated that she felt dizzy and physically ill. She then proceeded to vomit all over the clinician's office, ending the initial intake appointment rather abruptly.

What do these observations raise as far as issues to consider and hypotheses to test about the patient's current mental and physical state?

The assessor reviewed the hospital records for more information prior to the second appointment. The admission notes included a summary of the brief intake interview, with the client noted as "presenting symptoms of a manic episode including racing thoughts, psychomotor agitation, and no need for sleep in the days preceding hospitalization." The client was noted as having no known psychological history. The client was hospitalized, sedated, and after a few days, during which she mostly slept, she was released to home (where she lived with her parents) with a diagnosis of bipolar disorder and a prescription for lithium. No further evaluations were conducted during her hospital stay or at discharge.

What do these records suggest about the nature of the evaluation she received in order to reach the diagnosis she was given during the inpatient stay? What other considerations for her symptoms might be considered by the assessor? Should the assessor question the accuracy of any of the information obtained (including past history), given the context of the "assessment"?

At the next appointment, the assessor asked for more details about the client's symptoms as well as behaviors and events preceding the hospitalization. Instead of using the diagnostic descriptors in the hospital record, the assessor asked the client to "walk through" the days immediately prior to the hospitalization, including not only how she felt and behaved, but also including all aspects of her everyday routine and the environmental context for those days (who she was with, what sorts of stressors she might have experienced, etc.). She was also asked to "walk through" her days since her hospitalization, with the assessor wearing the biopsychosocial lens and asking about all aspects of her experience.

Through this comprehensive approach, it became clear that there were multiple factors contributing to the emergency room visit and to the client's general mental health, and none of them were related to bipolar disorder.

First, the client stated that she never said she did not *need* sleep, but that she *could not* sleep despite really needing to sleep, and that her lack of ability to sleep was due to intrusive thoughts and anxiety-provoking feelings that she experienced when she tried to lay down to sleep. When asked what those thoughts were, she indicated that they were flashbacks to a sexual assault she had experienced a few years prior; the flashbacks were precipitated by unexpectedly running into the perpetrator a few weeks prior to her hospitalization. She also reported other symptoms consistent with posttraumatic stress disorder (PTSD), dating back to the sexual assault itself (which led her to drop out of college because she didn't want to run into the perpetrator), but having grown recently worse due to her chance encounter with him in recent weeks.

Furthermore, the client reported that she had been drinking coffee all day long (at least four pots worth) in an attempt to keep herself from getting sleepy during the day, which was leading to jitteriness, shaking, and heart palpitations. She was also not eating well and had been eating mostly junk food in mild binges, alternating with starving herself for long periods of time to counteract the binges and the weight gain from the lithium. She denied having a history of similar eating behaviors, which was corroborated by interview with her mother.

Because the individual who conducted the initial intake evaluation in the emergency room jumped straight from one symptom to a symptom pattern ("looks manic") without considering other etiological contributions to the presenting problems, the client was misdiagnosed, and lifestyle factors and life events with major psychological and biological contributions to her presenting problems were completely missed.

The client was taken off lithium and began treatment for what was eventually diagnosed as PTSD; she continued to have sleep issues, although many of those symptoms were improved after consultation with a sleep clinic, where she addressed sleep hygiene issues and her caffeine intake. She was also referred for a general physical, and the physician suggested that some of her physiological anxiety-type attacks were due to hypoglycemia. Following a regular nutritional plan, cutting down on caffeine, and addressing her sleep went a long way toward addressing her "psychological" symptoms, and she felt they were just as important to her care as her psychological treatment for PTSD.

4

The Importance of Assessing for Noncredible Responding

It is the only hypothesis which covers the facts.
—SHERLOCK HOLMES, in *The Sign of the Four*

Back in 2001, as part of a neuropsychology listserv conversation, I was accused of "starting the funeral procession for neuropsychology." The accusation arose out of a discussion of the use of measures of noncredible responding within neuropsychological evaluations. The accuser opined that use of such measures in an evaluation, particularly when they actually indicated noncredible responding on the part of the person being evaluated, would mean that no one would "listen to anything else you have to say." I penned what I viewed as a well-reasoned and empirically supported reply to this accusation, based on the available research at the time; many of the arguments I presented then appear in this chapter.

It is optimistic to think that, given the explosion of research on the importance of assessing for noncredible responding and the validity of methods to detect it, as well as the publication of consensus statements advocating for the use of such measures in routine assessment, fewer assessors today would view routine assessment for this critical threat to the validity of an assessment as "death" for the field. In fact, given that the American Psychological Association (2002) code of ethics makes it clear that an assessor must consider the effects of specific contextual elements on the validity of the data collected in that specific assessment before the data are interpreted, consideration of noncredible responding is, in fact, necessary for ethical practice. However, even today, few training programs focus on training in the issue of noncredible responding and how to assess for it. This lacuna suggests a need for assessors to be reminded of both the importance of considering the validity of all data gathered as part of an assessment and the ever-growing research evidence that we can assess for noncredible responding in a valid manner.

Although most of the recent furor over the use of measures of noncredible responding arose around its use in neuropsychological assessment, it is important to note that psychologists have measured noncredible reporting within some self-report measures for decades (e.g., validity indices on measures such as the Minnesota Multiphasic Personality Inventory [MMPI] or the Personality Assessment Inventory [PAI]). Interestingly, however, most self-report measures of psychological symptoms/status do *not* include any measures of noncredible reporting; in fact, as can be seen below, most assessors still do not appear to consider the role that noncredible reporting/ performing might play in their assessments, whether those assessments include interview data, self-report questionnaires, or neuropsychological and other cognitive tests. Furthermore, even the use of validity scales on well-standardized and validated measures such as the MMPI has come under recent scrutiny, especially in the forensic setting. It's almost as if most assessors "don't want to know" and, when faced with the evidence that the individuals they are assessing might not perform or report credibly, the "messenger" is blamed (i.e., the measures of noncredible responding themselves are assumed to have no validity).

Assessing for the credibility of the data provided by the person being assessed, whether in his or her self-report, presentation, and/or test performance, is central to understanding whether data in the evaluation are valid to interpret. Although consensus statements and the American Psychological Association code of ethics remind us of the need to pay attention to this issue (American Psychological Association, 2002; Bush et al., 2005; Heilbronner et al., 2009), there seem to be several "stumbling blocks" for some assessors in regard to routine use of measures of noncredible responding in their assessment procedures. The purpose of the present chapter is to discuss those stumbling blocks and to raise the reader's awareness of the availability of, and need for, measures of noncredible performance in empirically based assessment. One stumbling block is unawareness of how common noncredible responding is. Another stumbling block is unawareness of the empirical support for measures of noncredible responding. A third major stumbling block is what Paul Green (personal communication, 2000) aptly named "invalidity shock" many years ago. A final major stumbling block, called up most often in neuropsychological assessment but relevant in all assessment, is the assumption that acknowledging the potential invalidity of data somehow weakens the value of the data provided in such an evaluation. Before discussing each of these stumbling blocks in more detail, a definition of noncredible responding is presented.

WHAT IS NONCREDIBLE RESPONDING?

Noncredible responding occurs when individuals present themselves in an inaccurate way during an assessment by behaving in a manner inconsistent with their actual abilities or concerns (as could be seen in their observed behavior or on actual performance tasks), and/or by reporting their history or symptoms in an inaccurate fashion (as might be seen in interview or on self-report questionnaires). Although noncredible responding could involve the presentation of self in an inaccurately positive light (e.g., as might be seen in contexts such as a parental evaluation for child custody or application for a job requiring high cognitive skills or no evidence of psychological concerns), a more common scenario in clinical assessment is the presentation of self in an inaccurately negative light. Contexts in which this is likely to occur include those involving any sort of external gain, such as to win a lawsuit, to receive disability or workman's compensation, to obtain access to prescription medications, or to avoid being held responsible for crimes committed. When there is evidence that a person being assessed has deliberately and consciously behaved in a noncredible fashion for the purpose of an external gain, that person is said to be malingering (American Psychiatric Association, 2013). However, individuals may also respond noncredibly with less than fully conscious awareness or deliberate action, and may be reinforced for doing so by internal gains, such as a psychological need for attention or care of loved ones, or to behave consistently with a sick role. The actions of these individuals would not meet the definition of malingering. However, it does not make the behavior any more credible and still invalidates the findings from the assessment. In many circumstances, it is difficult to determine whether the client's noncredible responding is conscious or unconscious or whether the motivations for the noncredible responding are external or internal in nature (or both). Furthermore, the level of conscious awareness and/or the nature of the motivations for noncredible responding can change over time and with context. Nevertheless, although it may be difficult to determine the "why," an assessor can accurately measure the "what" (noncredible responding) and can and should use data about the credibility of the client's responses when interpreting the results of the assessment.

As noted above, "noncredible responding" refers the behavior itself, not to the intention of the behavior. In addition, noncredible responding is not a characteristic of the person. "One is not a malingerer, but engages in malingering behavior periodically" (Rohling & Boone, 2007, p. 457). Because noncredible responding is a state of behaving and not necessarily a trait of a person, the behavior may manifest differently within different parts of the same evaluation, with different clinicians, or in different contexts such as when an evaluation has a different purpose. In addition, if the behavior is meant to communicate (whether conscious or unconscious) about specific types of symptoms, noncredible responding may be seen only when measures that appear to assess those specific symptoms are administered ("selective malingering"; Nelson, Sweet, Berry, Bryant, & Granacher, 2007). In other words, a person may (1) self-report symptoms in a noncredible manner while behaving in a credible fashion on cognitive measures; (2) perform noncredibly on cognitive measures but report accurately on self-report measures; (3) report noncredibly with regard to symptoms consistent with one disorder while reporting accurately on other symptoms; or (4) behave noncredibly on measures of one cognitive construct but not on others.

Noncredible responding, as seen in self-report and/or test performance, can be viewed as a communication. The client may be trying to communicate to the assessor that he or she deserves compensation, that he or she has been deliberately wronged, that he or she desperately needs help of some kind, and/or that this is the illness "lens" through which he or she views his or her current functioning and symptoms. On the other hand, the client may be deliberately attempting to deceive the assessor with his or her communications. Nevertheless, if what the client has communicated suggests inaccuracies in the communication, that communication is noncredible and not interpretable. Consider a patient who is getting a magnetic resonance imaging (MRI) scan and is asked to hold still. The patient may move due to pain, due to fear of the claustrophobic setting, or perhaps even due to less than conscious awareness of him- or herself and the surroundings . . . or the patient may deliberately move. Whatever the motivation, the movement artifact will render the MRI difficult to read and affect the validity of the data obtained.

HOW IS NONCREDIBLE RESPONDING MEASURED?

With regard to the assessment of noncredible performance, there are both stand-alone measures as well as measures embedded within other cognitive measures, and there are well-validated versions of both types of measures. Although many of these measures are focused on noncredible performance in the cognitive domain of attention/memory, there are also measures focused on reading skills, psychomotor processing speed, and perceptual–motor skills (Boone, 2007; Larrabee, 2007). Because most of these measures are used in the context of cognitive and neuropsychological assessment, they are discussed in more detail in Chapters 11 and 12.

With regard to the noncredible self-reporting of current symptoms, there are well-validated measures of noncredible symptom report in the form of embedded measures (e.g., the validity scales within broad measures of psychopathology such as the MMPI or the PAI), as well as stand-alone measures (e.g., the Miller Forensic Assessment of Symptoms Test [M-FAST], the M Test, the Structured Inventory of Malingered Symptomatology, Malingering Detection Scale, to name a view; see Boone, 2012, for a review). Some of these validity scales focus on whether the report of symptoms is consistent over time (i.e., whether the client consistently endorses items that have similar content, despite different wording). Some scales focus on the underreport of symptoms (i.e., not acknowledging symptoms that most people would acknowledge having). Finally, many scales focus on reporting a higher than normal number of symptoms or unusual symptoms that are not frequently endorsed by others, even those with medical, neurological, or psychiatric diagnoses. The validity indices specific to the MMPI and the PAI are discussed more thoroughly in Chapter 10. Unfortunately, whereas broadband self-report measures such as the MMPI and PAI have long included validity scales, most self-report measures of single psychological (and medical!) constructs do not include measurement of noncredible symptom report.

It is difficult to document the noncredible reporting of a person's past with formal measures. However, an assessor who gathers more than just self-report data from an interview (see Chapter 8) will be able to corroborate some aspects of a client's self-reported past. For example, as noted in examples in Chapter 3, clients may report their past academic performance as overly good or as overly bad, relative to the school record, including grades, performance on standardized tests with national percentiles, etc. But clients can also report their past symptoms and/or their medical history inaccurately (Greiffenstein, Baker, & Johnson-Greene, 2002). Consider the case of a client referred for psychotherapy to assist in the management of severe migraine-type headaches. The client was reluctant to participate in the initial intake interview, indicating that the severity, intensity, and frequency of his headaches was such that they would not respond to psychological treatment, and, because they were caused by a car accident in which he had sustained a whiplash injury, their etiology suggested that they would not respond to "standard" treatments for people with "run-of-the-mill" migraines. He insisted that he'd "never" had headaches prior to the accident, yet review of his medical chart showed repeated visits to the emergency room for severe migraine-type headaches in the several years prior to the accident, for which he received Imitrex injections. When confronted by the psychologist with this medical record, he simply stated, "Well, these new headaches are different."

Unfortunately, an area lacking in research is the potential for collaterals to report noncredibly about the person being assessed. An assessor must recognize that collaterals may also have motivations for both underreporting and/or overreporting the client's symptoms and functioning, depending on the context of the evaluation, and may also not report accurately on the client's history. For example, consider the case of an adolescent male who was burned over 80% of his body after climbing over a security fence in order to touch some electrical equipment on a dare. His parents reported that his current psychological and cognitive functioning was severely impaired, whereas his premorbid functioning was intact; in fact, his mother described him as "an angel" prior to the injury. However, existing school records documented a history of significant academic difficulties and severe behavioral and conduct problems (including placement at an alternative school for a period of time). Thus, consideration of other data (both formal testing as well as other extratest data, such as available records, is important to placing collateral report in context.

Noncredible Responding Is Common

The first stumbling block encountered by individuals who have not received training in the assessment of noncredible responding is that they don't understand how common it is. The reality, as pointed out by many researchers (e.g., Boone, 2007, 2012; Larrabee, 2007, 2012; Rogers, 2008a) is that noncredible responding is extraordinarily common and that most patients will engage in some sort of deception (either consciously or unconsciously) by either exaggerating, minimizing, distorting, or omitting parts of their "story" at one time or another.

Ways in which estimations of noncredible responding are obtained are quite varied, with some data arising from surveys of experts regarding how often they "see" this behavior in their practice and other data arising from actual outcomes on measures of noncredible responding. In addition, there are varied data on how often noncredible responding occurs on self-report measures versus on behavioral measures such as cognitive or neuropsychological tests.

Although many studies have documented that the presence of a financial incentive—such as in litigation, workman's compensation, or disability determination (Belanger, Curtiss, Demery, Lebowitz, & Vanderploeg, 2005; Binder & Rohling, 1996; Binder, Rohling, & Larrabee, 1997; Rohling, Binder, & Langhinrichen-Rochling, 1995)—is strongly related to noncredible responding, there is also a high base rate of noncredible responding even outside of a clear financial incentive context. As a few illustrative examples of the frequency of noncredible responding, it is estimated to occur in 10–40% of patients with various pain disorders (Fishbain et al., 2003; Gervais et al., 2001; Mittenberg, Patton, Canyock, & Condit, 2002), in 25–40% of patients with various medically unexplained disorders such as fibromyalgia and chronic fatigue syndrome (Larrabee, 2012; Greve, Etherton, Ord, Bianchini, & Curtis, 2009; Meyers, Millis, & Volkert, 2002; Mittenberg et al., 2002; Nelson, Sweet, & Demakis, 2006; van der Werf, Prins, Jongen, van der Meer, & Bleijenberg, 2000), in up to 28% of individuals with depression being evaluated in a forensic context (Green, Rohling, Lees-Haley, & Allen, 2001; Mittenberg et al., 2002; Stefan, Clopton, & Morgan, 2003), in up to 40% of patients with mild traumatic brain injury being seen as part of litigation (see Larrabee, 2012, for a review), and in at least 20% of both military and civilian individuals claiming PTSD (Elhai et al., 2004; Frueh et al., 2005). Overall, the base rate of for noncredible responding in individuals reporting psychological, physical, and/or cognitive symptoms and concerns is higher than the base rate of most actual disorders! Thus, a good decision maker will consider the potential "diagnostic" hypothesis of noncredible responding and behavior in any evaluation (given that most evaluations do have some sort of external or internal gain, but particularly when that context is very likely).

Measures of Noncredible Responding Are Valid

Another stumbling block to the regular use of measures of noncredible responding in assessment is that many people seem unaware or unaccepting of the large research base supporting the effectiveness and accuracy of many of these measures. Just a few of the texts that summarize the existing literature on the validity of measures of both noncredible reporting and noncredible performance include Boone (2007, 2012), Larrabee (2007, 2012), and Rogers (2008a). Most evidence for many of these measures shows that they are not only able to detect noncredible responding (i.e., have good sensitivity), but also that they do not have a high false-positive rate (i.e., have good specificity), although there are exceptions, and assessors should consult these texts and review the psychometric properties of any specific measure of noncredible responding they may be considering for use in assessment. As mentioned in Chapter 2 and as is discussed further in

Chapter 6, both sensitivity and specificity are important elements of accurate assessment. Specificity is considered to be of particular importance in this area of assessment, given the concern about negative interpretation of the motives of individuals who are judged to have responded noncredibly on assessment measures.

Invalidity Shock

Despite the fact that there is such a high base rate for noncredible responding and that there are valid measures for detecting noncredible responding within both self-report measures and cognitive performance domains, in addition to consensus statements (Bush et al., 2005; Heilbronner et al., 2009) emphasizing the importance of using such measures in all assessment, there is still resistance to their use from many assessors. Paul Green (personal communication, 2000) referred to this resistance as "invalidity shock." He opined that the use of measures of noncredible responding challenge core beliefs that assessors hold about the individuals they assess, including the following:

> "My clients report their history and symptoms accurately."
> "My clients always try their best on the tests I administer."
> "I can tell when a client is putting forth good effort."
> "If I establish good rapport, my client will put forth his or her best effort."
> "Questioning the validity of test results or self-report is harmful to the clinical relationship."

When an assessor holds the above core beliefs, but then sees evidence that the client has performed noncredibly, it is far easier for the assessor to "punish the messenger" rather than challenge the core beliefs. Thus, the assessor chooses to ignore or explain away the evidence of noncredible responding, and, in order to avoid experiencing such a challenge to his or her beliefs in the future, may avoid using such measures in subsequent evaluations. The first two core beliefs are in clear contradiction to the evidence reviewed in this chapter regarding the high base rate of inaccurate reporting of history and symptoms and evidence of invalid effort on behavioral measures among individuals presenting for assessment. Thus these two core beliefs are not consistent with scientific evidence and should be challenged. The third core belief, that an assessor "can tell" when a client is putting forth good effort, is also contradicted by research showing that, without use of well-validated measures of noncredible responding, psychologists are in fact inaccurate in making that determination (Faust, Hart, Guilmette, & Arkes, 1988; Heaton, Smith, Lehman, & Vogt, 1978).

The last two core beliefs are central to an assessor's concern about the nature of the relationship with the person he or she is assessing. First, some clinicians seem to feel that evidence of noncredible responding will lead to the conclusion that the behavior was somehow the assessor's fault. When one remembers that noncredible responding is a type of communication by the client, one can see that in fact "good rapport" may simply encourage more noncredible responding, rather than diminish it. When noncredible responding is done to deliberately communicate "I need this external gain," having a pleasant relationship with the person doing the assessment will not likely change the mind of the person who is deliberately and consciously making that communication. In the case of an individual who is convinced that everyday occurrences are evidence of impairment and illness, and this is the lens through which he or she views the world, being assessed by someone who appears to understand him or her may only enhance inaccurate communication of symptoms and distress. Finally, many assessors are concerned that raising questions about, or challenging, the accuracy of clients' self-reports or behaviors will harm the clinical relationship. Although it requires a great deal of clinical skill to confront individuals about inaccuracies in reporting or invalid performances on tests, it is a necessary clinical skill to develop to elicit the most accurate data possible for the assessment. Different approaches to discussing findings of noncredible responding are presented in Chapter 14.

An additional symptom to add to Green's list of symptoms of invalidity shock may be the countertransference that can develop when an assessor "takes personally" the client's noncredible responding, which certainly could harm the clinical relationship. Understanding that noncredible responding is not a reflection of the assessor's clinical skill or the degree of rapport with the client should minimize that component of harm to the relationship. In addition, the assessor should remember that noncredible responding is a communication and not necessarily a characteristic of the person being assessed, so evidence for noncredible responding does not necessarily indicate a "moral failing" on the part of the person being assessed. Furthermore, consideration of the reasons behind the communication may lead to important treatment decisions; remaining focused on the therapeutic value of the assessment may help mitigate a clinician's negative reaction to identification of noncredible responding.

When an assessor measures behavior, he or she should assess not only how the patient behaved, but also consider *why* the patient behaved in the way that he or she did. When a client performs in a noncredible fashion on self-report and/or performance measures, all that has been documented is that the data collected are not valid and thus cannot be used to reach an accurate understanding of the client's presenting problems. But the performance itself does not provide reasons for the noncredible behavior, and many hypotheses other than a conscious, deliberate attempt to feign or exaggerate one's condition for external gain (malingering) could be considered, some of which might lead to potential therapeutic intervention. For example, one hypothesis might be that the individual is deliberately behaving noncredibly to achieve an external gain. However, another hypothesis might be that an individual has such a strong identity as a patient, and is therefore convinced that he or she cannot do a memory task that appears to be incredibly difficult, that he or she performs in a noncredible fashion on the memory task. As already stated, the data in this case are still invalid in regard to interpreting the memory ability of the individual, but the explanation for *why* the patient behaved noncredibly doesn't appear in the invalid test result.

Use of measures of noncredible responding show the assessor only that there has been noncredible report or performance. A good assessor using such measures will not "stop there," but will develop and explore hypotheses about reasons for the noncredible behavior—hypotheses that include but go beyond malingering. If an assessor automatically assumes that noncredible responding is due to malingering (i.e., a conscious and deliberate attempt to deceive the examiner) without examining evidence for and against such an interpretation, such an assumption could bias the assessor in other decision-making areas, affect his or her rapport with the client, as well as influence recommendations for the client after the evaluation. On the other hand, an assessor who considers the context and the communication the client might be trying to make may be able to identify appropriate treatment recommendations or considerations.

In summary, a "scientific detective" must maintain a critical view of the information that is gathered from all sources and, at the same time, exhibit good clinical skills to maintain empathy and understanding for the person being assessed. The key is for the assessor to remember that he or she is checking for the validity of the data to determine whether they are interpretable. The assessor to consider if there is reason to suspect that the data are invalid to interpret. Failing to recognize noncredible behavior means colluding with clients who are behaving noncredibly, thereby reinforcing strategies that might be maladaptive for clients' own self-care, and is also harmful more broadly to society and to scientific understanding of psychological disorders.

Effects on the Way Data Are Viewed

When I was accused of "starting the funeral procession for neuropsychology," it was because the accuser believed that the use of such measures in an evaluation, particularly when they indicated noncredible responding by the person being assessed, would mean that no one would "listen to anything else you have to say." This argument is puzzling. If a child holds a thermometer up to a light bulb to make it read higher so that he can stay home from school, and the mom knows about it, she does not report that the child had a fever of 120—she knows the reading is invalid. If an individual receiving an MRI moves too much during the procedure and creates movement artifacts, the scan is not read because it is invalid. Neither the thermometer nor the MRI machine are blamed for the invalid data; nor is the individual who read the thermometer or the scan. It is OK for data to be invalid. It is not OK to interpret invalid data as valid. It is not the fault of the clinician or of the test(s) when the data are invalid.

It is appropriate professional and ethical practice to determine whether the measures of behavior are accurate indicators of the constructs they are supposed to assess (American Psychological Association, 2002). An assessor must judge whether the behavioral samples gathered are valid—that is, are reliable indicators of the patient's behavior across time and situations, and accurate indicators of that patient's ability in the domain being assessed. Even when a test is, in the abstract, judged to be a psychometrically valid measure of a construct (as is discussed in Chapter 6), in any $N = 1$ assessment situation, an assessor must consider effects of specific contextual elements on the validity of the data that were collected in that particular assessment before the data are interpreted. No matter how good of an interviewer or test administrator an assessor is, the data collected from a specific interview, observation of behavior, or from standardized tests can still be invalid, if in fact the person being assessed does not provide credible information or behave in a credible manner. When a patient responds in a way that invalidates that sample of behavior, the measure is no longer a reliable or valid indicator of that person's abilities or psychological status at that specific time. This noncredibility directly affects the assessor's ability to interpret any of the data gathered and to trust their accuracy, and accuracy is paramount to ethical practice (American Psychological Association, 2002).

Ironically, I was recently part of a different listserv discussion in which many researchers were expressing the opinion that a decline in the reputation of psychological assessment and diagnosis is due to the fact that many psychologists still do *not* use measures of noncredible performance in their practice, ensuring inconsistency in diagnosis across different assessors and leading to mistrust in clinical judgment.

IMPLICATIONS OF ASSESSING FOR NONCREDIBLE RESPONDING DURING ASSESSMENT

The scientifically minded assessor who was not already using measures of noncredible responding in assessment will hopefully be swayed by the evidence presented here of the need for, and value of, such measures as a standard part of assessment practice. However, there are some remaining issues that have been identified in the literature on noncredible responding that will be of value to the assessor to consider. The first is whether or not to warn an individual about the use of measures of noncredible responding within an assessment. The second is whether (and how, if one chooses to do so) to confront an individual during the course of an evaluation, once non-credible responding has been identified. Finally, an assessor needs to consider how to give feedback and how to write up test results in the context of evidence of noncredible responding. In the final section of this chapter, the first two of these issues are discussed; the third is addressed more fully in Chapter 14.

Warning

One debate in the existing literature on use of measures of noncredible responding in neuropsychological assessment has been whether an assessor should warn a client that such measures are included in the assessment. For some, the issue at hand seems to be one of providing full informed consent prior to the evaluation (American Psychological Association, 2002). I find this an interesting debate, given that it has only recently been raised, and yet measures of noncredible responding (e.g., in the form of validity scales on the MMPI) have been around for decades, with presumably little to no "warning" of their presence as part of a psychological evaluation.

It is indeed ethical practice for assessors to explain the nature and purpose of an assessment, the fees, any involvement of third parties, and the limits to confidentiality as part of informed consent for assessment (American Psychological Association, 2002). However, it is unclear whether informing an individual of the "nature and purpose" of an evaluation requires the assessor to mention in detail that the assessment includes measures specifically designed to detect noncredible responding. In fact, it doesn't require that the assessor mention in detail any of the constructs that will be assessed (or to name any specific measures of those constructs). An assessor assuming that one must mention only one of the many constructs being assessed, without mentioning all of the others, would not be acting consistently in relation to this definition of "nature and purpose."

In 2005, the National Academy of Neuropsychology (Bush et al., 2005) provided a consensus statement about assessment that suggested an assessor should request effort and honesty from examinees and that an assessor "may" inform examinees that such factors are directly assessed. Interestingly, a survey of neuropsychologists in 2004 suggested that, although half of those surveyed never provided such a warning, one-third always did (Slick, Tan, Strauss, & Hultsch, 2004), with little change in a subsequent survey that occurred after this consensus statement: 89% indicated that they only encourage best effort, 52% said they do not provide an explicit warning that measures of noncredible responding would be used in the assessment, and 22% reported that they did provide such an explicit warning (Sharland & Gfeller, 2007). The most recent consensus statement on this topic (Heilbronner et al., 2009) simply recommends that psychologists and neuropsychologists encourage optimal effort by the individuals they assess.

An important consideration for a scientifically minded assessor is whether such a warning has an effect on the validity of the data obtained during the evaluation. Research on this topic suggests that warning individuals being assessed about the use of measures of noncredible responding tends to make noncredible responding less extreme, making it harder to detect those who are more sophisticated in portraying themselves in an inaccurate manner (Johnson & Lesniak-Karpiak, 1997; Suhr & Gunstad, 2007; Youngjohn, Lees-Haley, & Binder, 1999). Thus, data suggest that an explicit warning about the presence of such measures may be contrary to good practice.

Given that assessors should use measures of noncredible responding in every evaluation, it behooves each assessor to be consistent in either warning or not warning those whom he or she assesses, regardless of referral question. As indicated in consensus statements (Bush et al., 2005; Heilbronner et al., 2009), it is adequate to simply request that the person being assessed provide his or her best effort and accuracy in both performance and self-report, in order to conduct a valid assessment of his or her concerns. However, if an assessor chooses to explicitly warn about the use of measures of noncredible responding, that warning should be clearly stated (and written) in the informed consent, and the assessor should consider the impact of this warning on the interpretation of test results.

To Continue or Discontinue? To Confront?

Another important issue is how an assessor should handle an assessment situation in which there is evidence of noncredible responding. When an assessor notices evidence for noncredible responding, should the person being examined be confronted about it? To some extent, this depends on when the evidence of noncredible responding becomes evident. For example, it may not be clear until later scoring that performance on the validity scales of a personality instrument such as the MMPI or PAI suggests that the measure was completed in a noncredible manner. However, if a stand-alone measure of noncredible responding is administered early in an evaluation, the score might be known right away before more measures are administered.

Another issue, similar to that occurring in conjunction with warning about noncredible responding, is what effect such confrontation might have on the rest of the evaluation. Just as when an examinee is warned about the use of measures of noncredible responding ahead of an exam, which might lead to more sophisticated and subtle attempts to behave noncredibly, confrontation after the first noncredible performance in an evaluation might do the same. In addition, the clinician must consider how to confront the client, as it may affect the working relationship. A client may choose to discontinue the evaluation entirely or to rescind consent to send the report to the referral source. Osmon and Mano (2009) and Bush (2009) provide some guidance in how one might approach this issue.

Yet another important consideration is that confrontation of an examinee immediately after failure of a measure of noncredible responding (particularly a stand-alone measure) could breach test security (an ethical violation; American Psychological Association, 2002) because it may make it obvious to the person being assessed that the measure just administered was meant to detect noncredible responding.

It is important for an assessor to remember that no one indicator of noncredible responding indicates that the individual has behaved noncredibly on every single test administered or in every self-report completed during an entire evaluation. Noncredible behavior may be present only on tasks the person being assessed perceives as being most related to his or her concerns (a selective communication, as noted earlier in this chapter), or as being particularly difficult or distressing. Thus, it is best to assess for noncredible responding throughout the evaluation, using both embedded and stand-alone measures (Heilbronner et al., 2009). This option renders the question of confrontation somewhat moot, as the nature of the noncredible responding (whether consistent or inconsistent, what types of communications seem noncredible) necessitates the use of more than just one indication to document well.

Furthermore, even within the context of evidence of noncredible responding, normal-range performances within an assessment battery may still be interpretable, with important clinical implications. For example, consider the validity indicators on the MMPI. Certainly in the context of underreporting measures (L, K), performance in the nonclinical range on the other measures is difficult to interpret. However, in the context of over-reporting measures (F series, RBS, FBS), nonclinical range scores on other measures may suggest lack of psychological complaints in those domains. Similarly, in the context of poor performance on a measure of noncredible performance that is focused on memory, normal-range performance on other cognitive measures (or even other memory measures) is at least interpretable as evidence of no impairment, even if the score may underestimate the person's true ability level.

Just as in warning, confronting a client about his or her noncredible responding requires an assessor's best clinical judgment. It is recommended that, if an assessor chooses to confront the person being assessed, he or she record that the confrontation took place, the client's reaction to that confrontation, and the impact of the confrontation on the validity of any consequent data collected during the evaluation.

5

Cultural Context in Assessment
An Empirical Approach

> The fact of her foreign birth and of her alien religion always caused
> a separation of interests and of feelings.
> —SHERLOCK HOLMES, in *The Adventure of the Sussex Vampire*

It is important for assessors to have cultural competence. According to Sue and Sue (2013), elements of cultural competence include (1) being aware of one's own cultural background and how this might influence clinical practice, (2) having knowledge of diverse cultures in order to understand possible cultural effects on clients' presentations and behaviors, and (3) considering the implications of both self- and other-knowledge on interactions with clients (Sue & Sue, 2013). The development of cultural competence occurs over time and via understanding of research findings in this area, as well as experience applying that empirical knowledge in clinical practice.

The goal of the present chapter is to provide an understanding of the need for assessors to consider cultural and diversity issues when conducting assessments, using the existing empirical literature to guide recommendations. It is hoped that, by the end of the chapter, assessors will respect the need to consider cultural diversity in its most compelling form, by focusing on the unique individual being assessed. The chapter begins with a consideration of the key components of Sue and Sue's (2013) cultural competence model as applied to the assessment context, and then discusses cultural diversity issues in specific stages of the assessment process, guided by existing research findings. However, in order to understand the existing empirical literature on this topic, it is it is important to first define culture and cultural diversity.

WHAT IS CULTURAL DIVERSITY?

Cultural influences can stem not just from race and ethnicity, but from any salient demographic, ethnographic, or group-identity factor, including gender, age, SES, geographical location, sexual orientation, religious affiliation, disability/ability status, or relevant subcultures (e.g., being a member of the military, being in prison, identifying with a particular political party), to name just a few. Most existing research on the effects of cultural diversity on assessment focuses on only the first few of these factors, and yet any or all may be critically relevant to a given assessment, depending on its context. For example, one of my students once described a situation in which he incorrectly assumed that a client of his would likely hold spiritual beliefs and values consistent with a highly conservative religious viewpoint, merely on the basis of the client's state of birth and racial background. However, the client was actually a Wiccan, and this initial cultural misunderstanding led to some difficult moments during early treatment sessions.

In addition, it is the rare individual who is defined or influenced by only one such diversity factor. When an assessor considers the complexity of different combinations of cultural factors, it becomes clear that no two people from "group A" are likely to be comparable to one another, and that any generic research findings about group A may or may not apply to the individual currently being assessed, even if he or she is a member of group A.

To accurately apply knowledge from cultural diversity research requires an appreciation of that diversity at its most individual level, reminding assessors to focus on the unique individual in front of them, while at the same time developing testable hypotheses about the role any specific cultural variables may play in that individual's presenting concerns. Culturally and linguistically appropriate services (CLAS) standards emphasize that clinicians must not only consider diversity variables such as race and ethnicity when assessing and treating individuals from minority groups, but should also avoid stereotyping these individuals by overgeneralizing cultural knowledge to any specific individual (Stone & Moskowitz, 2011). Thus, the goal of this chapter is not to present summaries of findings from existing cultural diversity research, but rather to emphasize appropriate use of these findings in the decision-making process of assessment when faced with the $N = 1$ case. Research findings in the diversity literature, much like research findings in any human science area relevant to understanding human behavior, should be used merely to develop initial hypotheses that must then be further assessed for, and examined as to their relevance to, the specific client's presenting concerns.

COMPONENTS OF CULTURAL COMPETENCY
Cultural Self-Awareness

The first factor in Sue and Sue's (2013) model of cultural competence, cultural self-awareness, is the understanding of one's own cultural identity and the ways in which it might influence clinical practice. This understanding is crucial for an assessor to consider because cultural influences are the lenses through which humans view much of their lives, including their professional experiences. If assessors are not aware of the ways in which their own cultural lenses may cloud the gathering of data during interview and testing and/or their interpretation of that data at the time of data integration, they may bias their understanding of the data and the decisions they make during an assessment. Developing such awareness requires conscious effort and thought and a great deal of introspection; it can be difficult to really see the personal lenses one is wearing because they are so transparent to the wearer (i.e., they are so automatic that is can be hard to recognize them). One way to begin this introspective journey is to read empirical literature about cultural diversity and then to stop and consider one's own background from a sociocultural perspective, beginning with the family of origin and then moving outward to the broader environment and its influences on one's identity, values, and beliefs.

An example of the way in which personal cultural lenses can alter the way assessment data are perceived occurs almost annually in my adult assessment course. Inevitably, at least one graduate student will interpret a client's school records as providing evidence of academic impairment, when those school records actually show that the client received all B and C grades throughout their K–12 education. From the standpoint of the graduate student culture, in which academic (over)achievement is a valued characteristic, the occasional C grade is viewed as "unacceptable" and evidence for impairment in functioning in a client, when it is, in fact, quite normative.

In addition to considering how their personal cultural lenses may alter how they view assessment data, assessors must also consider whether their own background or identity might have an impact on the clients they are assessing, watch for evidence of such an impact, and then address it appropriately during the evaluation. This issue is particularly relevant to the interview, potentially affecting what a client says and how he or she communicates it. However, it is also potentially related to the gathering of test data. For example, I recall the days early in my own clinical training when the older adults I was screening for dementia would call me "little missy" and express concern that I could not begin to understand their situation because I was too young (alas, those days are long past). Sometimes such concerns are expressed overtly, but the assessor who is fully attuned to the potential for such factors to affect rapport and communication during an evaluation will be ready to generate initial hypotheses about the potential relevance of such factors and address them as needed in the session.

Knowledge of Diverse Cultures

The second factor of cultural competence mentioned by Sue and Sue (2013) is knowledge of diverse cultures. Although it is important for assessors to know what research has shown about general characteristics of people from particular backgrounds, it is also important to remember that there is great heterogeneity within cultures that may make a particular cultural issue relevant for one person in that culture and not for another. As noted above, part of this heterogeneity arises because there are so many complex combinations of potentially relevant cultural elements in any one unique individual, and part arises because members of groups are diverse in their personal identification as a member of that group. Thus, mere knowledge of a person's racial/ethnic background, religion, and/or sexual orientation does not provide information about any specific values or beliefs that individual client holds or the sociocultural advantages/disadvantages to which that individual client may have been exposed. Furthermore, an assessor should keep in mind that what might be a relevant cultural consideration for one type of assessment question might not be relevant for another. For example, being raised in a family that held particular beliefs about children and discipline might be relevant when the referral question is about the client's own parenting skills, but may be irrelevant if the client has concerns about cognitive problems after a head injury.

An assessor cannot assume that all individuals of a particular subgroup, be that subgroup based on race, ethnicity, religion, SES, or other factor, are inherently similar to each other; members of a particular group may in fact be more similar to the dominant culture in their beliefs, values, ways of expressing themselves, and/or life experiences. In fact, many factors that individual studies might deem as "etic" to a specific culture, can, when seen across many different cross-cultural studies, be viewed as more "emic" in that they are in fact common to many cultures. An extremely important variable to consider when individuals being assessed come from

cultural backgrounds other than the dominant culture in which an assessment is taking place is their degree of acculturation (Mpofu & Ortiz, 2009).
Acculturation is not just adaptation to the language of the new culture, but
also understanding the norms, values, and worldview of that culture and
adopting it within oneself. I have trained many a new student who immediately assumed that intelligence and achievement tests would be biased
against an "international student" (based merely on the students' marking
of an initial contact sheet), only to find that the student was educated in
English from preschool on, spoke English as his or her language in every
setting except with parents, and would have been uncomfortable with being
tested in his or her "native" language.

This example also illustrates the importance of determining group
membership based on more than observation and/or simple self-report,
such as on an intake questionnaire, because such methods will not reveal
important sources of heterogeneity, such as membership in multiple important subgroups or strength of identity association with any particular subgroup. In addition, it is important for the assessor to remember that group
membership may reflect a more relevant but less observable diversity variable (e.g., SES). I am reminded of a diversity workshop I once attended,
in which the presenter was inaccurately attributing several stereotyped
characteristics exclusively to a specific minority group. My colleague and
friend, sitting next to me, was a member of that particular minority group
and recognized that most of these stereotyped characteristics applied to me
but not to him. He concluded with a bit of a smile, "I guess I'm more white
than you are." Thus, although it is important for an assessor to consider
the potential significance of diversity variables arising in a specific assessment situation, based on existing diversity research, the assessor must also
consider these as initial hypotheses for which more data must be gathered,
often by interviewing the person and asking directly, but also by gathering
outside information about individuals from their environmental context.

Application of Self- and Other-Awareness to Decision Making in the Assessment Context

The third aspect of Sue and Sue's (2013) cultural competence model is the
application of self- and other-diversity knowledge to the clinical situation. In
the assessment context, the assessor should consider the relevance of cultural knowledge to the decision-making process itself. A vital component of
applying cultural knowledge in the assessment context is to consider how
cultural knowledge can either increase or decrease decision-making biases.

One example of the role of cultural knowledge in the decision-making process is the consideration of diagnostic hypotheses from the very beginning of an evaluation, which might derive from base rates for specific diagnoses in specific diverse groups. There may well be relevant base-rate relationships with particular diversity variables, such as the risk for dementia increasing with increased age, or the differential risk for certain disorders in males and females. However, the empirically oriented assessor must be sure that he or she is actually using a *relevant* diversity variable when considering its impact on diagnostic hypotheses (e.g., whether different base rates are related to being a member of a particular racial/ethnic group or actually related to SES).

The bottom line is that, if an assessor starts with the assumption that the diversity lens of which he or she is most overtly aware is the most (or only) relevant lens through which to view the client, this stereotyped view will unduly influence the entire decision-making process, and the assessor will potentially have done the client a disservice. Stereotypes can arise from at least two sources: accurate understanding of the relationship of certain characteristics to certain subgroups, and inaccurate beliefs about the relation between certain characteristics and certain subgroups. Stereotypes are often used as heuristics in decision making (see Chapter 2), and thus influence the judgments of both laypeople and professionals, especially in situations that require quick decision making with little information (Dovidio & Fiske, 2012; Stone & Moskowitz, 2011). Because some stereotypes are, in fact, based on accurate information, they *may* improve decision making. A client's age, gender, SES, or race can indeed accurately reflect variable base rates for specific diagnostic hypotheses, which may then influence questions asked or tests administered in a way consistent with good inductive and/or deductive reasoning. However, the decision maker must be aware of (1) whether the individual actually belongs to, and associates or identifies with, the subgroup in question; (2) whether that subgroup membership and identity provide data *relevant* to the assessment question at hand; and (3) whether there are other important characteristics or issues relevant to the person being assessed that also influence use of other decision-making heuristics. In the situation where a decision maker (1) is so highly attuned to only one feature of the client, (2) has inaccurately perceived the client to be a member of or to value that particular subgroup membership as part of his or her identity, and/or (3) is using inaccurate understanding of the relationship of certain characteristics to that subgroup, he or she is conducting the assessment through distorted lenses that can bias decision making and make it less accurate.

DIVERSITY CONSIDERATIONS FOR SPECIFIC ASSESSMENT COMPONENTS

Interviewing

With regard to how diversity knowledge might influence the ways in which an assessor interviews a patient, the assessor should consider not only the content and/or wording of questions, but also the importance of nonverbal communication behaviors such as facial expressions or eye contact—all of which may have an impact on rapport with clients and the ways in which they choose to answer questions they are asked. Certainly language issues are always important to consider, and in fact the Standards for Educational and Psychological Testing strongly recommend that assessors only assess individuals in the assessors' native language (assuming good fluency) or in a second language in which they are highly proficient (American Educational Research Association, American Psychological Association, & National Council on Measurement in Education, 1999). Beyond language fluency, the assessor should consider the effects of the client's education level on his or her word choice during an interview, or of how dialects or cultural/sub-cultural expressions and idioms could influence understanding, even when the two individuals are speaking the same general language. Different backgrounds may influence clients' ways of talking about their symptoms, including descriptions of their symptoms as well as their understanding and explanation for the perceived causes of their symptoms. Thus, assessors should be careful to provide definitions of terms that they use in interviewing, to make sure everyone is "speaking the same language" with regard to issues presented during the interview. Furthermore, assessors should ask clients to provide definitions and examples when they discuss their problems, which can help determine whether the assessors' definitions of the terms used match those of the clients and can help clarify clients' perceptions of the etiologies of their concerns. For example, a client may attribute a certain behavior to his or her cultural background and therefore not see it as problematic; the assessor should not accept this interpretation at face value but should consider it an initial hypothesis that requires further exploration, including examination of whether that behavior has been maladaptive for the client, whether in fact that behavior is an acceptable part of the client's culture, and whether others from the identified culture might view that behavior as problematic in the present circumstances.

Diversity variables may influence not only what and how clients communicate, but also their willingness to do so, perhaps based on their beliefs about the acceptability of psychological services or on having negative feelings about health care providers generally (Dovidio & Fiske, 2012). In addition, as noted above, features of the specific examiner may make an individual more or less willing to provide information. Some of those features may be fixed, such as an assessor's age or gender. Others may be in the assessor's control, such as amount of eye contact, posture, gesturing, speed of speech, whether a directive or more open-ended approach to questioning is used, etc. Thus, an assessor should be attuned to the client's comfort level during the interview, consider as hypotheses whether there are relevant diversity-related variables (or psychologist–client mismatches) that may be contributing to perceived difficulties with rapport, and examine the validity of those hypotheses through further assessment with the client.

It is also important to remember that ill-considered application of research knowledge (i.e., taking this information as "universal" for certain diverse groups rather than truly considering the unique individual at hand) can be as harmful as not taking the time to consider potential implications of diversity literature for the case at hand. I am reminded of one of the most important teaching moments I experienced, at the hands of a patient's husband. While shadowing a medical student, I was "informed" by him of the diversity literature on "Native Americans" and how that was going to be reflected in his approach to interviewing the patient and her husband (who were Native Americans, according to the medical student) and to introducing me to the patient so that I could conduct some testing. The medical student indicated that he had encountered some "culturally related resistance" upon trying to work with the patient and her husband earlier in the day, which he attributed to their cultural background and their reaction to his "status" as a white male professional. I became as uncomfortable as the patient by the medical student's stereotyped attempts to apply what he thought he knew about diversity to the situation at hand. He was forgetting to treat his patient as the unique individual that she was, instead naively applying the stereotyped knowledge he had gained in texts about "Native American" culture. After the medical student left, I had to spend time repairing the breach in the relationship that had occurred secondhand, through the medical student's well-meaning but misguided attempt to apply diversity knowledge. I knew I had made progress when the patient's husband, who had been sitting in the corner with little to no facial expression or body movement up to that time, suddenly said, "That doctor? He's an a**hole. I don't want him back in here. Ever." Given the many aspects of diversity (sex, gender identity, race/ethnic status, social class, age, to name just a few) that may or may not be relevant in a particular assessment situation, it should not surprise an assessor that it is difficult to take the perspective of any other person and to truly consider how best to apply that knowledge to data gathering.

INFLUENCES ON TESTING AND TEST DATA

There is a clear belief among laypeople (and some clinicians) that psychological tests are biased against certain diverse groups (Phelps, 2009; Reynolds & Suzuki, 2013). For example, Furnham and Chamorro-Premuzic (2010) examined students' ratings of whether certain assessment methods were accurate and fair in student selection. General knowledge tests and intelligence tests, as well as drug tests, were judged to be the least accurate and least fair to student selection, whereas panel interviews and references were thought of as the fairest. Overall people viewed "face-to-face assessment" as fairer and more accurate than test data. Some of the charges raised against psychological measures include that the measures use content that is inappropriate for individuals from minority groups, that items are scored in a fashion that is biased toward majority group opinion, that tests do not use enough individuals from minority groups in their test development and/or normative samples to allow for minority group influence on the final test content and interpretation, that tests do not measure the same constructs in diverse groups, and that tests do not predict outcomes equally well for diverse groups.

Many of these charges are not supported by empirical evidence. For example, with regard to whether items are biased against group members, research has shown that this judgment cannot be made on an armchair basis by either laypeople or even "experts" (Camilli & Shepard, 1994; Jensen, 1980; Miele, 1979; Reschly, 2000; Reynolds, Lowe, & Saenz, 1999). Furthermore, most major instruments that are well validated are careful to include representative numbers of diverse populations to reflect diversity variables of relevance to the construct being assessed, and some measures even oversample individuals from minority groups in order to specifically test for item- or other test bias. In addition, research that examines whether tests show construct equivalence in diverse groups suggests that they do, and research shows that measures are equally predictive of important outcomes in individuals within diverse groups (see Reynolds & Suzuki, 2013, for a review). In general, the research shows that well-validated psychological measures are not biased against racial or ethnic minorities born in the United States, but in fact when there is any evidence of bias, it favors minorities by overpredicting their outcomes (Edwards & Oakland, 2006; Jensen, 1980; Kaiser, 1986; Neisser et al., 1996; Nisbett et al., 2012; Valencia, Suzuki, & Salinas, 2001; Wigdor & Garner, 1982).

Some of this continued social belief in bias in psychological testing seems to be based on the fact that group differences (i.e., different mean scores) still exist on some psychological tests (particularly ability and achievement tests; see Reynolds & Suzuki, 2013, for a review). However, the mere presence of group differences does not provide evidence of bias; furthermore, it depends on how the groups are defined and whether the researchers are controlling for the relevant variables. For example, the well-documented 1 standard deviation (*SD*) difference between blacks and whites on intelligence tests shrinks (although it does remain a reliable difference) when SES is controlled for (Jensen, 1980; Kaufman, 1973; Kaufman & Kaufman, 1973; Reynolds & Gutkin, 1981; Weiss, Chen, Harris, Holdnack, & Saklofske, 2011), and differences between black and white children have decreased over the past few decades, suggesting shifts over time in other variables that contribute to this group difference (Nisbett, 2009). The issue of psychometric bias and how to examine for it is discussed more fully in the next chapter, and details about psychometric bias in regard to specific types of psychological measures are presented in Chapters 9–12.

Another way in which tests have been suggested to be biased is in an assessor–client mismatch on important cultural variables, with the contention that examiners who are from a dominant culture might obtain lower scores on ability measures when assessing individuals from a minority culture (Sattler, 1988). However, reviews of studies examining this literature have not supported such a contention (Reynolds & Suzuki, 2013).

Assuming that a diversity variable automatically affects the validity of a test is another way in which decision making can be inappropriately influenced by the misapplication of diversity knowledge. For example, consider the case of a 17-year-old senior in high school who was referred by her father for evaluation of a possible learning disability. She received very high grades throughout school (almost a straight-A average), and for 2 years prior to the evaluation had taken all the possible AP courses available in her well-resourced school. However, in her junior year she received two "B" grades in math courses; as she was planning to eventually major in premed and attend medical school, her father felt these two B's were a sign of a potential learning problem. Both parents had advanced degrees and were in the upper-income bracket in their community. As the assessor began to explain the testing procedures, the girl's father interrupted, saying that he would not permit anyone to administer his daughter any "IQ" test because they were "biased against blacks." An assessor who also "felt" that was true, rather than relying on empirical data about the tests to be administered, may have opted to administer a less psychometrically valid instrument, or even chose to not administer an ability test at all, which would have been detrimental to decision making in the case. Instead, the assessor explained the existing research evidence suggesting that the intelligence measure to be used was, in fact, very valid to use with individuals similar to his daughter, and the evaluation was able to continue.

Training and Suggestions

Although it is important for assessors to be consciously aware of the stereotypes that exist about diverse groups, experts in the training of cultural competence emphasize an important pitfall of cultural competence training: Professionals may learn only stereotyped knowledge about cultures, which (whether positive or negative) leads to more "distorted lens" decision making rather than minimizing it. Thus, as emphasized repeatedly above, cultural competence training also requires a caution against overgeneralizing the abstract knowledge base when interacting with diverse clients.

Stone and Moskowitz (2011) suggest strategies for assessors to use to reduce cultural bias in their assessments. First, they suggest that the assessor make a conscious effort to keep the assessment goal of being accurate, fair, and unbiased in mind, rather than letting an overtly obvious diversity variable trigger a stereotype about a client that then "overshadows" other potential hypotheses. Second, they suggest that an assessor consciously call up all the potential cultural categorizations that may apply to a specific client, not just those that may have been most salient; including the diversity variables listed at the beginning of the chapter, as well as any other identities mentioned by the client, such as social or political identities, major interests and activities, etc. This strategy will help an assessor focus less on research findings for only one diversity variable that may or may not be relevant for that particular client or for the specific assessment context. In addition, the strategy will help an assessor identify ways in which he or she shares commonalities with a client and ways in which he or she differs, which in turn might point to ways in which self- and other-cultural issues could influence communication during all stages of the assessment. A third way to counteract the tendency to stereotype an individual being assessed is to purposely focus on counterstereotypical attributes and behaviors. Similar to what is required in good deductive reasoning generally, the assessor should consider evidence in support of *and* against hypotheses about the contribution of any particular diversity variable to the assessment question at hand. In addition, it is a good clinical skill to try to take the perspective of one's client—to do that successfully, an assessor must not assume, but must elicit sufficient details to imagine and appreciate the client's unique situation.

With regard to the assessment process itself, a clinician should start every assessment with an explanation of the purpose for the assessment, the general evaluation procedures to be followed, and to begin the process of establishing rapport; while doing so, the clinician may develop initial hypotheses about variables that may serve as barriers to the assessment, including, but not limited to, those tied to diversity. Then, in the process of assessing the individual, these hypotheses can be explored, both by reviewing the research knowledge relevant to any of the cultural hypotheses that arise in the specific case and by directly assessing for more information that would support or disconfirm their importance in that individual case. In the process of gathering additional data, use of tests that have been shown to be valid for the relevant cultural groups to which the client belongs, as well as not putting too much weight on formal test results but integrating them together with other data, will help mitigate any failures to consider the relevant variables as well as inappropriate consideration of irrelevant ones.

6

"Knowing What's under the Hood"
Psychometric Considerations

You know my methods, Watson.
    —SHERLOCK HOLMES, in *The Crooked Main*

In the world of empirically based "assessment," assessors still derive most of their data from formal tests. The advantage of test scores relative to data gathered by other methods is that assessors have data available on the validity of inferences drawn from test scores. It is important to keep in mind that a test is simply an objective and standardized measure of a behavioral sample. Although there is no question that test scores are valuable sources of assessment data and perhaps deserve priority placement in the weighting of confidence assessors might give to incongruent assessment data across different sources, it is important to remember that test data are only as good as their user.

One of the important assessment-related decisions an assessor must make is which, if any, tests to administer to a client. That first decision, which tests to administer to a given client, is comprised of additional decisions involving (1) determining which constructs need to be measured, (2) examining how good any particular measure is at assessing the constructs of interest, (3) considering the appropriateness of that measure in the context of other measures and other data available to make the assessment decision, and (4) evaluating whether that measure is appropriate for the client in the particular assessment situation at hand.

As discussed in Chapters 2 and 3, the first step, the act of determining the relevant constructs in any particular assessment case, is vulnerable to various decision-making biases, and is not an assessment step that should be taken lightly. However, assuming an assessor has already made good decisions about which constructs to measure in a particular assessment situation, the next step of deciding which tests, if any, to administer, requires knowledge of the psychometric properties of the tests under consideration. As Acklin (2002) put it, "The assessment psychologist must not only be able to drive the car but also know what is under the hood" (p. 15).

CONSTRUCT VALIDITY

To understand the psychometric properties of any given test, an assessor should first start with a theoretical understanding of the construct that test is supposed to measure. Once the assessor understands the construct, how it should theoretically "behave," what it should (or should not) be related to, how it might differ in certain groups—then it will be clear what sort of data are needed to judge the test's construct validity. Of course, as scientific understanding of constructs evolves over time, so do the measures of those constructs; no one study can provide adequate construct validity for any given measure. Examining the validity of the score inferences from different measures thus requires a thorough literature review and often goes well beyond the actual test manual.

What follows is not a comprehensive review of all the different types of reliability and validity analyses that are part of construct validity and that are often discussed in chapters such as these. Instead, the goal is to present the decision-making process that underlies the consideration of the construct validity of the measures an assessor would consider using in any assessment situation.

Reliability within the Context of Construct Validity

An important aspect of construct validity, though not usually conceived of in such a way, is the reliability of the measure. "Reliability" refers to the consistency of the score; for most assessment purposes, the assessor needs to be able to trust the scores obtained in an $N = 1$ situation, and thus an unreliable measure likely has too much error associated with it to be valid for most assessment purposes. When a score is reliable, it is minimally vulnerable to random fluctuation, leading the assessor to have more confidence in the score obtained on that particular administration and to be able to trust that the obtained score is a consistent representation of the individual's likely score on that measure on another occasion.

However, the types of reliability most relevant to the test(s) under consideration for any given assessment depend on the constructs the assessor is measuring. When the construct of interest is stable over time, then the test–retest reliability for a measure of that construct should be strong; when the construct is known to be unstable generally, one would not expect a measure of that construct to stay particularly stable over time. For example, for a personality characteristic thought to be stable over time, such as neuroticism, an assessor would expect a measure of that personality characteristic to show a strong correlation between Time 1 and Time 2 administration, separated by even up to several months in time. Such data would give the assessor confidence in interpreting a score administered at one time, if he or she needs to draw inferences about that characterological trait. However, if the assessor is interested in measuring changes to anxiety symptoms in response to phobic triggers, he or she may want a measure that doesn't show a lot of temporal stability, and thus would not care whether the test showed strong 2-month test–retest reliability; in fact, that might be a liability, given the construct being examined and the purpose of the assessment, which is to detect change in response to stimuli. Keep in mind, however, that such a measure would be psychometrically inappropriate if the goal of the assessment were to assess more characterological anxiety symptoms or syndromes or to aid in the determination of some anxiety disorder diagnoses, given its sensitivity to change.

Similarly, when a construct is relatively homogeneous or the goal is to assess a very narrow aspect of a particular construct, the measure should show high internal consistency and interitem correlation within the measure. However, if the goal is to assess a more heterogeneous construct or to use a measure that provides a broad representation of the full bandwidth of a construct, then it is likely that measures best suited for the purpose will have lower (although still "adequate") interitem correlation and internal consistency ratings, or will have subscales reflecting the heterogeneous nature of the construct (with each subscale showing strong internal consistency, particularly if subscale scores will be interpreted).

Other types of reliability may be less important in judging the construct validity of the measure, but they are still important for judging the consistency of the test data in the $N = 1$ setting of an assessment. For example, when a test requires subjective judgment in its scoring, then the assessor needs to examine data on the interrater reliability of the measure, in order to trust that the data from the present assessment session is likely to be reproducible.

Unfortunately, as pointed out by Charter and Feldt (2001), clinicians often lack confidence in their ability to understand the implications of reliability for test interpretation. One likely reason for this lack of confidence is that there are still no clear guidelines on what level of reliability would be needed in order to consider a measure adequate for a particular purpose. In this era of empirically based treatments and assessments, assessors can feel a need for a standard cutoff above which a measure would be judged to be "adequately" reliable. For example, many authors have purported that any internal consistency reliability below .9 is too imprecise for clinical judgment situations. An examination of the psychometric properties of many instruments (not just psychological) would show that this is a tough hurdle to overcome! There are too many factors that can influence a reliability estimate to suggest that there is one cutoff point for "adequate" reliability.

In addition to the nature of the construct the measure is supposed to assess, and whether the measure is supposed to assess a full or narrow range of that construct, other factors that can affect reliability include the length of the test itself or even the population being given the test. For example, a test might show a full range of scores in a normative sample, but in a patient sample there may be a restricted range of scores on the same measure, limiting the reliability estimates that can be obtained for use of the measure in that population. Charter and Feldt (2001) also point out that reliability standards are unlikely to be successful because they have such a varied effect on the accuracy of clinical decisions. For example, if an assessor needs to select a very small group of individuals and is thus using a cutoff score further from the test mean, a higher reliability would be required for accuracy in identification relative to use of a cutoff that is closer to the mean. Another factor that can influence how reliable the instrument "needs" to be is how much weight is being put on making certain types of errors over minimizing others (false positives or false negatives). So, although measures still require generally good reliability, the cutoff score can be altered to minimize one type of error over another, and a less reliable instrument can then still be quite accurate in detection.

As decision makers, assessors must consider the reliability data that are available (i.e., relevant to the construct being assessed, the way in which the test under consideration is supposed to reflect that construct, and the overall purpose of the evaluation) and use that information to guide decisions about administering any given tests. As Charter and Feldt (2001) note, "In many cases there is no alternative evidence that is more reliable than the test score in hand. To say that the scores are 'not reliable enough' hardly helps. If a decision about an examinee must be reached, what is the clinician supposed to do?" (p. 536). They emphasize that, in the clinical setting, decisions are expected to be made. "Only idealistic academicians can pretend that if reliability standards are not met, no decision should be made. In most situations, abstaining constitutes a decision and leads to the adoption of one or another action" (p. 537). In truly integrative assessment, lower reliabilities may be acceptable because test findings are treated as only one part of the evidence and require further confirmatory support from other data before definitive conclusions are drawn.

Thus, although assessors should be empirically guided when considering the psychometric properties of the test instruments under consideration, they do in fact need measures of the constructs that are vital to an assessment case, and they do in fact need to make decisions about those constructs and problems. Using the best available data (while actively considering the limitations of that data during interpretation) is a scientifically guided approach, and considering the weight of that particular data point in the context of its reliability (and its "weight" relative to other ways to assess the construct). An important way that an assessor can and should acknowledge any limitations to reliability in the instruments used to make assessment decisions is to use, and truly consider, the confidence intervals around a particular test score when deciding the value of the inference he or she can draw from the score (Crawford, Garthwaite, Longman, & Batty, 2012). Not only should the confidence intervals surround the scores when they are reported (American Educational Research Association, American Psychological Association, & National Council on Measurement in Education, 1999), but assessors should consider them even at the time of test interpretation and integration, in order to acknowledge the potential for error in the scores obtained.

Other Components of Construct Validity

"Validity" refers to the accuracy and appropriateness of a test score inference for a particular construct in a particular context. As previously noted, reliability is part, but not all, of validity; a test score can be quite consistent and reproducible, with minimal random error, and yet still inaccurately reflect the construct it purports to measure. Validity is examined relative to a specific construct in a specific context and is not a product of the test itself, but a product of the inferences drawn from the test. Establishing the construct validity of a test is also part and parcel of determining the validity of the construct itself, and an overall approach to assessing for construct validity is not different from the scientific methods for developing and confirming theories (Chronbach & Meehl, 1955). Construct validation establishes the truth-value of a construct: That is, one's measure of the construct relates in theoretically predictable ways to other variables; measures of that construct thus should behave in theoretically predictable ways to other variables as well.

Because construct validity involves validating a theory as well as measures of the theory, there are many explanations for "validity" findings from any given study. So, as pointed out by Smith (2005), if a specific study tests the hypothesis that construct X is expected to be related to constructs Y and Z, but it is not, it may be that (1) the theoretical relationship between X, Y, and Z is not correct; (2) the measures of any of the constructs X, Y, or Z are inadequate; and/or (3) the study was poorly designed. Smith goes on to point out that, even if X is related to Y and Z in any one study, it may not be because the theory about the relationships among X, Y, and Z is correct; rather, it may reflect design or measurement issues that created confounds in the study (e.g., the measures of X, Y, and Z actually overlap so much that they measure the same construct). Thus no one study can support the construct validity of any measure or detract from it. To analyze the validity of any given measure, multiple studies utilizing multiple measures and designs that test multiple hypotheses are needed. An assessor wanting to review such evidence for a test under consideration should conduct a thorough and updated literature review on any particular measure (going well beyond the clinical manual), in order to make an informed decision about whether that measure is appropriate for the assessment situation at hand.

As with reliability, it is still not clear what is "good enough" evidence of validity to support clinical use of a measure (Hunsley & Mash, 2008a). Furthermore, the criteria for a measure to be empirically validated may differ as a function of the purpose of the measure (e.g., whether the measure is meant to be a screening tool, diagnostic, or relevant to treatment monitoring) (Hunsley & Mash, 2005). Thus, although a measure may have psychometric adequacy as a screener for potential diagnosis of depression, it may not be a useful measure for reaching a diagnostic decision or for assessing treatment-related changes in depressive symptoms. Recent texts (Antony & Barlow, 2010; Hunsley & Mash, 2008b) review the validity of various psychological measures with regard to their purpose and are useful overviews for assessors to consult when deciding on an instrument to use for a particular assessment purpose. In addition, in determining the construct validity of an instrument, an assessor also needs to consider for whom the test has been validated because deciding whether or not a test is appropriate for a specific client includes knowing whether the empirical data (and norms) for the test are relevant for that client.

Analysis of the Internal Structure of a Test

Some aspects of construct validity are related to how well the internal structure of a measure reflects the theoretical construct being measured.

As noted above, such evidence can include reliability data such as stability over time or internal consistency, but also includes examination of content validity and factor analysis.

A point that cannot be emphasized enough is that analysis of the content validity of any given test, just like the analysis of any other component of validity, must consider the purpose of the test. For example, items might be chosen to specifically screen for a potential psychological condition or diagnosis, thereby reflecting only certain highly sensitive components of that construct. That measure is then inappropriate as a measure for the purpose of diagnosis, as it might not cover the breadth of content that fully reflects the construct, or perhaps not work as a measure for case conceptualization or treatment planning, as it might not provide enough depth of coverage within particular facets of the construct to serve that assessment purpose. Thus, to examine both item relevance and item representativeness in a content validity analysis, the assessor must consider the intended use of the measure. As noted by Ayearst and Bagby (2010), different measures of the same construct could in fact result in different scores because they represent the construct differently. For example, the Beck Anxiety Inventory (Beck & Steer, 1990) has items whose content reflects somatic symptoms of anxiety, whereas the Penn State Worry Questionnaire (Meyer, Miller, Metzger, & Borkovec, 1990) includes items whose content reflects a cognitive component of anxiety (worrisome thoughts). Of course, analysis of the content of items, even when judged by a panel of experts, is insufficient evidence of validity on its own.

Structural validity analysis allows for examination of whether a particular test shares the dimensional structure of the construct it is purported to measure. Factor analytic techniques are typically used to examine this aspect of internal validity. A discussion of how best to conduct such an analysis is beyond the scope of this text; for a concise review of relevant methods and limitations to the use of factor analysis for this purpose, see Ayearst and Bagby (2010) or Wasserman and Bracken (2013). In the process of making decisions about the use of a given instrument, such data can help inform the assessor about the use of measures or perhaps subscales of the measures, and how much variance in the latent construct is accounted for by the test, as well as how much overall variance is accounted for by any given subtest (or, if the structural analysis was at the item level, by any given item). As noted in Chapter 5, an important aspect of structural validity relevant to understanding whether a test has validity for use in diverse groups is the demonstration of factorial invariance (i.e., similar structural validity findings within diverse groups).

External Evidence for the Construct Validity of a Test

Other analyses of construct validity are external to the measure; the most predominant of these are how much a measure relates to other measures of the same construct (convergent validity) and evidence that the measure can distinguish accurately between clinical and nonclinical groups (diagnostic validity; Garb, Lillienfeld, & Fowler, 2008). Less often examined, but equally important, is evidence that a measure does *not* relate to measures of different constructs to which it shouldn't relate (discriminant validity), as well as evidence that the measure can distinguish accurately *among* clinical groups. Other evidence important to overall construct validity is how the measure behaves in terms of hypothesized relationships to external criteria (criterion validity), either concurrently or prospectively (predictive validity) measured, or how scores on the measure change in ways consistent with the construct being measured with regard to other factors, such as age, gender, or response to treatment/intervention, for example. As noted in Chapter 5, evidence for construct validity in diverse subgroups is also important (i.e., does the measure correlate in the same hypothesized ways with other important variables?; does it predict outcomes equally well in diverse subgroups?).

As noted above, the most common evidence available for the external validity of many tests is the correlation of those tests with other measures of the same construct. When looking at such data, an assessor needs to carefully consider whether the relationship seen between the measures reflects the shared construct variance, or whether there is a confound of shared method variance (e.g., both measures are self-report). This is of particular importance when there is a lack of discriminant validity evidence for a measure; that is, an examination that the measure does not, in fact, correlate with measures that should have no theoretical relationship to the others. Campbell and Fiske (1959) recommended that discriminant validity analyses include correlations with measures of various response biases (e.g., social desirability), which not only examine method variance issues but also remind the evaluator of the importance of considering response bias when examining the self-report (on questionnaire) of an individual being assessed (see Chapter 4).

However, it is equally important to consider the relationship of the measure to other psychological constructs. As an example, consider a client who is feeling generally distressed and as though everything in his or her past was negative, the present is negative, and the future will be negative (what I refer to, when teaching students, as the "my life sucks" lens). Such an individual will show highly correlated scores in self-report measures, reflecting high number of current stressors, lack of social support, more depressive symptoms, more health complaints, and poorer quality of life, but these relationships may merely reflect a generalized bias toward answering questions in a negative direction, rather than reflecting accurate causal relationships among any of these constructs. Chapters 4 and 10 suggest ways to address this kind of response bias in the clinical setting. In general, however, as with other validity analyses, evidence of convergent and discriminant validity cannot be provided by any one study, but must accumulate across many studies, often well beyond that available in the clinical manual.

Regarding diagnostic validity, the most typical type of analysis conducted is the examination for cutoff scores that distinguish a particular clinical group from those who do not have the disorder (i.e., a nonclinical comparison group). There are many important considerations in understanding diagnostic validity information when making a decision about whether or not to use a particular measure; these considerations include base rates, the purpose of the evaluation, and the nature of both the criterion and the comparison groups used to analyze diagnostic validity.

First, base rates matter. The accuracy of the measure depends on the overall base rate of the disorder. When the base rate of a disorder is low, measures are best used to rule out a condition, but not to rule it in. However, when the base rate of a disorder is high, measures are best used to rule a disorder in but not to rule it out (Ayearst & Bagby, 2010). Assessors must consider the base rates for the disorder in the studies for which cutoffs were determined; if the setting in which the assessors work has a much different base rate for the disorder under consideration, the measure's diagnostic validity is unknown. To assist clinicians in making that decision, many researchers have begun to publish data that reflect the accuracy of a given measure's prediction at different base rates for the disorder in question.

A second important consideration is the purpose of the assessment. If the clinician is conducting a screening evaluation, which is meant to be followed by more comprehensive evaluation should the screening results be positive, the assessor may choose a test that demonstrates good sensitivity at the sacrifice of a high rate of false positives because the assessor knows that a more comprehensive evaluation will follow that will address the lack of specificity. However, an assessor who makes diagnostic conclusions from scores on an instrument well validated as a screening instrument, but with poor specificity for actual diagnosis, is making a poor testing decision. Given that managed care has led to an increased demand for shorter evaluations and conclusions to be drawn from more preliminary evaluation data, this point is of particular concern for many assessors, who must be mindful of the many potential negative effects of a false-positive "diagnosis" based on the results of screening tests that are more appropriately used to refer for further evaluation, rather than to draw diagnostic and prognostic or treatment conclusions (Bufka & Camp, 2010; Newman & Kohn, 2009).

A third important issue is whether data are available on the diagnostic validity of the instrument for any relevant subgroups to which the person being assessed is a member. Most of the evidence for the diagnostic validity of psychological measures is in comparison to a healthy control group, whereas the decision in many clinical situations is not whether a client has a certain diagnosis or not, but to differentiate between several diagnostic possibilities that may overlap with one another. Thus, although having diagnostic validity for distinguishing "diagnosis X" from not having any diagnoses, few measures have demonstrated their ability to discriminate accurately between different clinical diagnoses.

In Chapters 9–12, examples from psychological and cognitive assessment illustrate how a scientifically minded assessor should make decisions about the appropriate tests to administer to a particular client, based on review of important construct validity data available for each measure under consideration.

Aspirational Goals: Incremental Validity and Cost Effectiveness

An important consideration in the overall decision about an assessment battery is not one measure in isolation, but any one measure in the context of all the other measures (and nonmeasure data) available to help make assessment decisions and to make an assessment cost-effective. Ideally, the assessor can determine whether any given measure adds incremental validity beyond what would be known from other test or nontest data, as well as whether it is appropriate to administer a measure to provide confirmatory evidence or even complementary evidence beyond pure incremental validity (Weiner, 2013). Incremental validity, or the extent to which an individual measure will add to the accuracy of prediction made on the bases of other test and nontest data, is an aspirational goal in situations in which diagnostic validity is of particular value because it directly speaks to the cost effectiveness of a test. However, incremental validity can be very difficult to establish, given the complexity of establishing diagnostic validity generally for any measures (or for nontest data, for that matter). As a result there are, as yet, no guidelines for "how much" incremental validity would be necessary to justify the administration of a measure in a specific assessment context. In addition, as noted by Weiner (2013), using measures that provide additional complementary or confirmatory information is sound assessment practice, given that any one measure of a construct does have error associated with it and cannot fully capture the constructs of interest.

Normative Data

The fourth step in the psychometric decision-making process is to determine whether a measure is appropriate for the individual being assessed in the $N = 1$ setting. One aspect of that decision, as previously mentioned, is whether or not there are relevant data regarding the construct validity of the measure for any groups or subgroups with which the individual identifies and that have relevance to the construct being assessed. In addition, however, appropriate normative data need to be available for interpreting that individual's score.

The basis for interpreting most tests is the relative standing of an individual's score against some normative comparison. Tests vary in the degree to which their norms are representative of the population of interest on potentially relevant domains such as age, gender, race/ethnicity, SES, and geographical region, but of course not all of these domains are relevant to every single construct being assessed, and the value of subgroup norms depends on the purpose of the evaluation. Tests also vary in the degree to which their norms represent clinical or nonclinical populations, which can lead to very different interpretations of findings. A depression score might be high for the overall population (which has implications for diagnosis) but low relative to inpatient norms (which may have implications for choice of intervention). Thus, the examiner making a decision about the appropriateness of norms available for any given test must consider the purposes of the assessment, as well as the individual being assessed.

In order to demonstrate the individual's relative ranking in whatever the normative group may be, scores are typically reported not as raw numbers, but in a metric meant to illustrate that relative standing, such as with percentiles or standard scores. When considering the interpretation of standardized scores of any type, the empirically oriented assessor remembers to always be mindful of the "raw data." When a measure's scores are not normally distributed (e.g., when test items are responded to infrequently, when the task has a truncated floor or ceiling, when test scores are skewed such as often occurs with timed scores), the "standardized" scores, if considered without consciously attending to the raw data, can be quite problematic and lead to misinterpretation (Donnell, Belanger, & Vanderploeg, 2011). As an example, the number of correct categories variable on the Wisconsin Card Sorting Task (Heaton, Chelune, Talley, Kay, & Curtiss, 1993) can range only from 0 to 6. The highest percentile score one can achieve is thus " > 16th percentile"; yet I have seen psychological reports that interpreted this score as abnormal, even when the raw data showed that the individual being assessed had achieved five or even six correct categories on the task.

The $N = 1$ Case

As reviewed above, a lot of data are required for an assessor to determine whether, in the abstract, a particular measure might be appropriate for use with a particular client in a particular assessment context. Although all of that evidence is important to the assessment decision of whether to *administer* any particular measure to a given client, only some of the data are relevant to *interpreting* any test score that results from that measure in a unique assessment situation. Because many factors can influence whether a test score is actually a reliable and valid inference for this particular client at this moment, an empirically guided assessor will remember to consider that information when deciding how to weight test scores in the final integration of data about that client. Some of these factors include issues external to the client, such as examinee and environmental factors, whereas others include issues internal to the client.

With regard to external issues that might affect the $N = 1$ reliability and validity of a test score, some of these factors are in the control of the assessor and therefore can be minimized. For example, when an examiner does not administer the measure in the manner in which it was developed and standardized, he or she must consider the implications of nonstandard administration for interpreting the resultant test scores. Thus, it is vital for assessors to be well trained and well experienced in the proper administration of all instruments they plan to use in their assessments. In fact, every assessor should occasionally review his or her own administration procedures, even when he or she has administered those instruments for many years. I have observed many an experienced clinician or psychometrician who has "drifted" away from the standardized administration rules of tests. In a manner similar to that used to minimize error in the use of behavioral observation scales, where there is observer drift over time by raters who use them, it is advisable for assessors using other types of instruments to review the standardized administration and scoring on a regular basis to prevent this type of error.

In addition, assessors should always double-check their scoring of the instruments they use to minimize examiner scoring error. Studies show that, on scoring-heavy tests, errors in scoring are made quite often, even by individuals with a great deal of experience who have confidence in their scoring, and that scoring errors can be minimized by double-checking the scoring or by having others double-check the scoring (Hetterscheidt, & Barnett, 2011; Hopwood & Richard, 2005; Keuntzel, Ryan & Schnakenberger-Ott, 2003).

As an extreme example of the potential effects of nonstandardized administration on test scores, consider a case in which a high school student was referred for reevaluation for a learning disability. The school had tested the student 2 years prior, but it was noted on the test protocol that the intelligence test had been administered over the course of the entire school year, with subtests (or sometimes only parts of subtests!) administered in 2- to 3-week intervals due to time constraints and lack of cooperation for more than brief periods of time by the adolescent. In addition, the test protocol showed that for many of the tasks, the administrator did not give the test in its standard fashion, starting at the beginning item on many subtests that actually required starting at an age-appropriate item, picking up in the middle of some subtests after weeks of delay. Furthermore, some scores had been calculated without consideration of time limits, with a note that the examiner felt "lack of cooperation" was causing the slow performance and therefore did not take it into account in scoring. However, in the actual report, none of this information was available for review, leading a reader who was not privy to the actual test protocol to assume that the scores reported were obtained on a standard administration. Although in this case client factors contributed to the lack of standardized administration, the assessor made no note of the potential effects of this way of administering the instrument on the scores that resulted, nor did it affect the assessor's interpretation of the data.

There are certainly times when an assessor must move away from a standard administration of a measure for a good clinical reason. For example, an assessor may need to compensate for a physical or sensory limitation or disability by slightly altering test administration procedures (e.g., administering a test orally if an individual cannot read). However, it can be difficult to know "how much is too much" nonstandardization; that is, how much of an impact the nonstandardized administration had on the interpretability of the resultant test scores. However, an assessor aware of the potential for nonstandard administration to affect $N = 1$ reliability and thus test interpretability will make note of any nonstandard administration and consider it when interpreting test results, as well as note the nonstandard administration in the report.

In addition to administration and scoring factors, assessors need to consider the environment in which the test was administered. For example, a room could be too noisy, too hot, or too cold. I recall a case in which the client became highly distracted by a spider in the corner of the exam room, necessitating the cessation of the evaluation until the spider could be removed, due to its impact on her ability to attend and concentrate and thus on the reliability of the scores obtained while the client was feeling anxious over the spider. Thus, an examiner should take careful note of these environmental factors and work to alter the environment if possible, delay testing to another day when the environmental factors can be addressed, or, if they cannot, consider those factors when interpreting the resultant test scores as well as noting those factors and their potential implications in the report.

Internal factors that affect the $N = 1$ reliability and validity of test scores include, but are not limited to, the client's fatigue/alertness, effort or motivation, presence of illness, and/or presence of high levels of distress. Some tasks may be more vulnerable to these types of effects than others. For example, the computerized interpretive guidelines for some continuous performance tasks specifically note that time of day can influence the interpretation of the data, due to circadian changes in basic alertness and arousal. A clinician who is staying attuned to client-related issues and takes note of them as the testing progresses is in a better position to be able to consciously consider the potential impact of these factors at the time of test interpretation. Thus, keeping in mind the importance of $N = 1$ reliability to the validity of test score inferences should remind the assessor of the importance of making and recording behavioral observations throughout an evaluation, and not just during the initial interview (see Chapter 7).

In addition, the assessor may need to make a decision to discontinue tasks or discontinue evaluation on a particular day, on the basis of observed client factors that, in his or her judgment, are impacting the reliability and the validity of the test scores obtained. I am reminded of a case in which a patient with a known intellectual disability and a seizure disorder was referred for a required reevaluation to continue to qualify for services. It was apparent after just a brief time that the patient was atypically confused, disoriented, and not very alert. A conversation with his guardian revealed that the guardian had not cancelled the appointment despite the fact that the patient had experienced three seizures the day before the assessment, finally requiring intervention in the emergency room to get them under control. Of note, the guardian actually made this decision consciously, as she believed that this gave the patient the best chance of "keeping his score low enough" to continue to qualify for services. After a discussion with the guardian about the professional and ethical implications of this issue, the testing session was rescheduled for another day when the patient was free of the aftereffects of seizures. In summary, $N = 1$ psychometrics are just as important to deciding on the validity (interpretability) of test scores as considering the psychometric properties of tests in the abstract.

7

Intake Interviewing
and Behavioral Observations

> I listen to their story, they listen to my comments, and then I pocket
> my fee.
>
> —SHERLOCK HOLMES, in *A Study in Scarlet*

An interview is usually an assessor's first direct contact with a client. Not only does an intake interview provide a firsthand perspective on clients' concerns and history, but it also provides a chance to observe clients as they discuss their concerns and history and react to assessors' questions. Thus, while the interview can provide valuable "raw data" as part of an assessment, it is equally important to consider what the limitations to interview data may be.

In many ways, an interview is only as good as the interviewee. It is during the interview that the lenses through which the client views his or her problem first become apparent, and where lack of information or inaccurate information provided by the client can unduly affect the rest of the evaluation. The interview is the client's reconstruction of events (Garb, 2007), which may not be accurate (see Chapter 4); the present chapter begins with a detailed discussion of the implications of this for the interview process.

In other ways, an intake interview is only as good as the interviewer. Many of the decision-making biases mentioned in Chapter 2 can present themselves during this first contact with the client, and the more unstructured the interview, the more likely it is that some of these biases will affect the reliability and validity of the overall data gathered during the interview process. However, structured interviews can also be subject to some of the decision-making biases reviewed in Chapter 2. To some extent, the "competition" between structured and unstructured interviews is a false one because, depending on the goal of the interview and the overall assessment, both may be used and can complement one another well. In fact, the combination of the two approaches, integrated flexibly to meet the needs of the individual client for a particular assessment purpose, reflects a scientist-practitioner approach to interviewing (Segal, Mueller, & Coolidge, 2012). The second part of the chapter focuses on the psychometric strengths and weaknesses of structured and unstructured interviews, ending with a recommendation for a best approach to take for the purpose of an intake interview.

Finally, the intake interview provides the first opportunity for the assessor to make behavioral observations about the client (i.e., not just *what* the client presents, but *how* he or she does so), which can not only help an assessor judge the validity of the self-report data provided by the client (see Chapter 4), but also be used as data as part of the integrative understanding of the client's concerns. This chapter therefore ends with a discussion of mental status and behavioral observations.

THE LENS OF THE CLIENT

If clients had a clear and accurate understanding of what their situation was and were always willing to communicate that understanding clearly and accurately, then the only information needed to be obtained in an assessment would be via the clinical interview. However, these two assumptions are not always valid. A client might highlight certain information over other information; might omit information, providing only part of his or her "story"; or might confuse the temporal order or causality of the problems by presenting a consequence of yet another more primary problem than the primary problem itself. Importantly, these things can occur even outside the context of deliberate and intentional noncredible responding (i.e., malingering), although certainly individuals who are motivated to consciously present themselves in a certain manner will also bias the information they give during an interview (see Chapter 4). Regardless of interview approach, it is important for a clinician to remember that self-reported information provided by the client may not be accurate.

There are several ways an interviewer can minimize inaccuracies and biases due to a client's "distorted lens." One way is to make sure that the client and the assessor share the same definition of the words and expressions used by the client. Research suggests that distortions of client report occur more frequently on psychosocial variables than on objective facts that can be corroborated by other records (Henry, Moffit, Caspi, Langley, &

Silva, 1994), although assessors should note that distortions of prior facts can and do also occur, which is why reviewing records can be important (see Chapter 8). For example, when a client says, "I feel depressed," what does he or she mean? Too often an interviewer jumps to the diagnostic criteria for major depressive episode without exploring what the *client* means by "depressed." The client may be using the term as laypeople do (what I refer to as "little d" depression when teaching students), using "depressed" as a simple adjective for something that is not necessarily clinically significant. Interviewers should make sure they have a sense of what clients actually mean by the terms they use, in order to understand the lenses through which clients are viewing their worlds. This can be accomplished by asking for definitions and/or for everyday examples of what clients mean by the terms they use, and by pointing out inconsistencies in their use of terms and their examples, if necessary. The interviewer can also use this discussion to develop hypotheses about the potential sources of these miscommunications, which might include sociocultural differences; deliberate misrepresentation (such as in malingering); or even distortions due to clients' deeply held belief that they have a particular condition or illness, among other possibilities.

Another way an interview can minimize the effects of distortion of self-report is by remembering that, just because the client says, "I think I have disorder X" does not mean he or she does, and that disorder X is not the only diagnostic hypothesis to test in the ensuing assessment (see Chapter 2). However, knowing that the client *thinks* he or she has a certain disorder should alert the assessor to the ways in which the client might distort his or her report of present symptoms and impairment, as well as his or her recall of the past, in ways consistent with this lens. Of note, there is evidence that retrospective recall of one's past is particularly vulnerable to inaccurate reconstruction (Garb, 2007). For example, in classic work by Mittenberg and colleagues (Ferguson, Mittenberg, Barone, & Schneider, 1999; Mittenberg, DiGiulio, Perrin, & Bass, 1992), it was shown that individuals with mild head injuries consistently underestimated how often they had experienced common cognitive, affective, and physiological symptoms prior to the injury (as compared to the rates in which such symptoms were endorsed by controls). In other words, the individuals with mild head injury seemed to be convinced that their injury was the cause of their current experience of such common symptoms, and therefore believed these symptoms occurred with less frequency in their past. This effect is likely not unique to mild head injuries and instead reflects a general distortion in recall of past symptoms when an individual believes things were better "before" (Gunstad & Suhr, 2001, 2002).

An additional way that an interviewer can minimize intake-related assessment bias is to use the biopsychosocial model to develop alternative hypotheses about the origins of and contributions to the presenting concerns of the client. Clients who have a patient identity will not only tend to report present and past symptoms in a distorted manner, but may also report only those life events and history consistent with their overall beliefs about the causes of and contributions to their perceived disorder. This can lead to a compartmentalized report of only isolated parts of their history, which a thorough biopsychosocial exploration should minimize. The biopsychosocial model presented in Chapter 3 is applied to the process of semistructured intake interviewing in following sections.

Another way that an interviewer can minimize the biases that can creep into an evaluation is to remember that, although coming first, the interview is just one piece of data that should be examined when drawing any diagnostic or treatment conclusions. The assessor should consciously hold him- or herself accountable for the assessment decisions the interview led to, and during the process of data integration, recognize whether any of the data, including that obtained in interview, is valid to interpret in the case. It has been shown (Brtek & Motavildo, 2002) that the validity of structured clinical interviews (with regard to diagnosis reached) increases when interviewers are held accountable for the decision-making process they used to reach the decision, rather than being accountable for the accuracy of the decision, regardless of the procedure followed. In fact, procedural accountability (discussed in more detail in Chapter 13) generally has positive effects on decision-making accuracy (see Brtek & Motavildo, 2002, for a review).

A final way that an assessor can minimize the inaccurate weight that might be placed on information obtained during an initial interview is to formally check for noncredible responding in the interview (see Chapter 4). Unfortunately, few structured interviews include any items or processes for detecting either a tendency to underreport or overreport symptomatology. However, some studies have examined such approaches (Rogers, 2008b), and other stand-alone interviews specifically designed to assess for overreporting of symptoms have been developed, although their psychometric strength is of question (for a review of such interviews and their psychometric properties, see Rogers, 2008b, and Boone, 2012). An area of research in this domain that has been relatively neglected is the potential for clients to noncredibly report on the degree to which they are *impaired* in their functioning, rather than their noncedible report of symptoms, per se; however, there is no reason to believe that report of impairment or disability would be any less vulnerable to noncredible responding than report of symptoms. For example, Lewandowski, Lovett, Codding, and Gordon (2008) demonstrated that both academic concerns and impairment were overrreported to the same extent as ADHD symptoms in college students.

As noted in Chapter 4, it can be difficult for an interviewer to balance empathy for the story the client is presenting at that initial contact, which is necessary for gaining rapport, with maintaining scientific skepticism about the accuracy of that information (i.e., consciously acknowledging the potential inaccuracy of the client's report). It might help for the assessor to remember that inaccuracy of self-report is normal and often adaptive behavior, even outside of the clinical context. People inherently construct explanations, rationalizations, and attributions for their behavior. However, believing that one can actually find an accurate explanation for people's behavior by paying attention only to their experiences and reports is using a "subpersonal" theoretical approach (what Pennington, 2002, refers to as the "phenomenological fallacy") in the interview, and is no different than starting an interview viewing the data through only one lens of the bio-psychosocial model or by wearing the very specific lens of one particular psychological theory to interpret the patient's story at the time of that initial data gathering. All such approaches invite decision-making biases (see Chapter 2) that can lead to inaccuracies in assessment. Overall, then, it is a good idea for assessors to consider the intake interview, regardless of whether it is structured or unstructured, as a way to generate hypotheses (i.e., inductive) that must be further tested with additional data, rather than as a way to draw conclusions (i.e., deductive).

TYPES OF INTERVIEWS

Unstructured Interviews

As mentioned above, given that little is known about the client at the point of the initial interview (with the possible exception of a referral question or some prior records or diagnoses—which, as pointed out in Chapter 2, may only serve to bias the assessor in this important first step), the goal should be more inductive than deductive. That is, the interviewer should gather information about the presenting concerns and the patient's current functioning and history, in order to develop potential hypotheses of "what is wrong" and what factors contribute to "what is wrong," in order to then determine what additional evidence is needed to determine the validity of any of these hypotheses.

For this inductive purpose, it may be appropriate to begin with a less structured interview approach that allows for more open-ended questions, to which the assessor can hear the open-ended responses to the vague and rather ambiguous questions asked. With such an approach, an interviewer is likely to hear more unique details about the presenting concerns and can note the client's spontaneous responses, which are likely to suggest what lens the client is wearing when considering his or her own concerns. If the assessor is using the biopsychosocial framework (see Chapter 3 and below) to examine data through multiple lenses, then various potential diagnostic and etiological hypotheses can be formed from the initial interview data, which can then be confirmed or disconfirmed with additional information.

At the same time, an interviewer needs to be mindful that this unstructured approach invites poor reliability (see Chapter 6), as two different interviewers may not ask the same questions, follow up on the same issues, or even ask the same questions by using the same wording. Thus, for the purposes of actually drawing conclusions in a deductive fashion, the unstructured interview is much more likely to lead to inaccurate conclusions.

Structured Interviews

Structured interviews were developed to improve the reliability of the clinical interview by providing a standardized set of questions to present to clients and to reduce clinical judgment about client responses. Their focus has always been diagnostic in nature; that is, using an agreed-upon set of diagnostic criteria for disorders and asking specifically about those criteria in a systematic way. Whereas unstructured interviews vary in the content and even the pattern of questions asked, and may be subject to the theoretical biases of the interviewer, structured interviews provide a consistent set of questions to be asked in a consistent manner, thus meeting the purpose of increased reliability over the unstructured interview format. However, structured interviews are still subject to decision-making biases that may make them inaccurate or their conclusions invalid. In fact, one can view a structured interview as little more than an orally administered test, rather than as an interview per se.

Diagnostic Bias in Structured Interviews

One of the first sources of bias in a structured interview stems from their development: Structured interviews are developed to assess some agreed-upon set of diagnostic criteria. To the extent that there are problems or controversies with the diagnostic system itself, those problems will be reflected in the structured diagnostic interview developed from them. Two such problems are (1) the categorical nature of dimensional constructs, which is the current model in most diagnostic systems; and (2) the nature of psychopathology itself and the decision to call something "abnormal."

Because current diagnostic systems are categorical in nature, the criteria require that clinicians be able to reliably determine into which "category" a client fits. When diagnostic criteria are developed to construct a disorder as homogeneously as possible (which is then reflected in the design of the structured interview), this homogeneity will lead to clearly defined categories that likely have a great deal of reliability, but will also leave many cases unaccounted for. However, when the diagnostic criteria are broad enough to capture heterogeneity within the disorder, the boundaries of the criteria will overlap with those of other disorders and make it difficult to distinguish between specific types of pathology (Widiger & Edmundson, 2011). To the extent that the underlying diagnostic system has strengths and weaknesses due to the chosen approach, a structured interview based on that diagnostic system will share that same problem.

A second problem arises when attempting to determine what psychopathology truly is. How do clinicians decide when something is "abnormal enough" to be categorized as a form of psychopathology? Such a decision carries major consequences; labeling something as abnormal gives it power because the diagnostic label usually suggests that it requires treatment or accommodation, should receive some sort of financial reimbursement or insurance coverage, or may have forensic/legal implications. For example, does someone who scored above average in all of his or her school records from kindergarten through high school, but now gets C grades in advanced premed coursework in college, truly meet criteria for a reading disability just because he or she wants to go to medical school? In the medical model of diagnosis, it is clear that many diagnoses are quite common and in fact many would not lead to any treatment per se (although seeing a physician about them would be reimbursed by insurance, e.g., seeing a physician for symptoms that lead to a diagnosis of a cold) (Maddux, Gosselin, & Winstead, 2012). In most diagnostic systems for psychopathology, the disorder is not diagnosed unless it leads to impairment in functioning, which should then lead to treatment; however, this aspect of diagnosis is often not considered by clinicians using structured interviews to diagnose psychological conditions.

Variability in Structured Interviews

Another important point to consider is that not all structured interviews are alike. Structured interviews vary greatly in their breadth and depth of coverage of any particular set of diagnostic criteria. For example, the Mini International Neuropsychiatric Interview (M.I.N.I.; Sheehan et al.,

1998) focuses primarily on (most but not all of) the anxiety disorders, eating disorders, mood disorders, substance abuse disorders, and psychoses. Although much shorter than more comprehensive structured interviews, it does not offer the breadth of coverage of possible psychopathology. In addition, it does not offer the depth necessary for establishing diagnosis; the M.I.N.I. only examines current symptoms and not lifetime symptoms, and only includes symptom criteria, not impairment criteria. As noted above, assessors generally seem to neglect the assessment of impairment/dysfunction as part of the diagnostic criteria they use, despite its importance in many diagnostic systems and in making treatment decisions.

Psychometric Review of Both Types of Interviews

Given the description of unstructured and structured interviews above, it should be clear that comparing the two methods is a bit like comparing apples and oranges. In fact, one can easily argue that structured interviews are not interviews but instead are standardized self-report measures in which the questions are administered orally rather than by paper and pencil (or by computer) and with the express goal of establishing whether a client reports symptoms (and sometimes impairment) consistent with an agreed-upon set of diagnostic criteria. However, research has often compared the two interview approaches psychometrically as if they do have the same purpose, and thus the next section of the chapter summarizes that literature from a decision-making perspective.

Standardized Process (Reliability)

Certainly for the purposes of establishing a diagnosis, reliability is important. In fact, it is often argued that structured interviews are more reliable than unstructured interviews because the questions and process are quite structured and force specific responses from patients that are relatively easy to interpret and "score" (Mullins-Sweatt & Widiger, 2009; Rogers, 2003; Zimmerman, 2003). However, data show that the relatively higher reliabilities obtained for structured interviews are *only* for the goal of identifying the presence or absence of psychopathology broadly; data regarding the reliability with regard to reaching the *same exact* diagnosis or syndrome are lower (Craig, 2013; Groth-Marnat, 2009). Similarly, higher reliabilities are obtained for identification of the presence or absence of overt behavior, but are relatively lower for covert and subjective psychological variables, such as exist in personality disorders (Craig, 2013; Groth-Marnat, 2009).

Furthermore, the degree to which structured interviews are truly standardized is of debate. There is still a lot of clinical judgment required for

many structured interviews that invites assessors to ask their own questions in their own ways, to make decisions as to whether or not to ask those
questions, or to decide whether client reports suggest "abnormality" to the
extent that the interviews should mark the symptom as clinically present or
not (Summerfeldt, Klooseterman, & Antony, 2010). Furthermore, research
has shown that reliabilities for unstructured interviews can be good so long
as clinicians carefully attend to the diagnostic criteria (i.e., using the interview carefully for the diagnostic purpose) (Garb, 1998a).

In the end, if the purpose of an interview were merely to establish
whether a client endorses a specific set of symptoms that is consistent with
a diagnosis, the more structured the interview, the more reliable it is likely
to be (although not necessarily more valid, given both are subject to distortion of self-report, as detailed above). But in an initial intake interview,
during which the process should still be inductive rather than deductive
and should be about exploring more than just endorsement of a set of symptoms, these data are less relevant for the assessor in making a decision
about interview approach.

Content Validity

The main source of data for establishing the validity of structured diagnostic interviews is their content validity, as judged by the experts that design
them; as noted above, such interviews are typically designed to cover a
specific set of agreed-upon diagnostic criteria (e.g., the DSM) for psychological disorders (Summerfeldt et al., 2010). However, as also noted above,
even structured diagnostic interviews vary in how much of the construct
of psychopathology they cover, including the range of disorders they cover,
whether they ask about only current symptoms or include lifetime symptoms, and whether or not they cover other aspects of the diagnostic criteria,
such as impairment criteria or exclusionary criteria. In fact, most structured interviews do little to consider etiological or developmental information that would be relevant to differential diagnosis. As an example, in the
Anxiety Disorders Interview Schedule–IV (ADIS-IV; Brown, Di Nardo, &
Barlow, 1994), examination of the "not due to medical conditions or substance use" criterion for most anxiety and depressive disorders involves
only a couple of questions asking the interviewee whether, during the time
period of having symptoms, he or she was taking any type of drugs, or if
he or she had any physical condition. As noted in Chapter 3, when a client
has not yet been diagnosed with the condition (or chooses not to communicate a previously received diagnosis to the clinician), such a brief and gross
approach to considering exclusionary factors would be highly inadequate.

Certainly such questions do not provide a thorough coverage of important rule-outs for diagnosis, which are also important etiological considerations that could lead to appropriate referrals for other treatment. Thus, relevant content for the purposes of diagnosis, as well as for the purposes of providing appropriate care, is not covered in many structured interviews, which is important for an assessor to consider when deciding on an approach to the initial interview with a client.

Diagnostic Validity

Criteria for diagnostic validity would include whether a particular type of interview is able to accurately detect the presence of a particular disorder, as defined by some criterion, and thus includes sensitivity and specificity analyses (see Chapter 6 for more discussion of these topics). Interestingly, it has been suggested that, because structured interviews provide higher rates of diagnoses than unstructured interviews (Zimmerman & Mattia, 1999a, 1999b, 1999c), they must have greater diagnostic validity (i.e., they are more sensitive to psychopathology). The suggestion is that disorders that are "missed" by a less comprehensive unstructured interview are correctly identified by the structured approach. However, there is little consideration that these diagnoses actually may be false positives or misdiagnoses, or reflect noncredible responding. In reality, it is difficult to reach generalized conclusions about the diagnostic validity literature for any given type of interview, given that validity is dependent upon so many factors, including (but not limited to) which disorder or disorders are being examined and the operational definition of the criterion diagnosis.

With regard to the first of these concerns, most diagnostic validity tests conducted are based on the assumption that clients have only one discrete disorder, despite the growing evidence that mental disorders aren't discrete clinical conditions and the fact that many individuals meet diagnostic criteria for more than one disorder. As noted above, there is only modest diagnostic agreement at the level of a specific diagnosis compared to the presence/absence of psychopathology (Craig, 2013).

With regard to the second of these concerns, most validity data for interviews (whether structured or unstructured) are relative to operational definitions of the construct that are very circular in nature. For example, in many studies, structured interviews are compared to clinician-derived diagnoses—but how were those diagnoses derived? Perhaps on the basis of unstructured interviews, other structured interviews, and/or other measurement tools, all of which themselves need validation information. The process is a circular one, given that there is no "gold standard" against which to compare the results from any interview technique. Although it has been a few decades since Spitzer (1983) proposed the LEAD standard (use of consensus diagnosis based on longitudinal observation by experts using all available data) as an optimum way for criterion diagnoses to be established, this is a time-consuming and expensive endeavor that is rarely used in the research literature and hardly at all in clinical practice.

A final important consideration in the examination of diagnostic validity, particularly in the clinical context in which cost effectiveness is an important consideration, is the incremental validity of the method under consideration. That is, does a structured diagnostic interview add incremental validity over other available data in order to establish a diagnosis? It has been observed that structured diagnostic interviews may not show incremental validity over brief symptom rating scales for the purposes of establishing whether a client is reporting symptoms consistent with a particular diagnosis (Hunsley & Mash, 2010). This should not be surprising when an assessor considers the fact that both techniques likely have the same content validity, and really only differ in their method of administration (i.e., paper-and-pencil vs. face-to-face questioning).

In the end, an assessor wishing to choose a specific structured interview for a specific *diagnostic* purpose should review all the literature available for the various structured interviews for that diagnosis or disorder; texts such as Antony and Barlow (2010) and Hunsley and Mash (2008b) provide good summaries of this information, although it should be noted that incremental validity data are likely lacking for many of the interviews commonly used. However, an assessor needs to remember that this information is relevant only for that specific deductive purpose (establishing whether a client reports symptoms consistent with a particular disorder in order to reach a diagnosis) and for a specific disorder, and thus may not be relevant for determining how best to approach a client during an initial meeting in which the goal is to develop hypotheses about the nature of the problems and the need for treatment (regardless of diagnosis). For that more inductive purpose, diagnostic validity information is irrelevant.

Construct Validity

To establish construct validity for any given interview method would require a large set of studies in which it was shown that the interview identified groups of individuals who behaved in ways consistent with the construct being assessed (see Chapter 6). Obviously, these kinds of data are difficult to summarize for any one specific structured interview for one specific disorder, and they are impossible to examine for unstructured interviews as a whole, given that unstructured interviews are not standardized. For example, to truly examine the construct validity of a particular structured interview for a particular diagnosis would mean examining whether the structured interview identified individuals who appeared to share the same underlying etiological factors, such as genetic vulnerabilities. The Schedule for Affective Disorders and Schizophrenia (SADS; Endicott & Spitzer, 1978) is a good example of a structured interview in which there is strong evidence of its ability to aid in the identification of genetic patterns in schizophrenia (Craig, 2013), although it should be noted that it is unclear whether other approaches (e.g., self-report questionnaires) might not also serve the same purpose equally well and be more cost-effective. Another potentially relevant aspect of construct validity might be whether the interview was able to identify individuals who respond the same way to pharmacological or nonpharmacological treatments. However, diagnosis itself is not a sufficient indicator of treatment need (Regier & Narrow, 2002), as "subthreshold" conditions often respond to the same treatments, and different disorders respond to the same treatments. Thus, as previously suggested, questions about the validity of constructs themselves (in this case, the construct of abnormality and psychopathology) also weaken the ability to examine the construct validity of the instruments designed to assess them.

Use in Diverse Groups

As noted in Chapter 5, it is important for assessors to consider whether it is appropriate to use assessment techniques with members from diverse subgroups. Unfortunately, there are limited data available on this topic with regard to interviews, regardless of whether they are structured or unstructured. There are some data to suggest that individuals from racial minority groups are more often diagnosed with more severe psychopathology based on interview data than individuals of more dominant groups. However, this difference might lie in the diagnostic constructs themselves, in the diagnostic thresholds used to establish diagnosis in different groups, in biased application of those thresholds, or in the interviews used to gather the data to make the diagnosis—and it may not reflect bias (i.e., it may reflect real differences) (Widiger, 1998). For example, studies show that, even when clinicians are unaware of race, African American males are judged to have more severe psychological symptoms based on their interview responses, suggesting that some of the diagnostic differences may be true (Winstead & Sanchez, 2012). Interestingly, Ford and Widiger (1989) found evidence of gender bias in personality disorder diagnosis, but no gender bias at the level of individual symptom ratings. Such a finding might suggest a biased application of diagnostic criteria during an interview (assessors making a quick inductive jump to a biased understanding of the diagnosis, based on gender stereotypes), whereas if the interviewer stayed focused on each individual symptom and examination of whether or not an individual displayed that symptom, there was less overall diagnostic bias. Thus, these results suggest there is a danger of diagnostic bias, and that perhaps an initial interview approach focused on examination of complaints, concerns, and behavior would lead to less overall bias than an interview approach focused on the goal of establishing diagnosis from first contact with the client.

DECISION-MAKING ISSUES

Unfortunately, in today's world of managed care, in which there is pressure to gather only the "required" information (which often seems to be presence or absence of a billable diagnosis) in the least amount of time, assessors may make many decision-making errors at the first moment of contact with the client. For example, such pressure might lead an assessor to conduct only a quick 5- to 10-minute "semistructured" intake interview focused solely on the first symptom (or even diagnosis) mentioned by the referral source or the client, asking only about other symptoms consistent with that particular disorder or symptom, or with a quick run-through of symptoms in every diagnostic category; such an unreliable approach is highly vulnerable to diagnostic decision-making errors (see Chapter 2). As noted by Mullins-Sweat and Widiger (2009), surveys of health care providers in practice show that they do not use diagnostic criteria correctly, which can lead to overdiagnosis, misdiagnosis, and inappropriate treatment.

Another assessor may respond to this time pressure and place a limited focus on only some of the psychometric data available for structured interviews, thus choosing to administer only a brief structured diagnostic interview (or even use computerized interviews to lower the direct contact time with clients), with little regard to the psychometric concerns raised above and without recognition of the continued need for good clinical judgment even in the structured diagnostic interview process. Interviewers who start only with a structured diagnostic interview may feel that they are on stronger psychometric ground, but it is important for those interviewers to note that they have chosen to start their assessment with deductive reasoning, including beliefs that there is, in fact, a diagnosis and that there is a specific diagnosis, with some high-frequency differentials to rule out (particularly when a very specific structured diagnostic interview is chosen). Thus, taking such an approach right at the point of an initial contact with a client is likely to create a decision-making bias from the moment the interview begins, and is also vulnerable to bias from the lens the patient wore when presenting for the evaluation. For example, consider the case presented in Chapter 1, in which the client appeared to meet diagnostic criteria for an anxiety disorder, based on structured diagnostic interview (and self-report measures focused specifically on diagnostic criteria for anxiety disorders). Although the diagnosis obtained in the structured interview was likely reliable, it was not valid.

A SEMISTRUCTURED INTAKE INTERVIEW USING A BIOPSYCHOSOCIAL LENS

At the point of an initial contact with a client, it makes the most sense to start with a semistructured interview approach using inductive reasoning processes to begin to understand the person in a developmentally oriented, biopsychosocial framework (see Chapter 3). The goal of such an interview is to develop *hypotheses* about what concerns (not symptoms) are most pressing for the client, the time course for development of those concerns (and possible contributing factors using the framework), as well as how those concerns are affecting the client in terms of his or her real-world functioning/impairment. Ultimately this approach should lead to hypotheses about how the concerns fit together into a potential diagnostic pattern (or don't fit), as well as hypotheses about potential treatments and interventions. These hypotheses should then be further examined with additional assessment data, including other self-report data, such as with a structured diagnostic interview or self-report measures (presented in Chapters 9 and 10); cognitive testing, if relevant (described in Chapters 11 and 12); and/or by gathering additional data from collaterals or existing records (as discussed in Chapter 8)—all with consideration of the validity of the data (see Chapter 4). Consistent with a scientist-detective model, the purpose of such an intake interview is to develop hypotheses about what the presenting problem might be and what factors are contributing to that problem, and then to avoid bad decision making by critically evaluating both support for and against each hypothesis as the interview continues and leads the assessor to the next steps in the assessment.

Table 7.1 presents the basic components of such an interview. The "structure" of the semistructured approach being presented here comes predominantly from the list of topics or components that should eventually be covered in the initial interview, but not necessarily in a particular

TABLE 7.1. General Structure for a Developmentally Oriented Biopsychosocial Intake Interview

Step 1: "Why are you here?"	Establish what brought the client to the assessment. Focus on reported concerns, behaviors, and real-life consequences, remembering to have the client define terms and provide examples.
Step 2: Temporal course of client's story	Examine the client's sense of when problems, behaviors, symptoms, consequences began; if the client has had similar concerns before (and what he or she did about those concerns in the past); whether the symptoms have come and gone or been unremitting since they began; and what kinds of events or factors may have surrounded the onset, if there are any clear ones. Clarify any prior assessment or treatment for the concerns (and consider getting those reports as part of rest of assessment).
Step 3: Biopsychosocial review	Although some aspects of a biopsychosocial review may have already arisen during Step 2, all aspects of the model should be revisited for comprehensiveness and consistency in the report. The aspects of the biopsychosocial review do not need to occur in any order, and the astute clinician will refer back to issues already raised by the client when ordering each part of the model. The interviewer should remember that any of these factors may be the presenting concerns, consequences of the presenting concerns (and perhaps reflective of impairment), or even causal to the presenting concerns. The interviewer should also note that some areas may be particularly relevant for one client's presenting concerns, but less relevant for another. The interviewer should at least briefly examine each of the areas, but some clients may not need the detailed level of questioning that is suggested below.
3a: Psychological history	The client may have psychological history beyond what he or she presented with as a primary reason for referral. The interviewer should ask about any prior psychological diagnoses, prior treatment (pharmacological or nonpharmacological), or any other times in which the client experienced psychological symptoms and perhaps was not diagnosed. Substance use/misuse/abuse history should also be established.
3b: Medical history	A scientifically minded and trained assessor should be aware of medical/biological/neurological contributors to psychological presentations and problems, and thus should ask not only about current and prior diagnoses and medications (as well as other treatments, surgeries, hospitalizations), but also about additional symptoms that might suggest need of formal evaluation for other disorders, as relevant to the presenting concerns. The assessor should also ask about the client's last physical exam.
3c: Daily routine	The interviewer should ask about relevant aspects of the client's daily routine, such as eating habits, sleeping pattern, exercise, hobbies and activities, and any recent changes in these.

TABLE 7.1. *(continued)*

3d: Early development	The interviewer should ask the client what he or she knows about his or her own early development, such as whether his or her mother had any complications during pregnancy or delivery, whether he or she was born full term, and whether he or she experienced any significant delays in developmental milestones such as learning to walk, talk, or toilet.
3e: Cultural history	The examiner should ask about the client's primary language, where he or she was raised, what his or her racial/ethnic identity is, gender/sexual identity, and other aspects of cultural diversity that seem relevant to the presenting concerns, based on knowledge of diverse cultures, which might include ways in which the client describes symptoms and functioning or to what the client attributes the causes of his or her difficulties.
3f: Family history	The examiner should ask whether members of the client's family have experienced similar problems and concerns (and, if so, what the effects were and whether they received any treatment for the condition). It is important to get actual details; just as clients might say they are "depressed," they may also say that many members of their family had depression, but with further examination the interviewer might find that no family members had ever been assessed or treated for the condition.
3g: Psychosocial supports and stressors	The interviewer should ask about the quality of the client's psychosocial interactions (family members, friends, etc.) to gain a sense of the importance of the client's personal experiences and concerns with his or her larger sociocultural environment (e.g., which might be consistent with the assessor's own cultural background).
3h: School history	The interviewer should ask about the client's academic history, including grades, performance on standardized tests, whether the client ever had an individualized education program (IEP) or 504 plan, whether the client was ever held back or skipped forward a grade, whether the client received any sort of academic interventions or informal accommodations, what types of courses the client took (honors, AP), and whether there were any behavioral problems during school.
3i: Work history	The interviewer should ask the client about number and types of jobs held, whether the client has ever been fired or received bad performance reviews, and reasons for any job changes (particularly if they were frequent).
3j: Legal history	The interviewer should establish whether the client has ever experienced encounters with the law.

order (with the sole exception of the first question, "Why are you here?"). Instead, the assessor should be guided more by what the client brings to the table as his or her primary concern, then following the client as his or her story is reported. Because such an approach requires a great deal of working memory skill for the interviewer, it is crucial for the interviewer to take detailed notes and to refer to those notes during the interview to check for issues that may have not been covered prior to the termination of the interview.

As the interview proceeds, the interviewer's questions can move from open-ended questions that follow the client's story to questions that are intermediately directive (e.g., requesting clarification, asking for specific examples, and confronting inconsistencies). Over time, as hypotheses become apparent, the interviewer can become even more directive in questioning in order to fill in missing gaps in information and to check for both confirmatory and disconfirmatory evidence for the various hypotheses that were raised—all the while keeping in mind that such evidence is at most preliminary, since it is entirely based on self-report. At its most direct and structured, then, the interview could end with diagnostically focused questions (including the "oral test" of a structured interview, which could be carefully chosen as the one with the best diagnostic validity for the particular diagnostic and differential diagnostic hypotheses that have been already identified). Along the way, it is also important for the interviewer to take note of what other evidence or information might be available from other sources (and ask the client about it right then) so that the assessor can gather that information (see Chapter 8). In addition, the interviewer should be taking note of *how* the client presents the information (as is discussed in more detail in the next section of this chapter).

As can be seen in Table 7.1, all of the lenses of a developmental bio-psychosocial framework are worn at the same time and are used to develop hypotheses about the dynamic and interacting contributors to the client's presenting concerns. In Steps 1 and 2, the assessor starts at the symptom and behavior level of analysis and seeks to be as descriptive as possible about the client's symptom(s). Are the symptoms actually unusual, or do they have a high base rate for individuals similar to the client and with consideration of the client's current context? Or are they developmentally appropriate and in the range of normal functioning, given the client's gender, age, and cultural context? When the client uses labels in statements such as "I am depressed" or "I have social anxiety," can he or she define what those terms mean and provide examples of symptoms and behaviors related to this illness representation? Do the symptoms cause impairment or dysfunction, and what evidence beyond the client's self-report is there for such impairment/dysfunction? When did the symptoms begin and have they changed over time? Are there several different symptoms or concerns clustering together (with the assessor specifically asking about other symptoms if they don't come up spontaneously but are part of the working hypotheses) that might be suggestive of particular psychological conditions (or even of other etiologies for the pattern identified)?

Next the assessor should consider the salient symptom or symptom sets and consider what known biological, genetic, environmental, psychological, sociological, cultural, and developmental factors are relevant to them, developing hypotheses about potential etiologies that can be examined by further questioning, referral to other appropriate health evaluation, seeking other information from collaterals, records, and via formal testing. Using this information, the assessor proceeds to build support for/against any of these interpretations, prior to then determining how well they fit any given diagnosis. For example, when considering the pattern of the symptoms over time, the assessor should be attuned to, and ask about, whether changes coincided with changes to the client's environment, social supports or stressors, health status, daily routines or behaviors, etc. This process might begin in Step 2, while listening to the client's story, but should continue in Step 3 to ensure that important areas of functioning have not been overlooked in the initial discussion of the client's story. It is important to note that these factors do not need to be considered in any particular order and that the level of detailed questioning needed for each area may vary, depending on the client's presenting concerns and the interviewer's initial hypotheses about potential etiologies and consequences of the presenting concerns.

BEHAVIORAL OBSERVATIONS

Let him, on meeting a fellow-mortal, learn at a glance to distinguish the history of the man, and the trade or profession to which he belongs. Puerile as such an exercise may seem, it sharpens the faculties of observation, and teaches one where to look and what to look for. By a man's finger nails, by his coat-sleeve, by his boot, by his trouser knees, by the callosities of his forefinger and thumb, by his expression, by his shirt cuffs—by each of these things a man's calling is plainly revealed. That all united should fail to enlighten the competent enquirer in any case is almost inconceivable.
—From "The Book of Life," an article by Sherlock Holmes quoted in *A Study in Scarlet*

Another important aspect of assessment, not only in the first contact with the client but throughout the entire assessment process, is observation of the client's presentation and behavior. Within the context of the initial interview, the assessor is considering "how the client said it" rather than "what the client said." The initial intake interview, particularly one that is less structured, is one of the few times that an assessor can observe the client in an open and ambiguous situation, seeing how the client organizes his or her verbal responses and how this coordinates with his or her nonverbal communication. However, the assessor should also observe how the client behaves and presents him- or herself throughout the rest of the assessment process, and how that behavior may change with time and/or differing assessment contexts. For example, a client may be cooperative during an interview but become angry after filling out a personality questionnaire; a client might seem relaxed at the beginning of cognitive testing but become flustered or frustrated when the cognitive test items get harder; or a client may become less alert and aroused during the course of an evaluation.

Not only should an assessor make such observations, but he or she should also *record* those observations. Taking notes about how a client behaved/presented as a corollary to his or her verbal or written (or even other behavioral) responses is helpful in later providing a context for interpreting those responses. For example, if an assessor judges that a client is showing limited motivation or cooperation, it can help that assessor to have actual behavioral documentation of that interpretation (e.g., recording number of eye rolls in response to questions).

It is important for assessors to remember that behavioral observations of this sort are made in a generally unstructured manner and thus have limited psychometric properties. Although there are some structured mental status observations, they are not commonly used; an exception is Folstein's Mini-Mental State Examination (Folstein, Folstein, & McHugh, 1975), which is focused only on cognitive symptoms and is discussed more in Chapter 12. However, many structured mental status observation forms are designed for use during the interview and typically ask about the assessor's *interpretation* of behavior and presentation (e.g., facial expression suggests anxiety, depression, anger; body posture suggests suspiciousness), rather than describing the actual facial expression, body posture, etc.

It is important for the interviewer to remember the decision-making bias of the halo effect (see Chapter 2). If an assessor develops a general impression of the person from first contact (be that impression negative or positive), the assessor is more likely to infer other characteristics about that person and interpret his or her subsequent behaviors based on this initial impression. Instead, an assessor should remember to make observations about the behaviors themselves and consider interpretations about the cause of those behaviors as merely hypotheses, subject to further confirmation or disconfirmation. For example, it may not be clear to an interviewer how much foot shaking by a client is "too much," as there are no normative data for such an observation within the dynamic context of assessment (i.e., foot shaking might change in response to the content of questions, to the difficulty level of cognitive challenges, to the need for the client to have a restroom or smoke break, etc.). There are also no data to suggest that certain behavioral observations would be specific to any one condition or disorder (e.g., foot shaking could indicate nervousness, boredom, restlessness, pain, anger, impatience, urinary urgency, nicotine craving). In fact, the behavior may be in the normal range for the person's cultural background (e.g., downcast eyes may be considered appropriate in a client's background; dramatic gestures may be consistent with a client's family communication style; a rigidly held posture might be viewed differently in a military veteran). Thus, as much as the assessor can, he or she should take notes about observed behaviors alongside the verbal responses being given (akin to what one might see in a script to a play). Table 7.2 provides a brief summary of some important behavioral observations for an assessor to consider noticing in the clients he or she assesses. This list is not comprehensive, but includes items that an assessor can observe without necessarily attributing a cause or reason for them.

TABLE 7.2. Important Behavioral Observations

Clothing	Is the client's clothing appropriate to weather/season? Is it appropriate to the context (considering cultural issues)?
Grooming and hygiene	Is the client's grooming and hygiene appropriate to the context (considering cultural issues)?
Posture	How does the client stand/sit? Does this change over time (e.g., with lengthy time sitting, in response to questions)?
Gait	How does the client walk? Does the client have good balance, walk at an overly slow or fast rate, stumble or shuffle?
Motor movements	What is the client's general motor activity level/speed of movement? Does the client make gestures, show tics, or have any other unusual body movements? Does the client have any physical limitations? Do any motoric behaviors change with time or context?
Speech	Is the client's speech rapid or slow? Is the client notably soft-spoken or loud? Is there evidence of slurring or misarticulation? Is the client's speech blunted or prosodic? Does the client make any other unusual vocalizations (verbal tics such as grunts, sighs, humming, whispering to self)?

(continued)

TABLE 7.2. *(continued)*

Facial expression	Does the client appear expressive with his or her face or make limited/no facial expressions? What facial expressions are made frequently (describe the actual facial expressions before attributing them to a specific mood or affect—e.g., grimace, smile, wrinkled forehead, tense thin lips)? Are those facial expressions congruent with the context of what the client is saying or what the client reports as his or her general mood?
Eye contact	Does the client make eye contact with the assessor? Does the client ever break eye contact and in what context? Has the clinician considered cultural context when considering eye contact with the client?
Level of attention/ alertness/arousal	Does the client respond in a timely fashion to requests and questions? Does the client appear awake and alert? Does the client yawn or even fall asleep?
Need for repetition	Does the interviewer have to repeat questions or directions often? Does this occur immediately or does the need for repetition come sometime after directions have been given? If it occurs immediately, does the client respond to a change in the direction (shortening it or using simpler vocabulary)?

8

Assessment Data
from Other Sources

I have devised seven separate explanations, each of which would cover
the facts as far as we know them. But which of these is correct can only
be determined by the fresh information which we shall no doubt find
waiting for us.
        —SHERLOCK HOLMES, in *The Adventure of the Copper Beeches*

Assessment involves the integration of information from a diverse
set of sources, most often scores from psychological measures and interview data, as well as observations of client presentation during interview
and test performance. However, assessment should also include other data
relevant to the referral question, such as information from the reports of
other relevant individuals who can share their perspective of the client's
concerns and/or history (collateral report) and from relevant historical
records. Unfortunately, efforts in establishing empirically based assessment procedures have thus far focused on the validity of the interpretation of psychological tests for particular purposes, as well as the diagnostic
validity of clinical interviews; there is almost no research focused on the
empirical value of these other aspects of psychological assessment. However, such a limitation should not lead an assessor to ignore that source
of information entirely. Just as research validity is limited by the use of
only one single method of measurement (monomethod bias) or by defining a
construct in a very narrow way (mono-operational bias) (Cook & Campbell,
1979), clinical assessment is also limited by such an approach. Data from
other sources may provide unique information, converging information, or
diverging information from that obtained by patient self-report. Drawing
conclusions from information obtained via a single method often leads to

inaccurate conclusions, and having to integrate data across multiple sources of information (particularly when that information does not completely converge) can help to minimize decision-making biases (Meyer et al., 2001). For example, Fennig, Craig, Tanenberg-Karant, and Bromet (1994) found that routine clinical diagnoses as part of usual hospital practice agreed with multimethod diagnostic conclusions (synthesized from semistructured interview, medical record review, interview of the treating clinician, and interview with a collateral who knew the patient well) only 45–50% of the time for a range of disorders, likely resulting in prescriptions for dramatically inappropriate medications for many patients. Similarly, studies comparing diagnosis of personality disorders by semistructured diagnostic interview to diagnosis by comprehensive integrative assessment methods showed that about 70% of the interview-based diagnoses were erroneous (Perry, 1992; Pilkonis et al., 1995).

Test scores and interview responses may take precedence in many assessors' minds because they have known psychometric properties. But when an assessor doesn't put data from those traditional sources into the larger context of the client's life, the assessor may not recognize the meaning of those data—Are the symptoms truly normal or abnormal? Do they actually cause impairment? How generalizable are the symptoms and consequent impairment? Is the self-report of current or past status accurate?— and may not develop a comprehensive understanding of potential etiologies for the symptoms (consistent with a biopychosocial model; see Chapter 2).

The present chapter reviews two of the most common sources of "other data" in clinical assessment: collateral report and records review.

COLLATERAL REPORT

Collateral reporters who can provide relevant information for an assessment vary depending on the presenting concerns as well as the client's broader context. For example, it would be unheard of to assess a minor without also gathering information from parents or guardians of that minor, but parents/ guardians and other relatives may also provide useful information in adult assessments. Other important potential collateral reporters include teachers, employers or coworkers, therapists or caseworkers, and other health care professionals. The intake interview is the most likely time that potentially relevant collateral reporters come to light, and an assessor should take note of such potential sources of information while gathering interview information from the client. Of course, obtaining information from these collateral reporters (particularly in adult assessment) requires the consent of the client (or, in the case of minors, the client's parents or guardians) (American Psychological Association, 2010).

Collateral information may converge with, provide unique information to, or may diverge from the information reported by the client. Whether the data converge, are unique, or diverge from the patient's report, an empirically minded assessor needs to consider the validity of the collateral's report. Some sources of error that might limit the validity of the collateral's report include (1) the nature of the constructs being asked about, (2) the collateral reporter's opportunity to observe the person being assessed with regard to those constructs, (3) the way in which the questions are being asked, (4) the collateral reporter's own individual differences that might lead to misperceptions of the behavior being reported upon, and (5) the collateral reporter's potential motivation to distort his or her report based on his or her personal relationship with the client.

An assessor needs to consider which constructs the collateral reporter is being asked to rate. If they are overt behaviors (e.g., "How often do you see this individual drink alcohol?"), then it is likely that the rating will be more accurate than if it requires an inference of some sort (e.g., "How anxious or depressed is this individual?") (Achenbach, Krukowski, Dumenci, & Ivanova, 2005). Just as when interviewing the client directly, an assessor should clarify with a collateral reporter the basis on which he or she is making an inferential judgment when one is presented (e.g., define terms, provide examples in daily life). An assessor should also consider whether the collateral reporter is making that inference or judgment simply because the client also self-reported it to the collateral, just as the client self-reported it to the assessor, rather than because the collateral actually observed the behavior or concern that led to the inference.

An assessor also needs to consider how often the collateral reporter has an opportunity to observe the behavior in question. For example, during the early school years, parents can observe their children in multiple contexts throughout the day; as they grow older, they may have less awareness of their child's behavior outside of the immediate home environment. Similarly, in elementary school, there may be only one or two primary teachers who can observe that child throughout the day and in many contexts; by high school, any one teacher may have knowledge of that child's behavior for only 45–50 minutes per day and in the context of one specific course. Studies show a higher degree of cross-collateral agreement when the collateral reporters have similar contact with the children (Achenbach et al., 2005). Even outside of child assessment, an assessor needs to consider how well the collaterals suggested by the adult client really have regular contact with the client. For example, in my experience, individuals with developmental disabilities often have caseworkers who have had virtually no direct contact with their clients (in quite a few cases, were only recently assigned to the client in question), and yet the caseworkers completed impairment ratings based on virtually no personal knowledge of their clients' functioning.

An assessor must also consider how he or she is asking the relevant questions. Simply asking a collateral reporter to provide information about the client is akin to conducting an unstructured clinical interview, with all its inherent weaknesses (as reviewed in the previous chapter). There are both standardized face-to-face interview methods for collecting data from collateral reporters (particularly other health care providers, teachers, and parents) and collateral report questionnaires for various specific disorders, symptoms, and conditions. These standardized methods have known reliability and validity (although the quality of such may vary) and also have normative data available in order to assist the clinician in determining if the collateral report is out of the range of "normal" for a particular issue. Of course, an assessor who chooses to use such standardized methods should carefully review the psychometric properties of the methods chosen to ensure that they are appropriate for (1) the constructs being assessed, (2) the client, and (3) the collateral reporter. The assessor must also remember that, even though there may be known reliability and validity data for the methods he or she chose to use, that does not guarantee that the collateral report is valid in the $N = 1$ case of the particular client being assessed, as there are still other sources of error for the assessor to consider.

An assessor must also consider the source of the information directly. Collateral reporters may have their own individual differences (personality, psychopathology, transient mood, expectations about others' functioning, cognitive weaknesses) that might lead to misperceptions of the behavior being reported upon. For example, it can prove frustrating when assessing an individual for potential dementia to find that the spouse of the client, who may be the most frequent observer of the client's daily functioning, is unfortunately not a very reliable reporter due to his or her own cognitive impairments (particularly when other family members do not see the client frequently enough to report reliably on the client's day-to-day functioning). Just as a client's transient psychological state may lead to distortions in his or her self-report of current and past symptoms and functioning, so too might the mental status of the collateral reporter be important to consider. Furthermore, the collateral reporter's own expectations about functioning may be of particular importance in considering the validity of his or her report, particularly when inferences were made. In other words, the assessor must also consider the lenses the collateral is using to view the client.

For example, consider the case of a 12-year-old male referred for eval-uation for a learning disorder. The school report indicated that the mother of the child reported that her son was "severely delayed" in learning to talk. Further questioning of the mother at the time of the evaluation, however, indicated that her firstborn child (a female) began speaking at 8 months, and her son began speaking at 13 months. From the mother's perspective, this was a "severe delay," but not from the perspective of developmental norms. As another example, consider the case of an 18-year-old senior in high school referred for evaluation for ADHD by her parents, who wanted her evaluated to receive accommodations prior to college. School records showed high achievement throughout, and teacher reports on standardized rating forms showed no academic, cognitive, psychological, or behavioral concerns. However, both parents rated their only child, who had no history of academic, disciplinary, or legal troubles, with maximum scores on cog-nitive and behavioral concerns on a well-validated, standardized collateral report measure. When asked about their ratings, with discussion of how their ratings fell above those typically achieved by children who were in detention centers or inpatient hospitals for behavioral problems, they sim-ply agreed that their child deserved to be rated that high. However, when asked for specific examples of behaviors consistent with such high ratings, the only examples they could provide were that "she does not take the trash out immediately when we ask her to," "she does not do her homework promptly, even when we remind her," and "she sometimes slams her door if we tell her to go to her room." They denied any other behavioral or oppo-sitional behaviors upon direct questioning, and yet still seemed convinced that their daughter's behavior was significantly out of the range of expecta-tions for a high school girl. Whether such distorted expectations came from the ways in which either of the parents was raised, sociocultural differ-ences, or other motivations, it was clear that their ratings on the collateral report instrument were not valid.

Finally, an assessor must consider that collateral reporters may have their own motivation to consciously distort their report of a client's symp-toms and/or functioning. Thus, an assessor must consider the collateral reporter's personal relationship with the client and listen for context that might suggest that this collateral reporter may either deny symptoms or impairment or exaggerate them. A collateral reporter may underreport symptoms or impairment, reflecting a desire to protect that individual from a potentially negative consequence. For example, consider the case of a mother with intellectual disability of mild severity, whose sister raised a concern about her parenting competency. The husband, motivated to protect his wife, might rate her as less impaired in her functioning than other collaterals might. Underreporting can also be of concern in collateral reporters who are antagonistic toward the client. This would be less likely in the context of clinical assessment, given that the client must provide consent to obtain information from collateral reporters, but it is not unheard of in the context of forensic assessment. For example, an employer rating an employee who is claiming a work-related cognitive injury might rate that employee as well functioning after the injury to minimize his or her own legal risk.

A collateral reporter may also overreport symptoms or impairment, especially if, like the client, he or she is consciously motivated to help the client obtain a secondary gain (i.e., malingering) or is unconsciously motivated to maintain a family or interpersonal dynamic as a care provider to someone who is ill (see Chapter 4). The assessor must consider whether the likely outcome of a diagnosis directly affects the collateral reporter (e.g., in the outcome of a lawsuit, obtaining access to stimulant medications if the child being assessed receives a diagnosis of ADHD), but also consider indirect effects (e.g., parents exaggerating their child's past and present academic and behavioral challenges to help them access accommodations or medications, or to assist them in avoiding negative consequences such as dismissal from university). Unfortunately, standardized collateral report questionnaires do not address the issue of noncredible responding in collateral report, and this is an area ripe for further scientific inquiry.

Given these many sources of error in collateral report, it should not be surprising that studies show generally poor to moderate correspondence of symptoms, behaviors, and impairment between child and parent reports, between parent and teacher reports, or between parent pairs or teacher pairs, and between adult and collateral ratings (Achenbach et al., 2005; Meyer et al., 2001). It is clear from such findings that an assessor should expect and anticipate disagreement and divergence within the data obtained across different sources, and should consider sources of error in all sources (not just the collateral report) when determining how best to integrate the information into the total assessment picture.

OTHER RECORDS

Another potentially valuable source of data in clinical assessment is records that may be available from other sources, such as educational/academic records, medical/hospital records, records from prior evaluations and/or treatment for the concerns being presented, employment records, or even legal records, depending on the referral questions and context. Knowledge of which records might be relevant to a case will likely arise during the course of the interview with the client, and of course access to these records requires the authorization of the client. Thus, a records review can be limited by the extent that the client is (1) willing to tell the assessor that the records exist, (2) willing to provide authorization to access the records, and (3) able to provide enough detail for the assessor to appropriately access the records (e.g., dates of prior hospitalizations, names of prior evaluators and dates seen).

Records can help the assessor examine the veracity of client (and collateral) report, such as how long a client was hospitalized for a prior condition, what prior diagnoses were given, what prior (or current) treatment was prescribed, whether the client is attending therapy, what the client's high school grade-point average (GPA) and ACT scores were, etc. For example, recall the case of the patient with the migraine headache described in Chapter 7, whose records indicated a very different history regarding premorbid headaches than that provided by the patient during the interview.

However, an assessor should remember that records as sources of assessment data also have their limitations. With regard to any reports generated from prior evaluations, it is important to remember that the information in those reports may have been gathered for a purpose other than the evaluative purpose for which it is being reviewed, and it may be outdated. For example, as I was writing this very paragraph, I received a request for the release of results from a 12-year-old evaluation of an individual with a developmental disability, for the purposes of determining continuation of services. I complied with the authorization but added a cover letter indicating that the report was likely outdated for their present purposes. In addition to these two limitations, there are other potential limitations specific to the source of the information, reviewed next.

Educational Records

Educational records are often important to review, particularly for individuals who are presenting for evaluation with cognitive or academic concerns. Educational records can not only provide verification of what has been reported by the client (and/or collaterals) regarding current or prior academic functioning, but they may also be a way to generally estimate premorbid cognitive/academic functioning in the case of suspected decline (see Chapter 11). Educational records are not limited to obtained GPA. An assessor can carefully examine grades across all courses (and also consider whether the courses taken were remedial, basic, college preparatory, honors, or AP courses). High school transcripts also often report on class rank, which can help an assessor determine whether the school tends to inflate grades (e.g., someone with a high GPA but for whom the class rank is 50th percentile). Occasionally an examiner is fortunate that a school provides a cover document with the transcript detailing overall school statistics such as percentage of students who matriculate to higher education settings or mean ACT/SAT scores for the graduating class, which can also help provide a general sense of the quality of the school.

School transcripts also often provide useful data on standardized test performance, such as annual proficiency exams, graduation exams, or even ACT and SAT scores. It is important for the assessor to carefully consider the interpretation of these scores. For example, annual proficiency exams may report both local percentiles (how the individual performed relative to other grade peers at that specific school, which is not a particularly useful number other than to indicate how that particular school might perceive that individual's performance) and national percentiles (which provide a more representative sample of grade peers). For tests such as the ACT and SAT, the assessor must remember that the percentiles reported are not based on a normative sample of age peers, but rather a more "elite" sample of individuals who are planning to attend college. However, particularly in the context of adults who are claiming learning or other disabilities that would require extended time on high-stakes testing (e.g., MCAT, LSAT, GRE), these records may provide an invaluable source of information on how that individual performed in a high-stakes and timed testing environment relative to peers who were also moving into non-normative academic settings. This is especially important when there should be developmental evidence of impairment, given the diagnostic hypotheses under consideration (such as ADHD or a learning disability).

School records may also provide some information about behavioral concerns. For example, yearly elementary school records may include qualitative comments from teachers, although it is likely that such comments were selected from electronic menus with a limited choice of potential descriptors. The value of such comments may be quite limited, particularly if they are limited to one teacher, one school year, or one particular course in one school year. Attendance records may also be of value to review, as they likely include information on tardiness and absences, which not only provide behavioral information but can help to put grades into perspective (e.g., if the client's grades in the first semester of sophomore year were poor, but attendance records showed that he or she missed many days that semester).

Clients may have also been formally evaluated in the school setting or may have received formal services and accommodations as part of an IEP or 504 plan. Accessing those records may also be useful. In such cases, it is critical that the assessor make a specific request for the results of the actual evaluation, including the raw data. School systems can fall prey to motivations to provide diagnostic labels to students, despite the lack of evidence for such diagnoses, in response to pressure from parents or in response to the high-stakes environment of having to show adequate yearly progress in their students (students labeled with learning disabilities can be reported in annual school reports based on "disability" status, to allow for alternative academic achievement standards or results, in order to demonstrate their yearly progress separately from the rest of the student body) (Kavale & Spaulding, 2008). In my experience, as well as that of several of my colleagues, it is not uncommon for adults to present for evaluation for academic and learning concerns, indicating that they had been diagnosed in school and received services throughout school, only to find that the sole evaluation that led to a "diagnosis" was conducted in second grade, with the parents waiving their rights to reevaluation in order to prevent potential removal of the diagnostic label and removal of accommodations. In addition, under response-to-intervention (RTI) models used to identify students suspected of having learning difficulties, students may end up "diagnosed," based on vague teacher judgments about their level of response to vague "interventions" for academic difficulties (Sideridis, Antoniou, & Padeliadu, 2008), rather than on the results of standardized testing. Thus, the assessor needs to access and review the actual data that were used to make a diagnosis and/or provide the accommodations.

Medical Records

As mentioned above, medical records can provide verification of the dates of services, prescriptions of medications, types of interventions received, and diagnoses given, as might have been reported by a client and/or collateral reporters. It is important for an assessor to take a careful and critical look at those data, even though they do show up in an official medical report or hospital chart. One major concern is the veridicality of prior diagnoses given. The assessor needs to look carefully not just at the diagnostic conclusion that was given in the prior record, but also upon what basis the diagnosis was given. As an extreme example, I once sent a request for records and reports pertaining to a prior psychiatric evaluation by a psychiatrist identified by a client as having conducted an assessment to diagnose the client with ADHD; the "record" that was sent in response to the request was simply a photocopy of a prescription script with the word "Ritalin" scribbled on it, with the psychiatrist's signature. I have also seen various psychological and neurological diagnoses given in prior records on the basis of the client's self-report during a brief mental status examination. Thus, assessors need to consider the value of those prior records not merely by what is reported, but upon *what basis* the diagnostic conclusions were drawn.

Assessors should also consider the results of research suggesting that health and mental health care providers may have their own motivations for inaccurately diagnosing clients. For example, surveys of physicians have shown that they are willing to enter false information into medical records, including exaggerating the severity of symptoms, altering what the client reported, or even listing symptoms clients didn't even have, in order to gain insurance coverage (Freeman, Rathore, Weinfurt, Schulman, & Sulmasy, 1999; Wynia, Cummins, VanGeest, & Wilson, 2000). Studies have shown that psychologists and other mental health care providers also report a willingness to alter the diagnosis of a client in order to receive insurance reimbursement (Danzinger & Welfel, 2001; Tubbs & Pomerantz, 2001), and vignette studies have shown that mental health professionals are influenced by payment plans (Lowe, Pomerantz, & Pettibone, 2007), even when they specifically indicate a belief that their diagnosis would not be affected by reimbursement (Gilbelman & Mason, 2002). In addition, studies examining differences in diagnostic patterns in actual clinical settings also point to the ways in which reimbursement policies can lead to inaccuracies in diagnosis. Kielbasa, Pomerantz, Krohn, and Sullivan (2004) found that psychologists were 10 times more likely to give diagnoses to their clients when the clients had insurance that would provide reimbursement for services, relative to when clients were self-paid. In a recent multisite study of the clinical diagnosis of autism spectrum disorders, the authors showed that variation in diagnosis was strongly related to the insurance coverage available for specific diagnoses within the states where the clinics were located (Lord et al., 2012). Bickman, Wighton, Lambert, Karver, and Steding (2012) also showed that clinician diagnosis was influenced by the type of reimbursement and services available to children being evaluated for both internalizing and externalizing problems; of note, research diagnosis (using multimethod assessment and integration of data) did not show such bias. Such studies only emphasize the need for assessors to carefully consider the value of outside records by examining more than just the final conclusions reached in those records, including receipt of the actual assessment data from the evaluations that were conducted.

9

Self-Report Measures of Single Constructs

It would be worth accepting as a temporary hypothesis. If the fresh
facts which come to our knowledge all fit themselves into the scheme,
then our hypothesis may gradually become a solution.
　　　　　—SHERLOCK HOLMES, in *The Adventure of Wisteria Lodge*

As noted in Chapter 7, an intake interview often provides the
assessor with hypotheses regarding a client's concerns; those hypotheses
require further assessment in order to determine whether they are truly
relevant to understanding the client's presenting problems. The initial
hypotheses may be diagnostic ("Is this an anxiety disorder?") or prognostic
("How severe are the symptoms relative to a comparison group?"; "How
impaired is the client's functioning?"), and/or may be related to potential
causes or consequences of the problems and concerns the client presents
with, which can have both diagnostic and prognostic/treatment implications.

Administration of well-validated self-report instruments that assess
these hypotheses is a useful next step in assessment. Such measures provide
a standardized way to assess areas of relevance to a client's concerns;
for example, they can help to determine the nature of the construct as the
client perceives it ("What does she mean by 'anxiety'?"), and whether the
amount/severity/distress associated with that construct is out of the range
of normal relative to appropriate comparison groups. Such measures not
only assess the frequency and severity of specific symptoms or symptom
sets, but also provide corroborating information for a diagnosis. In addition,
self-report measures can provide information about causes and consequences
of the presenting concerns—factors that could be relevant to

127

treatment planning or predictions of prognosis (keeping in mind, of course, that the method of assessment is still limited to self-report). Perhaps the best way to think of self-report measures is that they serve as a way to provide a standardized and quantified communication from clients.

Too often it seems that assessors make the choice to administer an instrument based on its familiarity to them (or perhaps its easy accessibility), with cursory attention to data about the "validity" of the instrument. However, as noted in Chapter 6, consideration of "what's under the hood" of a measure can be understood only in the specific context of a specific assessment situation for a specific client. This chapter presents a decision-making approach to the empirically guided selection of self-report instruments for use in clinical assessment. The chapter does not provide a comprehensive review of self-report instruments, but instead uses a few instruments to illustrate the decision-making process. Although the focus is on self-report measures of single constructs, there is also some discussion of a few additional measures whose subscales are interpreted in isolation (rather than in an integrative fashion, the way broad-based measures of personality and psychopathology do, as discussed in the next chapter).

In order to take an empirically guided decision-making approach to the selection of self-report instruments to use in a particular assessment, the assessor should ask him- or herself the following questions when deciding on which, if any, self-report measures to use in a given assessment. The assessor should ask these questions for every measure under consideration in a given assessment.

DOES THE SELF-REPORT MEASURE ASSESS THE RELEVANT CONSTRUCT?

The assessor should consider the constructs at hand when determining what additional data are needed. Use of the biopsychosocial model (see Chapter 3) can assist the assessor in determining what relevant additional data to assess, given the initial hypotheses. In addition, the assessor should remember that, in order to avoid confirmatory bias (see Chapter 2), he or she should consider measures of constructs that are relevant to all alternative hypotheses as well. For example, if the assessor has a particular diagnostic hypothesis, he or she might consider the need for more data to (1) confirm/disconfirm of the presence of a particular symptom of sufficient severity to be of clinical concern; (2) confirm/disconfirm other symptoms or patterns of behavior that would be consistent with that diagnostic hypothesis; (3) confirm/disconfirm other symptoms or patterns of behavior that would be consistent with alternative diagnostic hypotheses; (4) assess for past history of symptoms or problems that would be consistent with, or exclude the possibility of, that diagnostic hypothesis (or that provides support for or against diagnostic alternatives); (5) determine the client's perceived impairment related to the presenting symptoms or problems; and/ or (6) assess for the presence of potential causes/contributing factors to the presenting concern, some of which might help to confirm the diagnosis and some of which might suggest alternative etiologies that preclude the diagnosis under consideration.

As an example, assume one of the assessor's working hypotheses, based on the intake interview, is that the client is presenting with depression. What additional constructs should the assessor gather data on to help determine whether the client has depression? Are there useful self-report measures for those constructs? One component of the construct of depression is the symptom set and pattern that the client presents with and whether it is consistent with agreed-upon diagnostic criteria for depression (i.e., is the client reporting symptoms of sufficient number, severity, and length of time to be consistent with a particular diagnostic scheme?) To collect additional data relevant to this component, an assessor might consider the Beck Depression Inventory–II (BDI-II; Beck, Steer, & Brown, 1996), one of the most frequently used psychological measures of depressive symptoms (Camara, Nathan, & Puente, 2000; Santor, Gregus, & Welch, 2006). The BDI-II was designed to assess the severity of symptoms of depression the client has experienced in the past 2 weeks. Items for the original version of the BDI were chosen based on the reports and on observation of the behavior of depressed psychiatric inpatients; the revised version was modified to make the item set consistent with DSM-IV symptoms of depression. As noted in Chapter 7, the assessor might also consider giving a structured diagnostic interview such as the ADIS-IV—Lifetime Version (ADIS-IV-L; Di Nardo, Brown & Barlow, 1994), given that such interviews can be viewed as an orally administered self-report measure. An advantage of a structured diagnostic interview might be that, in addition to examining whether the client reports other symptoms of depression with sufficient severity and duration consistent with a diagnosis, structured interviews ask about symptoms of other common psychological disorders that are important alternative hypotheses. Although there are other self-report instruments that might also provide a more "cross-cutting" assessment of symptoms beyond just those consistent with one diagnostic hypothesis (e.g., the Symptom Checklist–90—Revised [SCL-90-R]; Derogatis, 1994), they are typically designed to be used as screeners only (see below), and thus their relevance for assessment for this particular purpose might be limited.

Continuing our example, another important aspect of the construct of depression is its effect on functioning; an assessor might wish to assess for specific common consequences of depression and/or assess whether the client perceives that he/she is impaired in functioning. One common factor associated with depression is suicidal ideation; scales such as the Beck Hopelessness Scale (Beck & Steer, 1988) and Beck Scale for Suicide Ideation (Beck & Steer, 1991) were specifically designed to assess for the presence of suicidal ideation and suicide risk. Scales related to satisfaction with life functioning and/or perceived impairment in functioning may also be useful to consider when assessing the construct of depression, not only because they are important to treatment planning, but also because diagnostic criteria for depression include consideration of a client's level of functioning. Hunsley and Mash (2008b) recommend use of the Quality of Life Inventory (QOLI; Frisch, Cornell, Villaneuva, & Retzlaff, 1991) in the assessment of depression. The QOLI was designed to measure perceived satisfaction with life across multiple areas of functioning that are deemed important by the person being assessed. Administration of the ADIS-IV-L also allows clinicians to collect clients' ratings of impairment and distress rather generically, unless the full semistructured interview is administered, in which questions about specific impairments associated with specific disorders can also be administered. DSM-5 (American Psychiatric Association, 2013) recommends use of the World Health Organization Disability Assessment Schedule–2.0 (WHO-DAS 2.0; World Health Organization, 2012), a measure of self-reported disability in six life domains, including community functioning, ability to get around, self-care, interpersonal interactions, completion of life activities, and participation in society. DSM-5 also recommends a "cross-cutting assessment" approach to gathering self-report of "problem areas" that may cross many diagnostic categories. These problem areas may be an essential part of differential diagnosis but are also important in planning treatment or making prognostic predictions. "Level 1" assessment includes one to three questions in each of several domains, including depression, anger, mania, anxiety, somatic symptoms, suicidal ideation, psychosis, sleep problems, memory concerns, repetitive thoughts and beliefs, dissociation, personality functioning, and substance use. Scores identified as "high" in a given domain should then be followed by "level 2" assessment, for which they recommend various other self-report instruments.

Other data important to assess for, given the construct of depression, include potential health/medical explanations for the symptoms, which might preclude a diagnosis of depression and potentially suggest the need for alternative treatments and interventions. However, such data are not readily gathered by psychological self-report measures, and thus would need to be assessed using other methods, such as a review of medical records or by referral to appropriate specialists for further examination.

DOES THE MEASURE SUIT THE PURPOSE OF THE PARTICULAR ASSESSMENT?

When considering the purpose of the measure, the assessor should consider not only aspects of relevant constructs the measure is assessing, but also the measure's clinical purpose. Is the assessor looking for an instrument that will screen for the potential presence of a condition, or for a measure that will assist in confirming the presence of self-reported symptoms consistent with a diagnosis? Is the measure meant to help "rule in" or "rule out" a particular diagnosis? Is the measure meant to assess for other symptoms, syndromes, problems, consequences, and/or history consistent with what is known about the diagnoses or conditions under consideration? Depending on the purpose of the measure, it will need to behave in different ways.

Consideration of whether an instrument was specifically developed to screen for a disorder versus to help confirm the presence of a disorder is a critical issue for an assessor to consider. Measures developed to screen for disorders are meant to be used with healthy, asymptomatic individuals where there is low probability for the diagnosis. They are typically designed to err on the side of identification of potential cases, in order to refer them for further examination and assessment. Thus, many of these measures have strong sensitivity, but poorer specificity (i.e., a high false-positive rate). In addition, accuracy of the measure overall depends on the base rate of the disorder in the population being assessed; thus, data on the accuracy of a screener in a community setting will not assist an assessor in determining its accuracy in a sample in which the base rate for the disorder is much higher. In addition, if the screener's accuracy has mostly been determined in samples of individuals with one particular disorder as compared to healthy controls, it will not be clear that the measure can accurately discriminate between individuals with one particular disorder versus other disorders, particularly when those disorders share symptoms and presentations. This is not a minor point for an assessor to consider, particularly if he or she is working in a setting in which very short assessments are encouraged (e.g., in primary care).

Continuing the example of depression, assume that the assessor is searching for an instrument to help confirm the presence of symptoms consistent with DSM criteria for depression. The purpose of the BDI-II is to assess for presence and severity of depressive symptomatology; although it is guided by DSM-IV criteria for depression, it cannot confirm a diagnosis, but only provide corroborative information (or help rule out consideration of depression as a diagnosis) (Dozois & Dobson, 2010). Because it assesses severity of symptoms and has strong reliability, it can also be used for the purpose of tracking changes over time (Persons & Fresco, 2008). The ADIS-IV-L, as mentioned above, is a semistructured diagnostic interview (i.e., an orally administered self-report measure) that assesses the presence and severity of symptoms across the anxiety disorders as well as mood disorders (e.g., depression), somatoform disorders, and substance abuse. Thus, while also examining the presence of current symptoms of depression (consistent with DSM-IV criteria), the ADIS-IV-L can provide information regarding presence and severity of symptoms of highly comorbid disorders as well, and (assuming the more comprehensive interview is administered) can provide information regarding past diagnoses.

Other popular measures of depressive symptoms are also focused on DSM criteria for depression, but were specifically designed as screeners. For example, the Center for Epidemiologic Studies Depression Scale—Revised (CESD-R; Eaton, Muntaner, Smith, Tien, & Ybarra, 2004), whose items focus on DSM criteria, was developed specifically as a screener for depression in the general community, and thus shows a large number of false positives and is not a sufficient measure for diagnosis of depression or to make treatment decisions (Bufka & Camp, 2010). Similarly, the Patient Health Questionnaire (Spitzer, Kroenke, Williams, & the Patient Health Questionnaire Primary Care Study Group, 1999) is a popular screening measure for depression (as well as other psychological disorders) in research settings as well as in primary care settings; however, even though its items are focused on DSM criteria, it too has problems with specificity (Bufka & Camp, 2010) that limit its usefulness for the purpose of reaching diagnostic conclusions. As an example of a more general psychopathology measures, the SCL-90-R (Derogatis, 1994) assesses for the presence and severity of symptoms in nine different dimensions, but is also designed to be a screening tool, not a diagnostic tool; in addition, the subscales are not psychometrically sound, and thus it is best as a screener for general psychopathology, rather than for depression (or for other differential disorders an assessor might be considering) (Bufka & Camp, 2010). Thus, if the purpose of the self-report measure were to raise preliminary hypotheses that would lead to further assessment, such scales might be adequate; for the purpose of providing additional information to test the veracity of a diagnostic hypothesis already under consideration, however, they fall short.

DOES THE MEASURE SHOW ADEQUATE PSYCHOMETRIC PROPERTIES AS A MEASURE OF THE CONSTRUCT OF INTEREST AND FOR THE ASSESSMENT PURPOSE?

As reviewed in Chapter 6, in order to determine the overall usefulness of the measure in question, the assessor needs to consider whether the measure is a valid measure of that construct, considering its purpose. Assuming that the assessor is interested in a self-report measure meant to help corroborate the interview data and further examine whether the patient reports a sufficient number of symptoms with sufficient severity and length of time to meet at least the symptomatic criteria for depression, then the assessor should examine a measure's content validity (Does the content match the diagnostic scheme in question?), internal validity, convergent and divergent validity (Do scores on the measure relate in meaningful ways to scores on other measures of the same construct, and relate less with scores on measures of unrelated constructs?), diagnostic validity (with consideration of *acceptable* rates of sensitivity and specificity, given the purpose is not to screen), and incremental validity (which might speak to its cost effectiveness).

Continuing the example of the BDI-II, as already discussed above, the content validity of the measure is strong. With regard to internal validity, the BDI-II shows strong internal consistency and good 1-week test–retest reliability (Beck et al., 1996; Dozois & Covin, 2004). Factor analyses show that the BDI-II generally measures two factors of depression: cognitive symptoms and somatic–affective symptoms; of note, however, there is no subscale interpretation of this measure for clinical purposes. The BDI-II also shows strong convergent validity, in that scores on it correlate highly with scores on other self-report measures of depression, as well as with interview ratings and clinician ratings of depression severity (Antony & Barlow, 2010; Groth-Marnat, 2009; Hunsley & Mash, 2008b). Not surprisingly, the BDI-III does not discriminate well between depression and anxiety, but this is true of most measures of depression and may actually be consistent with what is known about the constructs of depression and anxiety generally (Antony & Barlow, 2010). Although scores on the BDI-II cannot confer a diagnosis of depression, they do distinguish individuals with a diagnosis from those without, as compared to structured diagnostic interviews (Groth-Marnat, 2009), and multiple studies have examined various cutoff scores on the BDI-II with regard to diagnostic sensitivity and specificity, as compared to diagnoses obtained using structured diagnostic interviews in many diverse samples (see below).

With regard to incremental validity, there are little data available for the BDI-II (or, for that matter, for other alternatives, such as whether a structured diagnostic interview has incremental validity above and beyond any other data available). The original BDI has been shown to detect depression as effectively as longer and more costly structured interviews (Stukenberg, Dura, & Kiecolt-Glaser, 1990). Of course, incremental validity is just one part of the decision-making process of keeping an evaluation cost effective; the BDI-II provides information only about depression, and not on any other alternative diagnostic hypotheses, so that factor would need to be taken into account when deciding whether the BDI-II will offer "bang for the buck" in a given assessment. Although the ADIS-IV-L (or even shorter interviews) provides information for (some) highly likely alternative diagnostic hypotheses, it requires lengthy training and lengthy time to administer (up to 2–4 hours if both present and past history are assessed for) and so that aspect of cost effectiveness would need to be considered as well.

IS THE MEASURE APPROPRIATE FOR USE WITH THE CLIENT IN QUESTION?

In order to determine whether a particular measure is appropriate in a particular assessment situation, the assessor should consider not only whether the measure is valid to assess the relevant construct under consideration, but whether the measure is appropriate for the particular client being assessed. One aspect of this consideration is whether the measure shows construct validity when used for any particular group or subgroup to which the client belongs (when evidence shows that subgroup membership is an important consideration for that construct; see Chapter 5). The assessor should not limit the focus to racial/ethnic diversity when considering relevant subgroups, but consider the construct itself (i.e., what important subgroup differences in the construct might be accurately assessed by measures of that construct?). For the construct of depression, for example, the assessor should consider whether the measure is valid for use with community members, outpatients, or inpatients; whether it is valid as a measure for depression in individuals with psychological problems and/or for those with medical/physical problems, whether there are important differences in presentation with depression across different ages or for males/females, and whether there are important differences in presentation with depression in different racial/ethnic groups. Depending on which of these subgroups are relevant for the client in question, the assessor may be able to find additional information (often beyond the test's manual) to determine whether it is appropriate to use for that client. In addition, given that the measure under consideration involves the self-report of a client, the reading level of the measure is important to consider for clients for whom language fluency is limited and/or whose reading fluency/comprehension is suspect due to presence of a learning disability or low educational level.

Continuing the example of the BDI-II, with regard to reading comprehension, the BDI-II is written at a fifth- to sixth-grade reading level. In addition, the BDI-II has been translated into many different languages, including Spanish, Chinese, Turkish, and Japanese, among others (Byrne, Stewart, Kennard, & Lee, 2007; Byrne, Stewart, & Lee, 2004; Canel-Cinarbas, Cui, & Lauridsen, 2011; Kojima et al., 2002), and those translations have shown adequate psychometric properties, although there are few empirical studies of some of the translated versions. With regard to construct invariance, the BDI-II has shown good internal consistency and a generally similar factor structure in studies of college students, community members, outpatients and inpatients with psychological problems, and medical patients in many populations and across different age ranges and in different racial/ethnic groups (Beck et al., 1996; Byrne & Campbell, 1999; Byrne et al., 2004, 2007; Canel-Cinarbas et al., 2011; Dozois & Covin, 2004; Grothe et al., 2005; Joe, Woolley, Brown, Ghahramanlou-Holloway, & Beck, 2008; Kojima et al., 2002; Osman, Kopper, Barrios, Gutierrez, & Bagge, 2004; Penley, Wiebe, & Nwosu, 2003; Steer, Kumar, Ranieri, & Beck, 1998; Steer, Rissmiller, & Beck, 2000; Stukenberg et al., 1990; Van Vorhis & Blumentritt, 2007). In addition, the BDI-II has shown convergent validity (correlations with other measures of depression, with interviewer ratings) and diagnostic validity (relative to structured diagnostic interviews) in many different countries and populations (e.g., see Byrne et al., 2004; Canel-Cinarbas et al., 2011; Joe et al., 2008; Kojima et al., 2002; Van Vorhis & Blumentritt, 2007).

In regard to normative data, although the sample upon which the conventional "cutoffs" for interpretation of BDI-II raw scores were determined included both healthy males and females and male and female outpatients with depression, there was limited diversity with regard to race/ethnicity and no information regarding SES or other sociodemographic factors. However, other studies have examined mean scores and also clinically relevant cutoff scores on the BDI-II in a number of diverse populations across a wide variety of ages, from adolescence to older adults. Whereas the original study on the scale reported no difference in scores among different racial/ethnic groups (Beck et al., 1996), other studies have identified statistically significant differences in BDI-II scores in different racial/ethnic groups (e.g., see Byrne et al., 2007; Van Vorhis & Blumentritt, 2007). Of note, however, in the vast majority of studies such differences, although statistically significant, were of such low magnitude that they were not likely clinically meaningful and were also noted to reflect accurate differences in the construct of depression in those diverse groups.

As noted above, multiple studies have examined the use of the BDI-II in various settings (inpatient vs. outpatient psychiatric treatment, inpatient and outpatient medical treatment, community settings), in different ages (adolescent to old age), in males and females, in different countries, and in different racial/ethnic groups. Although some of these studies suggest slightly different cutoffs for the purposes of confirming a diagnosis of depression, the overall pattern of results suggests a general scalar invariance (i.e., the scores mean the same thing when they are high or low across diverse groups) for this dimensional scale (if the purpose is to determine general severity of depressive symptoms and implications for functioning). An assessor attuned to those potential differences in the interpretation of BDI-II scores will seek out relevant literature for the use of the scale in his or her setting and for specific populations; however, that assessor should also keep in mind that any one study of the BDI-II for a very specific population should not be viewed in isolation. In other words, the suggested cutoffs from one specific study may not generalize well to the different aspects of diversity represented by the specific client being assessed.

DOES THE MEASURE INCLUDE A WAY TO ADDRESS NONCREDIBLE RESPONDING?

As reviewed in Chapter 4, it is vital to consider the $N = 1$ validity of self-report data, and one way to do this is for self-report measures to include a way to assess for the invalidity of self- report as part of the measure. However, in a quick examination of many popular and well-validated self-report measures (as summarized by Antony & Barlow, 2010, and Hunsley & Mash, 2008b), it is extremely rare for self-report measures of single constructs to include a way to assess for noncredible responding. In fact, of the measures reviewed in these two texts (including structured diagnostic interviews), there were no measures of anxiety or depression, no measures of post-traumatic stress, no measures for sleep or eating problems, no measures of impairment/distress/quality of life, and no measures of pain symptomatology that included assessment of noncredible responding. In fact, the only measure to do so was one measure of substance use/misuse (the Drug Use Screening Inventory—Revised; Tarter & Kirisci, 1997). Although not reviewed by those two volumes, there are also few measures of noncredible symptom report within self-report measures for cognitive concerns (such as ADHD rating scales). Conners' Adult ADHD Rating Scale (CAARS;

Conners, Erhardt, & Sparrow, 1998) includes an Inconsistency Index (which assesses for inconsistency in responding to items with similar content), and attempts have been made to develop scales for the CAARS that assess for noncredible overreporting of ADHD symptoms (Suhr, Buelow, & Riddle, 2011). As mentioned in Chapter 4, there are also self-report measures well validated specifically to assess for invalid self-report, although their psychometric properties are not as strong as for the validity scales that are embedded within self-report measures of multiple constructs, as is seen in the next chapter.

10

Broadband Self-Report Measures of Personality and Psychopathology

> Still, it is an error to argue in front of your data. You find yourself
> insensibly twisting them round to fit your theories.
> —SHERLOCK HOLMES, in *The Adventure of Wisteria Lodge*

The trend for use of abbreviated and focal measurement tools in assessment settings may be misguided when considering the complexity of patient presentations across many assessment contexts (Sellbom, Marion, & Bagby, 2013; Sweet, Tovian, Guidotti Breting, & Suchy, 2013). Several broad-based personality and psychopathology measures have a wealth of empirical evidence supporting their value across different assessment settings. Such instruments can provide information about many different psychological constructs that may be directly related to the immediate reason for referral. For example, they might reveal unsuspected difficulties that contribute to the immediate reason for referral and should be addressed as part of client care. In addition, they can address differential diagnostic issues. Furthermore, they can identify both interpersonal and intrapersonal strengths and weaknesses to consider when making predictions about functioning and treatment recommendations. Measures that provide this much "bang for the buck" may be cost-effective in the long run. In addition, given the clear need to focus on validity of client self-report (see Chapters 4 and 9), it is important to note that, unlike the vast majority of single-construct self-report measures, several broad-based instruments have well-validated subscales designed to assess for inconsistent responding, as well as both over- and underreport of symptoms.

In this chapter, two popular and well-validated broad-based instruments are described to illustrate decision-making issues relevant to choosing multifaceted psychological instruments for use in assessment. Although there are many broad-spectrum measures available, focusing on two of the most frequently used measures will demonstrate how an assessor can compare and contrast the strengths and weakness of such instruments for use with a specific client and for a specific purpose. A measure consistently listed as one of the most utilized in assessment is the Minnesota Multiphasic Personality Inventory; here we focus on its most current version, the Minnesota Multiphasic Personality Inventory–2—Restructured Form (MMPI-2-RF; Ben-Porath & Tellegen, 2011). The other measure that is used in comparison is the Personality Assessment Inventory (PAI; Morey, 1991). In addition, because broad-based personality and psychopathology measures provide a multitude of subtest scores that need to be interpreted in the context of each other, the last part of the chapter addresses interpretation issues when using broadband instruments. This is especially important in an era where computerized scoring and interpretation are ever more common, particularly for broad-based scales such as the MMPI-2-RF and the PAI.

WHAT CONSTRUCTS DO BROADBAND PERSONALITY/PSYCHOPATHOLOGY MEASURES ASSESS?

Different broad-based personality/psychopathology instruments focus on different sets of diagnoses/syndromes/symptoms sets, and some use theoretical models of personality and psychopathology to guide the choice of which constructs to address. It is important for an assessor to consider the constructs being assessed by any one of these measures, and whether the measures are, in fact, assessing the constructs relevant to the particular assessment situation.

The MMPI-2-RF

Because the newest version of the MMPI is radically different from its predecessor, and because some assessors have still not moved from use of the MMPI-2 to the MMPI-2-RF, a bit of history on the development of the MMPI-2-RF and how it differs from the versions that preceded it will provide a context for understanding this instrument and the constructs it purports to measure. A detailed review of the MMPI history can be found in Ben-Porath (2012). In addition, understanding the empirical strength of the MMPI-2-RF over its predecessor may help assessors who have not yet transitioned to the new version make a scientifically guided decision to do so.

The original MMPI (published in 1940) was a radically different instrument from other personality and psychopathology instruments from that time period, which typically did not provide comprehensive coverage of personality and psychological factors associated with psychological disorders. In addition, because items for such measures were content valid only, they were vulnerable to noncredible symptom reporting. In order to generate a diverse set of characteristics seen across a wide range of personality and psychopathology characteristics in the development of the first MMPI, the initial pool of items was selected from symptoms and other descriptors of psychological traits associated with psychological diagnoses from that time period. Thus, the item content was congruent with a descriptive understanding of both normal and abnormal psychological traits for the time. However, rather than placing items on subscales based on their content, items were placed on subscales based on whether they empirically discriminated specific clinical conditions from nonclinical groups. This empirical method of scale creation was quite unique for its time. In addition, as the developers of the initial MMPI were still aware that test takers would respond to the face validity in the content of the items, the second major improvement over existing scales was the inclusion of Validity Scales.

Thus, the original MMPI was not tied to any particular psychological theory about personality or psychopathology, but was instead based on empirical findings, with content not considered relevant to interpretation. Interestingly, some content scales were presented in the 1960s, in response to users who were dissatisfied with the lack of content interpretation, but the content scales were not considered core to the interpretation of the instrument.

When the MMPI was revised between 1982 and 1989, the goals included retaining this empirically based model, updating the norms to be more representative than those of its predecessor, updating or removing items that were empirically unsound, and identifying new scales that would assess areas of personality or psychopathology identified as important in contemporary research. For example, the PSY 5 Scales were presented in a revised manual published in 2001; their development was based on research by Harkness and McNulty (1994), which demonstrated five major personality factors within the DSM personality disorders (aggressiveness, psychoticism, constraint, negative emotionality/neuroticism, and positive emotionality/extraversion). Thus, the evolution of the MMPI-2 toward a content- and construct-based instrument (at least with regard to scales beyond the original clinical scales) was beginning. However, the core clinical scales remained true to the empirical keying approach to development and interpretation.

The original MMPI and the MMPI-2 had some significant psychometric weaknesses. First, there was high intercorrelation among the scales, which led to analysis and interpretation of profile codetypes rather than to analysis of individual scales. The high intercorrelation was due to significant item overlap in the scales—a direct result of the way in which the scales were developed. Using the empirical keying approach meant that any item that distinguished a particular clinical group from nonclinical controls would be included on the scale for that clinical syndrome/symptom; if that item also happened to distinguish another clinical group from nonclinical controls, it would be included on the scale for that clinical syndrome/symptom as well. In addition, the scales showed significant heterogeneity. This was also recognized as a consequence of the empirical keying method of item selection during the measure's development. So long as an item empirically distinguished a clinical group from a nonclinical group, it would be included on the scale, which meant that the resultant scales did not necessarily reflect content components of a disorder or a construct; in fact, "subtle" items (items that had no content validity for a particular disorder or construct but that had empirically distinguished the groups) were included on the scales. Thus, two people with high scores on the same scale may actually have endorsed very different sets of items whose content would not even be considered related to the area of psychopathology purportedly being assessed. Over time and with continued empirical analyses, these psychometric weaknesses were deemed to be problematic. Thus, work had already begun in the early 1990s to further revise the core of the MMPI-2, using theoretical guidance.

Watson and Tellegen (1985) recognized that a lot of the item overlap on various scales of the MMPI-2 was likely due to a shared construct seen across many forms of psychopathology: demoralization. Frank (1974) identified demoralization as a factor that was related to the nonspecific findings in psychotherapy; "demoralization" was conceptualized as the shared factor that contributed to treatment seeking as well as to treatment change regardless of therapeutic approach. In general, demoralization was viewed as having too little positive affect and too much negative affect, psychological features that appeared regardless of the specific nature of the psychopathology present in a client. Tellegen and colleagues (2003) used the existing MMPI-2 items from scales 2 and 7 that loaded together to develop a scale reflecting demoralization. Then the core components of all the clinical scales (including 2 and 7) were identified, after removing the effects of demoralization using factor analysis. This led to "seed scales," which were further analyzed, retaining only the items that loaded best on their seed scale and removing items that loaded high on more than one seed scale, to maximize discriminant validity. Once seed scales had been identified, the rest of the MMPI-2 item pool was analyzed to identify items that could be added to the seed scales; to create internally consistent scales that showed convergent and discriminant validity, items were selected for inclusion on a seed scale if they loaded on that scale but did not load on others.

In addition to this empirical guidance for item selection, experts judged the content of each item with regard to its representation of the construct underlying the seed scale. Ultimately, this resulted in a new Demoralization scale, in addition to restructured versions of the original clinical scales 1, 2, 3, 4, 6, 7, 8, and 9 (scales 5 and 0 were omitted from the clinical scales so that the main set of Restructured Clinical Scales would be focused only on psychopathology). In order to provide further validation for the Restructured Clinical Scales, their external correlates were examined, primarily by using archival datasets from MMPI-2 data (although, as noted below, additional data have been published since that time).

Thus, the goal of this major revision of the MMPI was to take advantage of the wealth of existing data on the MMPI-2 item pool, but to use construct validation methods to create subscales that were psychometrically stronger and whose content was actually related to the areas of psychopathology being assessed. Detailed discussion of the steps briefly described above can be found in Ben-Porath (2012), Tellegen and colleagues (2003), and Tellegen and Ben-Porath (2011). This initial theoretically guided work led to publication of the Restructured Clinical Scales in 2003 (Tellegen et al., 2003). After some initial evidence for their validity and utility, these scales were added as supplemental subscales to the MMPI-2 in 2003, although it is safe to say that many clinicians who were not staying abreast of the empirical literature on the MMPI-2 may not have been aware of these new scales until publication of the MMPI-2-RF.

The entire MMPI-2 was restructured and published as the MMPI-2-RF in 2008, although assessors can still purchase materials for both the MMPI-2 and the MMPI-2-RF. In addition to further refinement to the Restructured Clinical Scales, there were additional changes as part of the MMPI-2-RF, including (1) addition of Higher-Order Scales, (2) creation of scales for constructs that were judged to be important in clinical practice but were not represented in existing clinical scales (Specific Problems Scales), (3) further revision of the PSY 5 Scales, and (4) revision of existing and inclusion of new Validity Scales. Some of these additional changes were construct-driven. For example, psychopathology research had shown the existence of higher-order factors of internalizing and externalizing psychopathology, and these had been identified in factor analyses of the MMPI-2; therefore, Higher-Order Scales were created representing these two constructs (as well as a Higher-Order Scale representing signs of thought disorder, which was deemed by experts to be a clinically relevant higher-order dimension worthy of including). The Specific Problems Scales were also constructed using a construct validation approach, starting with consideration of the entire MMPI-2 item pool and whether it contained clinically significant content not captured in the Restructured Clinical Scales or the PSY-5 Scales, as judged by a series of experts. Ultimately, potential scales representing clinically relevant constructs, as well as facets of Restructured Clinical Scales that might require separate assessment (such as substance use), were subjected to similar factor analytic procedures to make sure the scales were not loaded with items reflecting demoralization and did not include items that correlated with other scales. This process resulted in a series of Specific Problems Scales that were nonoverlapping with one another. Of note, although some Specific Problems Scales assess facets of the Restructured Clinical Scales, they are not subscales of the Restructured Clinical Scales. There is some item overlap among the Restructured Clinical Scales and the Specific Problems Scales, but within each set there is no item overlap. Details regarding these developmental steps can be found in Ben-Porath (2012) and Tellegen and Ben-Porath (2011).

Ultimately, the MMPI-2-RF is a much shorter instrument than the MMPI-2 (338 items vs. 567), with 51 total scales (nine Validity Scales, three Higher-Order Scales, nine Restructured Clinical Scales, 23 Specific Problems Scales, five PSY 5 Scales, and two Interest Scales). See Table 10.1 for a description of each of the subscales of the MMPI-2-RF.

The PAI

The PAI was published in 1991 (Morey, 1991) and was meant to provide descriptors of important personality and syndromal variables often seen in psychological settings for individuals 18 and over. The clinical scales were specifically meant to describe pathological characteristics associated with major psychological disorders using DSM as a guide, five additional scales reflect psychological constructs important in treatment decisions, and two additional scales assess basic aspects of interpersonal functioning. The scale was developed using classical construct validation approaches (Cronbach & Meehl, 1955). The constructs were chosen based on their relevance to the existing categorization of mental disorders at the time, as well as the significance of those constructs to psychological treatment. Thus, as with the MMPI-2-RF, the scales may be relevant to diagnostic questions but may also be relevant to contextual issues, prognostic issues, and treatment-related issues. In addition, as is true for the MMPI-2-RF, one major strength of the PAI is the inclusion of Validity Scales. At the time of its development,

TABLE 10.1. Summary of MMPI-2-RF Scales

Scale type	Scale	Description
Validity		
CNS	Cannot Say	Unscorable items; high scores generally indicate that the profile cannot be interpreted.
VRIN-r	Variable Response Inconsistency	Inconsistent responding to item content; high scores generally indicate that the profile cannot be interpreted.
TRIN-r	True Response Inconsistency	Tendency to respond true (or false), leading to inconsistent response to item content; high scores generally indicate that the profile cannot be interpreted.
F-r	Infrequent Responses	Items infrequently endorsed by a nonclinical population; the higher the score, the more likely that it reflects overreporting of symptoms and not genuine psychopathology.
Fp-r	Infrequent Psychopathology Responses	Items infrequently endorsed even by a clinical population; the higher the score, the more likely that it reflects overreporting of symptoms and not genuine psychopathology.
Fs	Infrequent Somatic Responses	Items infrequently endorsed even by individuals with health, medical, and physical concerns; the higher the score, the more likely that it reflects overreporting of health-related symptoms and not genuine psychopathology.
FBS-r	Symptom Validity	The higher the score, the more likely that it reflects overreporting of somatic and cognitive scales.
RBS	Response Bias	The higher the score, the more likely that it reflects noncredible memory complaints.
L-r	Uncommon Virtues	The higher the score, the more likely that it reflects underreporting rather than a traditional/ conventional upbringing.
K-r	Adjustment Validity	The higher the score, the more likely that it reflects underreporting rather than a traditional/ conventional upbringing.

TABLE 10.1. *(continued)*

Higher-Order

EID	Emotional/ Internalizing Dysfunction	Low scores reflect better-than-average emotional adjustment; high scores reflect considerable emotional distress.
THD	Thought Dysfunction	High scores reflect self-reported symptoms of thought dysfunction.
BXD	Behavioral/ Externalizing Dysfunction	Low scores reflect higher-than-average behavioral constraint; low scores reflect increasing severity of externalizing and acting- out behavior.

Restructured Clinical

RCd	Demoralization	Low scores reflect higher-than-average morale and life satisfaction; high scores reflect life dissatisfaction and unhappiness.
RC1	Somatic Complaints	Low scores reflect self-reported physical well- being; high scores reflect multiple somatic com- plaints and preoccupation with health concerns.
RC2	Low Positive Emotions	Low scores reflect a high level of psychological well-being, optimism, and social engagement; high scores reflect a lack of positive emotions, pessimism, social disengagement.
RC3	Cynicism	Low scores reflect high trust in others; high scores reflect cynical beliefs and distrust of/ hostility toward others.
RC4	Antisocial Behavior	Low scores reflect below-average past antisocial behavior; high scores reflect significant history of antisocial behavior, including substance misuse.
RC6	Ideas of Persecution	High scores reflect persecutory ideation and paranoia.
RC7	Dysfunctional Negative Emotions	Low scores reflect below-average negative emo- tions; high scores reflect above-average negative emotions such as anxiety, anger, and/or fear.
RC8	Aberrant Experiences	High scores reflect unusual thought and percep- tual processes, with increasingly higher scores potentially reflecting psychotic symptoms.

(continued)

TABLE 10.1. *(continued)*

RC9	Hypomanic Activation	Low scores reflect below-average levels of energy, activation, and engagement; high scores reflect above-average levels of energy, activation, and engagement.

Somatic/Cognitive

MLS	Malaise	Low scores reflect general well-being; high scores reflect reports of poor health and other nonspecific physical complaints.
GIC	Gastrointestinal Complaints	High scores reflect symptoms of gastrointestinal distress and potentially a preoccupation with such symptoms.
HPC	Head Pain Complaints	High scores reflect head (and potentially neck) pain complaints.
NUC	Neurological Complaints	High scores reflect vague neurological complaints.
COG	Cognitive Complaints	High scores reflect vague cognitive complaints.

Internalizing

SUI	Suicidal/Death Ideation	High scores reflect history (and potentially current) suicidal ideation and attempts.
HLP	Helplessness/ Hopelessness	High scores reflect belief that things are hopeless and cannot change.
SFD	Self-Doubt	High scores reflect self-doubt and lack of confidence.
NFC	Inefficacy	Low scores indicate self-reliance; high scores reflect passivity, indecisiveness, feeling ineffective in coping.
STW	Stress/Worry	Low scores indicate below-average stress or worry; high scores indicate above-average stress, worry, rumination.
AXY	Anxiety	High scores reflect anxiety symptoms.
ANP	Anger Proneness	High scores reflect anger proneness and low frustration tolerance.
BRF	Behavior-Restricting Fears	High scores reflect multiple fears that restrict normal activities.

TABLE 10.1. (*continued*)

MSF	Multiple Specific Fears	Low scores reflect lower-than-average report of fears; high scores reflect higher-than-average report of fears and harm avoidance.

Externalizing

JCP	Juvenile Conduct Problems	High scores reflect history of school behavior problems, potentially troubles with authority and in interpersonal relationships.
SUB	Substance Abuse	High scores reflect significant past and current substance use.
AGG	Aggression	Low scores reflect lower-than-average aggressive behavior; high scores reflect acts of physical aggression, violent behavior, and losing control.
ACT	Activation	Low scores reflect low levels of energy and activation; high scores reflect episodes of heightened activity and energy.

Interpersonal

FML	Family Problems	Low scores reflect conflict-free past and current family environment; high scores reflect past and/or current family conflict and lack of support.
IPP	Interpersonal Passivity	Low scores reflect assertiveness, being opinionated, possibly being viewed by others as domineering and self-centered; high scores reflect submissiveness, unassertiveness, and passivity in relationships.
SAV	Social Avoidance	Low scores reflect gregariousness and outgoingness; high scores reflect lack of enjoyment of social events and interactions, introversion.
SHY	Shyness	Low scores reflect lower-than-normal social anxiety; high scores reflect high anxiety in social situations, shyness, and embarrassment/discomfort around others.
DSF	Disaffiliativeness	High scores reflect dislike of others, preference for being alone, lack of close relationships.

(*continued*)

TABLE 10.1. (*continued*)

PSY-5		
AGGR-r	Aggressiveness—Revised	Low scores reflect chronic passivity and submissiveness; high scores reflect chronically aggressive and assertive/socially dominant behavior.
PSYC-r	Psychoticism—Revised	Low scores reflect no past or current thought disturbance; high scores reflect long-standing unusual thought proceses and perceptual experiences.
DISC-r	Disconstraint—Revised	Low scores reflect history of overly constrained behavior; high scores reflect history of unconstrained behavior and sensation seeking.
NEGE-r	Negative Emotionality/Neuroticism—Revised	Low scores reflect lower-than-average negative emotional experiences; high scores reflect chronic experience of anxiety/worry, self-criticalness.
INTR-r	Introversion/Low Positive Emotionality—Revised	Low scores reflect high energy and a history of positive emotional experiences; high scores reflect a lack of positive emotional experiences, avoidance of social situations, chronically pessimistic and social introversion.

Interest		
AES	Aesthetic–Literary Interests	Low scores reflect no interest in activities or occupations that are aesthetic/literary in nature; high scores reflect above-average interest in such activities or occupations.
MEC	Mechanical–Physical Interests	Low scores reflect no interest in activities or occupations that are mechanical or physical in nature; high scores reflect above-average interest in such activities or occupations and can also reflect sensation seeking.

both conceptual and empirical methods were used to guide item decisions; not only did items need to show desirable psychometric properties, but they needed to reflect expert decisions on content coverage.

Thus, like the MMPI-2-RF, both content validity and convergent/divergent validity were considered important in the final decisions about items and subscales. With regard to content validity, both the breadth of content for a given disorder (e.g., anxiety) and the depth of coverage (e.g., cognitive symptoms, physiological symptoms) were considered. In order to have breadth of coverage, developers utilized the research literature and existing diagnostic schemes (DSM, International Classification of Diseases [ICD]), as well as clinical experience, to generate potential items. Of note, Morey did not use existing personality instruments to generate items. With regard to depth of coverage, rather than a true–false format as in the MMPI-2-RF, the PAI utilizes a rating scale, allowing for ratings of severity on each item. Experts judged whether items had the potential to be offensive or biased, were worded ambiguously or used slang, and were reasonably specific to the construct in question, before they were chosen for further analysis. During scale development, the goal was to select items that had maximal associations with indicators of the construct under consideration and minimal associations with other constructs measured by the test. The initial items were tested in nonclinical groups and patient samples with regard to item distributions, correlations, and response to social desirability and response sets, as well as potential gender and/or racial/ethnic bias. These methods of test development resulted in a final instrument with 344 items, including four Validity Scales, 11 clinical scales (nine with subscales), five scales of psychological constructs considered relevant to treatment (one with subscales), and two Interpersonal Scales. It is important to note that, unlike the MMPI-2-RF, the subscale scores are subscales of the clinical scale scores. See Table 10.2 for a description of the scales in the PAI.

DOES EITHER MEASURE VALIDLY ASSESS THE RELEVANT CONSTRUCTS OF INTEREST?

Once an assessor has made the decision to administer a multifaceted instrument rather than a single construct instrument, the decision then turns to which multifaceted instrument is most appropriate to assess the constructs the assessor wants to assess in that particular assessment setting and for that particular client. Given the multiple constructs that these two multifaceted instruments were intended to assess, evidence for their construct validity is much more complex than for single construct measures and is not comprehensively reviewed here. The manuals for each test provide detailed information that is briefly summarized below, supplemented by additional information from independent studies outside of that presented in the manuals, for illustration of the decision making an assessor should undergo when deciding which measure might be best for a particular client and for a particular assessment purpose.

TABLE 10.2. Descriptions of PAI Scales and Subscales

Type of scale	Scale	Description
Validity		
ICN	Inconsistency	High scores reflect inconsistent responding to item content.
INF	Infrequency	High scores reflect atypical responding.
NIM	Negative Impression Management	High scores reflect exaggeration of complaints and concerns.
PIM	Positive Impression Management	High scores reflect an attempt to portray an uncharacteristically favorable impression.
Clinical		
SOM	Somatic Complaints	SOM-C: High scores reflect perception of rare sensory–motor symptoms.
		SOM-S: High scores reflect perception of frequent health concerns and symptoms.
		SOM-H: High scores reflect preoccupation with health status.
ANX	Anxiety	ANX-C: High scores reflect ruminative worry and cognitive concerns.
		ANX-A: High scores reflect reports of tension, fatigue, and difficulty relaxing.
		ANX-P: High scores reflect report of physical signs of anxiety and stress.
ARD	Anxiety-Related Disorders	ARD-O: High scores reflect report of intrusive thoughts, rigid thinking, perfectionism.
		ARD-P: High scores reflect report of phobic fears.
		ARD-T: High scores reflect report of distress associated with prior traumatic experiences.
DEP	Depression	DEP-C: High scores reflect report of feeling worthless, hopeless, indecisive, having cognitive complaints.
		DEP-A: High scores reflect reports of sadness, anhedonia, lack of interest.

TABLE 10.2. (*continued*)

		DEP-P: High scores reflect report of low energy and changes to sleep and appetite/weight.
MAN	Mania	MAN-A: High scores reflect reports of high activity level, overinvolvement, disorganization, accelerated speed of thought and behavior.
		MAN-G: High scores reflect inflated self-esteem.
		MAN-I: High scores reflect frustration with others and irritability.
PAR	Paranoia	PAR-H: High scores reflect suspiciousness and hypervigilance.
		PAR-P: High scores reflect a belief that one is being treated inequitably or being persecuted.
		PAR-R: High scores reflect bitterness, cynicism, and holding grudges against others.
SCZ	Schizophrenia	SCZ-P: High scores reflect experience of unusual perceptions and or sensations and report of unusual ideas and/or magical thinking.
		SCZ-S: High scores reflect social isolation, awkwardness, and detachment.
		SCZ-T: High scores reflect report of cognitive difficulties and thought disorganization.
BOR	Borderline Features	BOR-A: High scores reflect poor emotional regulation.
		BOR-I: High scores reflect uncertainty about identity and lack of purpose.
		BOR-N: High scores reflect history of negative relationships.
		BOR-S: High scores reflect report of impulsive behavior with high risk for self-harm.
ANT	Antisocial Features	ANT-A: High scores reflect report of a history of antisocial and/or illegal activities.
		ANT-E: High scores reflect lack of empathy or remorse and tendency to exploit others.
		ANT-S: High scores reflect sensation seeking and low tolerance for boredom.

(*continued*)

TABLE 10.2. (*continued*)

ALC	Alcohol Problems	High scores reflect (past or current) problematic consequences of alcohol use, potential alcohol dependence.
DRG	Drug Problems	High scores reflect (past or current) problematic consequences of drug use and potential dependence.

Treatment Consideration

AGG	Aggression	AGG-A: High scores reflect reports of hostility, poor anger control.
		AGG-V: High scores reflect report of use of verbal aggression.
		AGG-P: High scores reflect report of use of physical aggression.
SUI	Suicidal Ideation	High scores indicate thoughts about suicide.
STR	Stress	High scores suggest difficulties with stressful life events that are impacting functioning.
NON	Nonsupport	High scores reflect little social support or social/ interpersonal conflict.
RXR	Treatment Rejection	Very low scores indicate a cry for help, over-whelming distress; average scores may be consistent with a lack of psychological difficulties (in those without clinical elevations on other scales) or an absence of motivation for treatment; high scores reflect individuals who do not acknowledge difficulties and see no need for change.

Interpersonal

DOM	Dominance	Low scores indicate a tendency to be passive in relationships; high scores indicate assertiveness, confidence, potentially domineering and controlling.
WRM	Warmth	Low scores suggest individuals who are more distant in personal relationships and may be viewed as aloof and reserved or interpersonally cold by others; high scores suggest individuals who are perceived as warm, friendly, or at an extreme needing a great deal of acceptance from others.

The MMPI-2-RF

The method of determining the content validity of the MMPI-2-RF was generally reviewed above when presenting the historical overview of this instrument, and the constructs assessed by the instrument were summarized in Table 10.1. It is worth nothing that empirical tests supported the removal of the subtle items that were part of the MMPI and the MMPI-2, as they appeared to add only construct-irrelevant variance (Ben-Porath, 2012).

With regard to reliability, the technical manual points out that the 1-week test–retest reliabilities and the internal consistency of the individual subscales of the MMPI-2-RF are improved over the MMPI-2, which is consistent with the goal for revision and resulted in tighter scales with smaller standard errors of measurement (*SEM*) (Tellegen & Ben-Porath, 2011). Some scales (especially some of the Validity Scales) were found to have lower internal consistency and thus have larger *SEM*, resulting in a need to consider a higher *T*-score before such scales can be interpreted as clinically meaningful.

With regard to the internal structure of the MMPI-2-RF, earlier factor analyses of the MMPI-2 consistently revealed two dimensions with internalizing and externalizing pathology, as expected, but not a dimension consistent with thought disorder, which was assumed to reflect the fact that there was so much scale overlap. However, factor analyses of the MMPI-2-RF Restructured Clinical Scales show three factors: an internalizing factor (consisting of RCd, RC1, RC2, and RC7), an externalizing factor (consisting of RC4 and RC9), and a thought disorder factor (consisting of RC3, RC6, and RC9), consistent with expectations for the general structure of the revised instrument (Tellegen & Ben-Porath, 2011).

A major strength of the MMPI, which remains true of the MMPI-2-RF, is the extensive external validity for the subscales, providing empirical correlates for the interpretation of high (and sometimes low) scores on the scales. These empirical correlates include likely diagnoses, other symptoms and problems the client may be experiencing, ratings of client functioning, and likely scores on other measures of psychopathology and health functioning. Much of the empirical correlate data for the MMPI-2-RF is based on rescoring of MMPI-2 protocols into the MMPI-2-RF subscales using archival data (including samples of individuals in outpatient treatment at community mental health centers, individuals receiving inpatient treatment in psychiatric facilities, individuals receiving treatment at VA medical centers, individuals undergoing disability evaluations, and defendants in criminal cases) and is summarized in the technical manual (Tellegen

& Ben-Porath, 2011). However, additional studies conducted with new samples who completed the MMPI-2-RF in its new form (including healthy controls, outpatients in medical and mental health settings, and individuals in inpatient psychiatric care) have also provided empirical correlate data that overall indicate good external validation for the subscales (Anderson et al., 2013; Avdeyeva, Tellegen, & Ben-Porath, 2012; Forbey, Lee, & Handel, 2010; Ingram, Kelso, & McCord, 2011; Sellbom, Anderson, & Bagby, 2013; Tarescavage, Wygant, Gervais, & Ben-Porath, 2013; Thomas & Locke, 2010; van der Heijden, Egger, Rossi, Grundel, & Derksen, 2013; van der Heijden, Rossi, van der Velt, Derksen, & Egger, 2013). Assessors who are considering using the MMPI-2-RF in specific types of settings should consider looking for other independent studies in which the participants are sampled from similar settings, to help make the decision regarding the appropriateness of the instrument for that type of setting.

The PAI

As with the MMPI-2-RF, the content validity of the PAI was presented above, when giving the history of the development of this scale, and a summary of the constructs assessed by the PAI was presented in Table 10.2. It is important to note that, despite scale and subscale names, scores on the PAI do not correspond directly to clinical diagnoses.

From the standpoint of reliability, the scales of the PAI show reasonable internal consistency (generally above .75), although many of the subscales fall below .70, and this should be considered when interpreting subscale scores. Approximately 1-month test–retest reliabilities were tested in two samples—75 community-dwelling adults and 80 college students—and were generally .80 and above for the main scales, but lower for the subscales. Overall, reliability analyses suggest that the scales show adequate reliability, but that much caution should be used when examining and interpreting the subscale scores, due to their lower reliability (Morey, 1991, 2003).

With regard to internal validity, factor analytic studies suggest a three-factor model when the clinical scales are used and four factors when all scales are used. The first two factors are consistent with the higher-order factors of psychopathology often identified in research (subjective distress/internalizing symptoms and antisocial/behavioral acting out), and the third factor consists of egocentric/narcissistic/callousness characteristics. For clinical samples, the fourth factor is invalidity, whereas for healthy controls the fourth factor is social detachment and social sensitivity (Morey, 1991).

With regard to evidence for external validity, the 2007 manual (Morey, 2007) provides detailed external correlates for several samples collected specifically for the initial development of the scale. In addition, many other independent studies have been conducted in clinical and nonclinical samples since the scale was first presented. Although that extensive literature cannot be adequately summarized here, a brief overview suggests that there are data to support use of the PAI in criminal/legal settings (Boccaccini, Rufino, Jackson, & Murrie, 2013; Hendry, Douglas, Winter, & Edens, 2013; Magyar et al., 2012; Percosky, Boccaccini, Bitting, & Hamilton, 2013; Ruiz, Cox, Magyar, & Edens, 2014), in the employment context (Lowmaster & Morey, 2012), with inpatient and outpatient clinical samples (Sinclair et al., 2012; Slavin-Mulford et al., 2012, 2013), with medical patients (Hill & Gale, 2011), in military psychiatric settings (Calhoun, Collie, Clancy, Braxton, & Beckham, 2011) and to assess various interpersonal/personality characteristics in both normal and clinical populations (Ansell, Kurtz, DeMoor, & Markey, 2011). A relatively recent text also provides a good summary of the use of the PAI in various clinical settings (Blais, Baity, & Hopwood, 2011). As with the MMPI-2-RF, an assessor wishing to consider use of the PAI should look into the independent literature beyond that summarized in the manual to examine validity evidence for the particular clinical setting in which the assessor may consider using the PAI.

IS EITHER MEASURE APPROPRIATE FOR THE PARTICULAR CLIENT BEING ASSESSED?

As noted in Chapter 5, it is important to consider not only the validity evidence for a scale, but also consider evidence of the validity of the scale for diverse individuals.

The MMPI-2-RF

The MMPI-2-RF is appropriate for use in individuals ages 18–80 and requires a four-and-a-half- to fifth-grade reading level. There is also a tape-recorded version for those who cannot read the items and a Spanish language version available.

Although the normative sample is dated, the norms were broadly representative of the U.S. census in 1990 and included an equal number of males and females from ages 18 to 90, with approximately 82% European Americans, 11–12% African Americans, and 7% other racial/ethnic group members. The normative sample slightly overrepresented European Americans and slightly underrepresented Asian Americans and Hispanics, given the census data for the time.

Meta-analyses of the MMPI-2 show few differences in scores in racial/ ethnic minorities in the United States (African Americans, Hispanics/Latinos) and few gender differences on the scales; as noted in Chapter 5, mean differences between groups is not evidence of bias if there is evidence that the scores are accurate in diverse groups. Data on empirical correlates of MMPI-2-RF scale scores were provided for several archival samples that were generally balanced in gender (except for the VA samples) and included members of diverse racial/ethnic groups, to varying degrees. Generally, empirical correlates of MMPI-2 scale scores showed that they did not vary by racial/ethnic status, although there was some evidence that acculturation can be important to the validity of scale interpretation for Asian Americans (Groth-Marnat, 2009). In addition, many of the independent studies of the empirical correlates of the MMPI-2-RF that have been conducted since the test's release have included diverse samples. However, there have been no studies specifically examining whether there is internal or external validity evidence for diverse groups. With regard to reliability, although test–retest and internal consistency analyses were conducted with diverse samples, including clinical groups, there were no separate reliability analyses of specific subgroups, with the exception of gender.

Whereas the normative data available for the MMPI-2-RF consist of healthy controls, the interpretive manual also includes data on samples of clinical comparison groups so that assessors can examine whether scores for an individual client are typical for individuals who have particular diagnoses that might be under consideration for that client (Ben-Porath & Tellegen, 2011; Tellegen & Ben-Porath, 2011).

The PAI

The PAI is also appropriate for use with individuals 18 and over (the standardization sample includes individuals up to age 89) and has a fourth-grade reading level. There is also an audio version available for individuals who cannot read the items. The PAI has a Spanish translation and has also been translated into other languages, but with little empirical evaluation of their validity (Morey, 2007).

The PAI manual reports data from three standardization samples. One was a sample of 1,463 community-dwelling individuals that were culled to 1,000 people fully cross-stratified by 1995 U.S. Census data with regard to gender, race (European American, African American, other), and age. The second was a sample of 1,265 individuals who were being seen for psychological treatment in 68 different clinical settings; although not specifically matched to census data, statistical analyses demonstrated that their demographic and clinical characteristics were generally consistent with epidemiological data available at the time for psychiatric samples. The final sample consisted of 1,051 college students sampled from seven universities. The clinical normative sample provided in the manual was meant to allow assessors to determine whether an individual client was showing unusually high or low scores relative to a clinical sample with the same (hypothesized) diagnosis.

With regard to potential bias in the test, at the time of test development an expert panel reviewed every item to judge items that might potentially reflect cultural issues rather than psychopathology. In addition, items that appeared to behave differently in subgroups were also eliminated (i.e., if items did not show similar relationships with indicators of psychopathology in diverse age groups, race/ethnic groups, or for males/females). Data from the PAI manual suggest there are some mean score differences at high age levels and at very low education levels, but that mean scores are not related to gender or race/ethnicity (Morey, 2007). In addition, scale and subscale internal consistencies did not vary much as a function of gender, age, or race/ethnicity. As with the MMPI-2-RF, there are few data available on internal (structural) or external validity data separately for diverse subgroups, although many studies examining these psychometric properties did consist of diverse samples.

HOW DO THE MEASURES ASSESS NONCREDIBLE RESPONDING?

As mentioned at the beginning of this chapter, one of the strengths of some multifaceted measures is their inclusion of measures of noncredible responding. As noted in Chapter 4, this issue is absolutely vital to determine the interpretability of the self-report of any client being assessed.

The MMPI-2-RF

The MMPI-2-RF has one of the most complete set of measures of noncredible responding in psychological measurement. There are scales of nonresponsiveness (unscorable items because they were omitted or both true [T] and false [F] were marked [CNS]), inconsistent responding (random responding [VRIN-r] or fixed true or false response bias [TRIN-r]), overreporting bias (F-r, Fp-r, Fs, FBS-r, RBS), and underreporting bias (L-r, K-r) (Tellegen & Ben-Porath, 2011). Just as in the Restructured Clinical Scales, most item overlap in the Validity Scales has been eliminated, although there is still some minimal overlap on a couple of the scales (FBS-r and

RBS). Whereas F-r focuses on items rarely answered in the scored direction by the normative population, Fp-r focuses on items rarely answered in the scored direction by individuals with psychopathology, and Fs focuses on items rarely answered in the scored direction by patients in treatment for various physical disorders. FBS-r is useful in identifying individuals reporting noncredible somatic and/or cognitive symptoms in the context of litigation, and RBS is useful in identifying individuals likely to fail on behavioral measures assessing for noncredible performance (particularly in the memory domain) (Ben-Porath, 2012; Ben-Porath & Tellegen, 2011).

Beyond data provided in the clinical manual (and through the long history of its predecessor, the MMPI-2), independent studies have provided further validation of the Validity Scales of the MMPI-2-RF for the assessment of noncredible responding in a variety of clinical samples, including PTSD (Goodwin, Sellbom, & Arbisi, 2013; Mason et al., 2013), malingered cognitive symptoms in individuals filing for disability due to head injury (Tarescavage, Wygant, Gervais, et al., 2013; Youngjohn, Wershba, Stevenson, & Thomas, 2011) as well as other disability (Wiggins, Wygant, Hoelzle, & Gervais, 2012), individuals with psychopathy (Marion et al., 2013), patients with medically unexplained pain and other somatoform disorders (Greiffenstein, Gervais, Baker, Artiola, & Smith, 2013), and both civilians and veterans being evaluated for traumatic brain injury who failed behavioral measures of noncredible responding (Jones & Ingram, 2011; Jones, Ingram, & Ben-Porath, 2012; Rogers, Gillard, Berry, & Granacher, 2011; Schroeder et al., 2012).

The PAI

The PAI Validity Scales include a measure of inconsistency in responding (ICN), a measure of items that are infrequently endorsed by both healthy and clinical samples (INF) and likely suggestive of overreporting, a scale reflecting exaggerated and distorted negative impressions of oneself (NIM), and a social desirability scale (PIM). Using patterns of responses on the Validity Scales of the PAI and on other clinical and treatment scales, users can also calculate several other potential indicators of both overreporting and underreporting validity, including the Malingering Index, the Rogers Discriminant Function Index, the Defensiveness Index, and the Cashel Discriminant Function (Morey, 2007). As with the MMPI-2-RF, beyond the data presented in the manual, there have been additional investigations of the validity of the PAI Validity Scales, including use in feigned ADHD (Rios & Morey, 2013), feigned mental disorder (Rogers, Gillard, Wooley, & Kelsey, 2013), feigned PTSD (Thomas, Hopwood, Orlando, Weathers, & McDevitt-Murphy, 2012), mild traumatic brain injury (Whiteside, Galbreath, Brown,

& Turnbull, 2012), malingered pain-related disability (Hopwood, Orlando, & Clark, 2010), and feigned cognitive impairment (Whiteside et al., 2010).

SUMMARY OF THE MMPI-2-RF AND THE PAI

Overall, from the standpoint of construct validity, there is ample evidence that both instruments provide valid and reliable assessment of psychological constructs known to be important to diagnostic as well as treatment decisions in clinical practice in a wide variety of clinical settings (and in nonclinical settings as well). Although some constructs overlap, each scale also assesses unique constructs, making comparisons of them a bit like comparing apples and oranges. In fact, only one study has compared the PAI to the MMPI-2-RF for a specific assessment purpose. Locke and colleagues (2011) administered both instruments to patients who were being evaluated on an epilepsy monitoring unit and found that the PAI Somatic Complaints subscales were better than another PAI scale and any MMPI-2-RF scales for distinguishing patients with epilepsy from those with psychogenic seizures. Unfortunately, there are no data available on the incremental validity or cost effectiveness of either instrument in clinical assessment. Both instruments appear to be appropriate for use with diverse populations, although more data are needed in this regard. In addition, both have the strength of including well-validated Validity Scales to aid in the interpretation of scores, although the MMPI-2-RF is much more comprehensive in its coverage of validity issues related to specific types of referral questions. Given that there are few data to compare the two in terms of their usefulness, an assessor should instead consider (1) which constructs are most important to assess for the client at hand and whether those constructs are assessed by either instrument, (2) whether there is evidence for the valid use of that instrument in the setting in which the individual is being assessed, and (3) whether aspects of diversity relevant to the client and the referral question are represented in the normative data, and/or whether there is evidence for the appropriateness of that instrument for clients from similar (relevant) backgrounds.

DECISION-MAKING ISSUES WHEN USING BROADBAND MEASURES WITH MULTIPLE SUBTESTS

An assessor needs to consider multiple issues when using psychological tests, some of which are not unique to multifaceted tests. However, with a higher number of scores from scales (and subscales) on multifaceted instruments, the chance of making decision-making errors does increase. Following is a discussion of important issues to consider when using such instruments.

What Is a Clinically Elevated Score?

Elevated scores are certainly not unique to multifaceted tests, but are also important to consider when using single-construct tests that generate only one score. An assessor needs to take into consideration the normative sample, as well as the guidelines given by the test developers; in addition, a smart assessor will examine the research literature for additional data available for samples similar to the person being assessed, to aid in this determination. When the instrument has multiple scores, the assessor must additionally incorporate the impact of considering multiple scores concurrently in the decision-making process.

For example, the MMPI-2-RF manual (Ben-Porath & Tellegen, 2011) suggests that most scales can be interpreted when the *T*-score falls at 65 or higher, which is about the 92nd percentile or higher (for scales that can be interpreted when low, a *T*-score of 38 or lower is recommended, which is equally unusual at the other end of the distribution). However, the manual points out that the recommended cutoffs given to examine external correlates of the scales are "heuristic guidelines rather than rigid demarcation rules" (Ben-Porath & Tellegen, 2011, p. 21). The manual also notes that for certain groups, an assessor may want to consider the mean and *SD* of scale scores for different clinical samples that are provided for interpretive guidance.

The PAI manual suggests that *T*-score elevations above 60, which fall at about the 84th percentile in the normative group, can be interpreted as elevated, but that *T*-scores falling at 70 (96th percentile) are indicative of problems that are likely clinically significant. In addition, the scoring profile also provides a "skyline" for clinical interpretation, which demarcates the score on each scale that falls 2 *SD* or higher above the mean of the clinical standardization sample. The manual recommends that assessors consider which frame of reference is most appropriate for the particular assessment question at hand to determine whether a scale score is clinically interpretable. For example, if one of the 11 Clinical Scales, AGG, or SUI fall at or above a *T*-score of 70 (96th percentile relative to nonclinical comparison group), then it is suggested that evaluation of scales and subscales should shift to a clinical focus, evaluating data in relation to the clinical standardization sample to compare the severity of symptoms. As another example, the scale RXR (lack of treatment interest) may mean something quite differently in individuals who have no elevated scores on any other scales and who were completing the measure outside of a treatment-seeking context, as compared to individuals who have clinical symptoms or are currently in a clinical treatment setting.

What Do Elevated Scores Mean?

For each individual scale on both instruments, there is a list of all predetermined clinical correlates or descriptors that are more likely than not to appear in someone with that high a score on that scale. Critically, that does not mean that every single correlate applies to all people with elevated scores on that scale in all contexts; such descriptors do not consider the unique circumstances of the individual or of the evaluation setting, and the descriptors are considered in isolation of elevations on any other scales.

In order to consider these scale elevations and their potential meaning for an individual client, an assessor needs to (1) "get under the hood" by examining the actual data that led to the elevated score (i.e., item analysis), (2) consider the base rates of having *any* scale elevations in the context of the number of scales being administered, and (3) take an integrative look at elevations across different scales because no scale should be interpreted in isolation.

Know Your Raw Data

It is important for an assessor to examine the raw data upon which the standardized scores were obtained. For example, on the MMPI-2-RF, there are several scores for which endorsement of only a few items in the clinical direction would result in a *T*-score of 65 or above. The SUI scale requires endorsement of only one item to reach this clinical elevation. The AXY and DSF scales require endorsement of only two items to reach this clinical elevation, and HLP, SFD, RC3, and BRF scales all fall in the clinically elevated range with endorsement of only three items. Thus, it is important for an assessor to consider this fact when interpreting elevations on these scales.

In addition, both the MMPI-2-RF and the PAI suggest that there are critical items for an assessor to consider for follow-up and further evaluation if they are endorsed. For the MMPI-2-RF, elevations on scales RC6, RC8, SUI, HLP, AXY, SUB, and AGG should alert the assessor to the need for examining the specific content of the scale for the items that were endorsed (Ben-Porath & Tellgen, 2011). On the PAI, several critical items are identified that examine content relevant to important clinical issues, such as the presence of delusions and hallucinations, potential for self-harm or aggression, substance abuse, traumatic stressors, unreliability of behavior, and additional indicators of invalid responses (Morey, 2007).

Base Rates of Elevations

The important point that an assessor must remember when interpreting scores from multifaceted tests is that each scale score cannot be interpreted in isolation. Although a T-score of 65 or greater on one isolated MMPI-2-RF or PAI scale occurs in only 8% of the normal population, the probability of an individual having at least one score elevated to this level, out of multiple scale scores, is much higher and dependent not only on how a clinical elevation is defined (see above) but also on how many scales are being examined at the same time. Odland, Martin, Perle, Simco, and Mittenberg (2011) addressed this point using the MMPI-2 as an example. Their analyses demonstrated that 36% of the normal population would score a T of 65 or greater on at least one of the 10 MMPI-2 Clinical Scales when the 10 were considered together, and 67% of the normal population would score this high on at least one scale when considering all the clinical and supplemental scales together (with 39% scoring this high on at least two). In fact, when considering all of the MMPI-2 clinical, supplemental, and content scales together, 33% of the normal population would show elevations on five or more scales. This issue is not unique to the MMPI-2 but would be true about any multifaceted scale. Thus, to determine the clinical interpretability of a client's elevated score on one of multiple scales, an assessor needs to consider the context of other scale elevations, not each score in isolation, and to integrate this interpretation with other assessment information.

Integrative Analysis

Given the issues raised above, an assessor needs to consider not just each scale score on a multifaceted instrument in isolation, but rather use a more integrative approach to interpreting the overall profile of scores on the instrument.

For example, the MMPI-2-RF manual recommends a somewhat hierarchical approach to the interpretation of scale scores. The Higher-Order Scales are meant to capture a broad range of symptoms in three common dimensions of psychopathology and that represent some of the most common codetypes on the MMPI-2: Emotional/Internalizing Dysfunction represents the codetypes 27/72, Behavioral/Externalizing Dysfunction represents the codetypes 49/94, and Thought Dysfunction represents the codetypes 68/86. However, because the other substantive scales are not subtests of these Higher-Order Scales, it is important to know that the other scales can be interpreted when they are clinically meaningful, even if the Higher-Order Scales that represent them are not elevated. Elevation of the Higher-Order Scales is more of a general indication of overall functioning and the prominence of symptoms within a particular dimension of functioning (Ben-Porath & Tellegen, 2011).

Descriptions of each scale include scores at which the scale can be meaningfully interpreted, the empirical correlates of certain score ranges, diagnostic considerations, and treatment considerations. The manual (Ben-Porath & Tellegen, 2011) also recommends a general structure for interpretation of scores in seven scale groupings, including (1) validity, (2) somatic/cognitive dysfunction, (3) emotional dysfunction, (4) thought dysfunction, (5) behavioral dysfunction, (6) interpersonal dysfunction, and (7) interests. Within these groupings, subgroupings are based on Higher-Order Scales, Restructured Clinical Scales, and Special Problems Scales that are specifically related to the subgroupings. For example, within the domain of emotional dysfunction, demoralization, and the Specific Problems Scales of SUI, HLP, SFD, and NFC are meant to be interpreted together, and RC7, STW, AXY, ANP, BRF, and MSF are interpreted together. However, within the descriptions of the interpretation of each scale score, there are also times in which integrative interpretations might cross these subgroupings. For example, when RC1 (Somatic Complaints) is high, but RC3 (Cynicism) and SHY (Shyness) are low, this cross-grouping integration is associated with potential for a somatoform disorder. Figure 10.1 shows a graphical display of the recommended structural groupings for interpretation of the MMPI-2-RF scales, combined with the comments across groupings, to guide the integrative interpretation across all scales.

When interpreting PAI scales, Morey (2003) recommends focusing initially on the full-scale scores that have a T-score of 70 or greater, based on the normal standardization sample, and then examining the clinical standardization sample for any high scores. In addition, for any full-scale scores that are elevated and that have subscales, the subscale elevations should be examined to help provide clarity to the meaning of the full-scale elevations. For example, if the DEP scale is clinically elevated, an assessor should examine DEP-C (cognitive symptoms of depression), DEP-A (dysphoria/distress), and DEP-P (vegetative). As noted above, however, because the PAI subscales have questionable reliability, examining subscale scores should be done with caution. It is recommended that, for diagnostic considerations, an individual would need to score clinically high on each of these subscales to have a pattern consistent with a diagnosis of depression. In

(a)

CNS	VRIN	TRIN	F	Fp	Fs	FBS	RBS	L	K

EID	THD	BXD	RCd	RC1	RC2	RC3	RC4	RC6*	RC7	RC8*	RC9

MLS	GIC	HPC	NUC	COG	SUI*	HLP*	SFD	NFC	STW	AXY*	ANP	BRF	MSF

JCP	SUB*	AGG*	ACT	FML	IPP	SAV	SHY	DSF	AES	MEC

AGGR	PSYC	DISC	NEGE	INTR

Step 1: record all T scores from profile sheets onto this form.

Step 2: circle or highlight all those that are clinically meaningful (using MMPI manual, and remembering to look whether they are interpretable as high or low).

Step 3: copy those that are clinically meaningful over onto page 2 (high scores above the scale label, low scores below).

Step 3a: any scales with an asterisk next to them have critical item content: if the scale is clinically elevated, specific items should be examined for need for immediate attention.

Step 4: use page 2 to help you integrate results and conceptualize case, together with other assessment data.

FIGURE 10.1a. First part of an interpretive worksheet for the Minnesota Multiphasic Personality Inventory–2–Revised Form (MMPI-2-RF).

(b)

Validity Scales

	1	1		2	2,3	3		
CNS	VRIN	TRIN	F	Fp	Fs	FBS	RBS	L	K

1. 70 plus, check other validity scales; 80 plus can't interpret
2. When high, be careful interpreting somatic scales
3. When high, be careful interpreting cognitive scales

Somatic/Cognitive

1	2				
RC1	MLS	GIC	HPC	NUC	COG

1. See RC3 and SHY
2. See EID and its facets, RC9, ACT

Thought dysfunction

			1
THD	RC6	RC8	PSYC

Emotional dysfunction part 1 and 2

				1		2,3,4	2,3,4
EID	RCd	SUI	HLP	SFD	NFC	RC2	INTR
						2,3	2,3

1. See IPP
2. See MLS
3. See RC9, ACT, DSF, SAV
4. See Interests scales

	1					
RC7	STW	AXY	ANP	BRF	MSF	NEGE

1. See SAV, SHY

Behavioral dysfunction

	1			2		2	2	
BXD	RC4	JCP	SUB	RC9	AGG	ACT	AGGR	DISC
				2		2		3

1. See IPP, FML
2. See RC2 and INTR, MLS, ACT, DSF, SAV
3. See IPP

Interpersonal functioning

1	2	3,4	3		4,5
FML	RC3	IPP	SAV	SHY	DSF
6				7	

1. See RC4 and facets
2. See NFC, AGGR
3. See RC7 and facets, NEGE
4. See RC2, INTR, RC9, ACT
5. See THD and facets
6. See RC1 and SHY
7. See RC1 and RC3

Interests

1	
AES	MEC
2	2

1. See DISC, RC9, ACT, RC4
2. See RC2 and INTR (when both low)

Scales within each of these sections should always be considered together as a group. Footnotes indicate when unusual scores (elevations above, low scores below) need to be considered in the context of scores from other sections of this interpretive guideline.

FIGURE 10.1b. Second part of an interpretive worksheet for the Minnesota Multiphasic Personality Inventory–2–Revised Form (MMPI-2-RF)

addition to analysis of the full-scale scores (and then their subscales, when necessary), a profile code interpretation is also available, which is based on the two highest full-scale scores in which both scales have T-scores of at least 70. However, the PAI manual reminds the interpreter that using only the codetypes for interpreting the PAI profile ignores information from the rest of the clinical scales, and this may mean that meaningful clinical differences between two people with an identical codetype are overlooked. The manual also reminds the user that, because of reliability issues, an assessor must be careful to consider whether the overall configuration would also meet criteria for alternative codetypes, considering at least a T-score range of 5 around the two highest scores to determine whether another codetype might apply, accounting for error in measurement.

The Use of Computerized Interpretations

The American Psychological Association (2010) code of ethics reminds assessors that, when they use computer-based assessments/interpretations of tests, they retain responsibility for the application, interpretation, and use of the computerized interpretations. Thus assessors need to know how the computerized interpretations were generated and the evidence for their accuracy; what normative samples they were based on (e.g., if not the same as the noncomputerized test); and whether there is evidence that the test, when administered in a computerized format, is equivalent to that delivered in another format. For example, consistent with Standard 6.12 of the standards for educational and psychological testing (American Educational Research Association, American Psychological Association, & National Council on Measurement in Education, 1999), the computerized interpretation for the MMPI-2-RF allows the assessor to compare a specific client to the normative group or to other clinical comparison groups. Interpretive statements are provided for each scale score elevation, and, most importantly, the *source* of the interpretive statements are also referenced (content interpretation, empirical correlation, or inference for all treatment considerations), allowing an assessor to critically evaluate the scientific basis for each interpretive statement.

Even when such evidence exists, however, an assessor needs to remember that computerized interpretations are based on what is typical/ expected of persons who have those test scores, but are not profiles of the unique person who is being assessed in the specific assessment situation. Thus, any clinical correlate or descriptor for a given score is something that is more likely than not to be true of any given person, but that doesn't mean *every* clinical correlate or descriptor applies to all people with that score. None of the unique circumstances of the individual or evaluation are considered in the computer-generated interpretation, and computer-generated reports cannot take the place of a qualified test user who considers extratest data and integrates all the information into the interpretation of the test results. Of course, this is also true when an assessor uses a clinical manual to interpret test scores, but when computerized scoring automatically generates the interpretation, it can increase the likelihood that an assessor will blindly rely on that interpretation. In my clinical experience, it is unfortunately still not that unusual to see paragraphs directly lifted from computerized interpretations of tests and placed into reports, or the computerized printout attached as an amendment to the assessment report, with those data used in isolation as the interpretation of the test itself. Such a method is not consistent with an empirically based process of assessment and interpretation. Instead, an assessor should consider the computerized interpretive comments simply as hypotheses that require integration with other test (and nontest) data before they can be considered valid for a given client, and if the assessor does use information from a computerized narrative, that information should be cited and synthesized with other data in the final interpretation of the profile.

11

Intellectual and Achievement Testing

Things must be done decently and in order.
—SHERLOCK HOLMES, in *The Adventure of the Empty House*

When a client has concerns about his or her cognitive functioning and/or has poor functioning that might be due to cognitive impairment, direct assessment of relevant cognitive skills is essential to the assessment. Such variables cannot be assessed accurately by self-report. This chapter begins with a discussion of measures of performance commonly administered when questions arise about cognitive functioning, with a primary focus on intelligence tests, but also some coverage of achievement testing. Chapter 12 discusses neuropsychological assessment.

As in previous chapters, the focus here is not to comprehensively review all available measures of intelligence and achievement, but rather to focus on a decision-making process an assessor could undergo when deciding which intelligence measure to give to a specific client in a specific assessment situation. Given its popularity with psychologists, the Wechsler Adult Intelligence Scale—Fourth Edition (WAIS-IV; Wechsler, 2008b) serves as the main example. Surveys show the WAIS is the first choice as a measure of intelligence among clinical neuropsychologists (Rabin, Barr, & Burton, 2005), forensic psychologists (Archer, Buffington-Vollum, Stredny, & Handel, 2006), clinical psychologists (Camara et al., 2000), and adult assessors in general (Groth-Marnat, 2009; Sattler & Ryan, 2009; Weiss, Saklofske, Coalson, & Raiford, 2010). Other measures of intelligence, including the Woodcock–Johnson Tests of Cognitive Abilities–III (WJCOG; Woodcock, McGrew, Schrank, & Mather, 2007) and the Stanford–Binet Intelligence Scales, Fifth Edition (SB5; Roid, 2003), compared and contrasted to the WAIS-IV on each important decision-making question to illustrate the thoughtful consideration of their similarities/differences and strengths/weaknesses prior to deciding which instrument is most appropriate for a given purpose.

The first step in the decision process, as pointed out in previous chapters, is for an assessor to carefully define the construct he or she is planning to assess.

WHAT IS THE CONSTRUCT OF INTELLIGENCE?

Intelligence is a complex construct, and there are no clear, agreed-upon operational definitions; in fact, different definitions and theories have guided the development of different intelligence tests, many of which are not reviewed here. In 1997, Gottfredson offered a working definition of intelligence, describing it as the "ability to reason, plan, solve problems, think abstractly, comprehend complex ideas, learn quickly, and learn from experience" (p. 13). Although individuals can generally agree upon such a definition of intelligence, it is easy to imagine a wide variety of measures that might assess these components of intelligence. In fact, each part of this definition is a separately definable cognitive construct that also lacks agreed-upon operational definition. For example, Gottfredson's definition includes the ability to "learn quickly." Most measures of learning and memory involve the repeated rehearsal of previously novel information (short stories, word lists, word pairs, complex abstract drawings) that is too large for the immediate attention span to hold, followed by a sufficient delay to measure retrieval of that information. However, in the Cattel–Horn–Carroll (CHC) model of intelligence (see below), the factor Glr (long-term storage and retrieval) includes both measures of immediate and delayed visual/auditory learning and measures that tap retrieval of remote information from semantic memory, rather than from recent and novel information presented during a testing session, within the same factor (Schneider & McGrew, 2012). Yet, from a neuropsychological perspective, these are highly dissociable cognitive constructs. Most measures of intelligence do not include measures of learning and recall of new information, likely because such measures typically have non-normal distributions precluding their usefulness as measures of a construct, for which one expects to be able to distinguish the full range of the normal curve; instead, such measures are included in neuropsychological batteries (as discussed in Chapter 12).

There is also no agreed-upon "structure" for the construct of intelligence, although many researchers argue strongly for the hierarchical CHC model of intelligence (Schneider & McGrew, 2012), which is generally composed of g, or general intellect, at the highest level, as well as several higher-level fluid g factors, several higher-level crystallized g factors, and more specific sensory and motor abilities. This model is not theory-driven but rather is a taxonomic structure of intelligence built from decades of psychometric research on measures of cognitive abilities (Schneider & McGrew, 2012). Although specific measures of *some* components of the CHC model exist, there are no measures or test batteries that assess the whole model; furthermore, it is unclear how strong the evidence is for the CHC model in its entirety. However, most intelligence tests used in clinical practice today generally endorse a hierarchical structure to intelligence, with a single g factor as reflected in a total score, and then more specific, underlying cognitive abilities or factors (usually one or more crystallized factors and one or more fluid factors) assessed by index or even subtest scores.

Finally, an important part of the construct of intelligence, at least in the clinical context, is the fact that intelligence should be related to successful functioning in the real world, in both academic and nonacademic settings. Therefore, there is a predictive component to the construct beyond its psychometric structure, which is important for an assessor to consider when deciding which measure of the construct of intelligence is most appropriate to use for a given purpose and for a specific client. The fact of the matter is that all cognitive ability measures, even when purported to assess narrow or specific cognitive skills, assess multiple cognitive constructs to varying degrees. Although this complexity can make it difficult to model an overall structure to intelligence or to parse out the key components of intelligence in a specific cognitive battery, it is what makes measures of intellect particularly predictive of real-world functioning (i.e., give it ecological validity). Furthermore, whereas measures of specific cognitive abilities are subordinate to the general intelligence factor, they may be predictive of specific real-world outcomes and thus account for criterion variance beyond that of general intelligence. In addition, data on specific cognitive patterns within tests may be diagnostically useful (although it should be noted that evidence for the diagnostic value of specific cognitive patterns within any current intellectual measure is weak at best).

DOES THE WAIS-IV MEASURE ASSESS THE CONSTRUCT OF INTELLIGENCE?

Wechsler (1939) provided a working definition of intelligence similar to that provided by Gottfredson (1997), as mentioned above. Wechsler described intelligence as a global capacity (i.e., g) that was an aggregate of qualitatively differentiable (but not independent) cognitive elements, which together reflected a person's rational thinking, purposeful action, and overall ability to effectively interact with his or her environment. Generally, Wechsler viewed g as an important construct to assess by including measures of many different types of underlying cognitive skills (using both verbal and nonverbal modalities for assessing them) within a scale. Thus, the assumed "structure" to intelligence in the Wechsler tests is a hierarchical one. The original scale, the Wechsler–Bellevue Intelligence Scale (Wechsler, 1939), addressed a clinical need for a measure of general intelligence with both verbal and nonverbal material that followed this hierarchical model. In its current edition, the WAIS-IV, revisions were made to better reflect the "state of the science" with regard to the intelligence construct, enhancing the measure of fluid reasoning, working memory, and processing speed. In so doing, the revisions responded to the growing evidence base for core components of hierarchical models of intelligence (e.g., CHC), as well as the evidence base for the importance of certain cognitive areas in assessment of cognitive changes associated with neurodevelopmental and neurological conditions and with aging (Wahlstrom, Zhu, & Weiss, 2012; Wechsler, 2008a; Whipple Drozdick, Wahlstrom, Zhu, & Weiss, 2012). Thus, both structural components of intelligence and clinical value/ecological and diagnostic validity are important parts of the intelligence construct as defined by the current WAIS.

The core components of the WAIS-IV comprise four indices and 10 subtests: Verbal Comprehension (with three core subtests of Similarities, Vocabulary, Information), Perceptual Reasoning (with three core subtests of Block Design, Matrix Reasoning, and Visual Puzzles), Working Memory (with two core subtests of Digit Span and Arithmetic), and Processing Speed (with two core subtests of Symbol Search and Coding). There are five supplemental subtests, including one for Verbal Comprehension (Comprehension), two for Perceptual Reasoning (Figure Weights and Picture Completion), one for Working Memory (Letter–Number Sequencing), and one for Processing Speed (Cancellation). In addition, users can (when appropriate in a given case) report a Full Scale IQ score or alternative composites, including the General Ability Index (comprised of Verbal Comprehension and Perceptual Reasoning) and the Cognitive Proficiency Index (comprised of Working Memory and Processing Speed) (Wechsler, 2008b).

For comparison, the WJCOG is based on the CHC model of intelligence. The WJCOG is comprised of 20 tests (10 standard, 10 expanded), each of which is purported to measure one or more narrow or specific cognitive abilities within the CHC model (but do not assess the model in its entirety). There is a diagnostic supplement with 11 additional cognitive tests, but most existing data focus on the 20 better-known tests (Schrank & Wendling, 2012). Of the seven broad abilities consistent with the CHC model, there are two subtests of Comprehension-Knowledge (Verbal Comprehension, General Information), three subtests of Long-Term Retrieval (Visual-Auditory Learning, Visual-Auditory Learning Delayed, Retrieval Fluency), three subtests of Visual-Spatial Thinking (Spatial Relations, Picture Recognition, Planning), three subtests of Auditory Processing (Sound Blending, Incomplete Words, Auditory Attention), three subtests of Fluid Reasoning (one of which is cross-loaded; Concept Formation, Analysis-Synthesis, Planning), four subtests of Processing Speed (Visual Matching, Decision Speed, Rapid Picture Naming, Pair Cancellation), and three subtests of Short-Term Memory (Numbers Reversed, Auditory Working Memory, Memory for Words). The cluster scores for these CHC factors are weighted combinations of the subtests that are part of the cluster, based on factor analytically derived weights. In addition to these seven cluster scores, an additional eight cluster scores (Verbal Ability, Thinking Ability, Cognitive Efficiency, Phonetic Awareness, Working Memory, Broad Attention, Cognitive Fluency, Executive Processes) are calculated from various test permutations, which, according to the technical manual, are based on "logical collections of tests" and thus do not have any psychometric validity. The General Intellectual Ability score is calculated based on a weighted combination of test scores based on the overall CHC factor analytic model (Woodcock, McGrew, Schrank, et al., 2007).

The SB5 is a revision of the earlier versions of the test to specifically align with Carroll's (1997) hierarchical model of intelligence (now incorporated into the CHC model). Thus, there is a g score as reflected in the composite index, as well as verbal and nonverbal measures of Fluid Reasoning (Matrices, Verbal Absurdities/Analogies), Knowledge (Picture Absurdities, Vocabulary), Quantitative Reasoning (Nonverbal Quantitative Reasoning, Verbal Quantitative Reasoning), Visual-Spatial Processing (Form Patterns, Position and Direction) and Working Memory (Block Span, Memory for Sentences/Last Word). Assessors can also calculate a nonverbal IQ (combining the nonverbal measures across the five factors) and a verbal IQ (combining the verbal measures across the five factors). The SB5 diminishes the role of psychomotor processing speed in their instrument; this construct is not assessed specifically by any of the subtests, and each subtest minimizes the degree to which processing speed might interfere with performance by having very extended time limits for items (Roid, 2003).

In summary, each of these three measures uses a hierarchical model of intelligence composed of measure(s) of g, followed by factors/clusters/indices representing various fluid and crystallized components, and then with subtests meant to represent varied specific cognitive domains relevant to an overall structure of intelligence and/or to answer specific clinical needs.

IS THE WAIS-IV APPROPRIATE, GIVEN THE PURPOSE OF THE ASSESSMENT?

For the purpose of providing a full measure of intellect, an assessor should consider not only the content of the specific measure or measures under consideration, but also the psychometric data regarding the construct validity of the measure(s) (reviewed below). However, sometimes assessors seek to provide only an estimation of intellectual level or need to estimate premorbid intellect after likely cognitive changes due to injury or illness. Different measures are more appropriate for these purposes.

Screening/Estimating Intellect

If an assessor's purpose is to provide a quick screen for estimated intellect, the WAIS-IV, WJCOG, and SB5 would not be appropriate choices, given the extended amount of time it would take to administer any of them. However, the Wechsler Abbreviated Scale of Intelligence—Second Edition (WASI-II; Wechsler, 2011) provides a screening of intellectual ability in four subtests that would be appropriate in settings in which an in-depth intellectual evaluation cannot be conducted. The four subtests—Vocabulary, Similarities, Block Design, and Matrix Reasoning—can result in an overall estimate of cognitive ability, a Verbal Comprehension estimate, and a Perceptual Reasoning estimate. A two-subtest version, comprised of only Vocabulary and Matrix Reasoning, can also be administered and results in an estimate of general cognitive ability only. The specific subtests chosen for use in the abbreviated version were those that loaded the strongest on an overall intellect factor. Although the WAIS-II subtests are similar to those in the WAIS-IV, they are not the exact same measures; they parallel the counterpart measures in both the WAIS-IV and the Wechsler Intelligence Scale for Children—Fourth Edition (WISC-IV; Wechsler, 2003). However, if the WAIS-II scores result in a need to administer a full WAIS-IV or WISC-IV, these four subtest scores can be substituted for the corresponding scores on the full instrument.

With regard to the other two full measures of intelligence, the WJCOG has a three-subtest battery (Verbal Comprehension, Concept Formation, Visual Matching) meant to provide an estimate of intelligence (Brief Intellectual Ability) (Woodcock, McGrew, Schrank, & Mather, 2007). For the

SB5, the first two subtests, Verbal Knowledge and Nonverbal Fluid Reasoning, serve as both "routing" tests to determine the start points for all remaining subtests, but also can serve as an estimation of intellect (Abbreviated Battery IQ) (Roid, 2003).

It is important for assessors to note that all of these screening instruments are *only* screening instruments and are not comprehensive measures of the construct of intellect. Therefore they should not be used as "stand-ins" for more comprehensive assessment of intelligence when the assessment situation calls for such.

Estimating Premorbid Intellect

The estimation of an individual's premorbid intellect (or other cognitive skills) is a vital assessment question for assessors working with individuals who have potentially acquired cognitive deficits as a result of injury or illness. It is a myth that an assessor can accurately estimate a client's premorbid intellect by using the highest subscale score obtained by the client on an individually administered intelligence test. As is discussed in detail below, individuals frequently have significant variability in their scores across different cognitive abilities that comprise typical measures of intelligence, and use of only the highest subscale score to estimate premorbid functioning is likely to lead to a spuriously high overestimate of premorbid intellect. However, it is possible that examination of patterns of scores on cognitive tasks that are more crystallized in nature (and thus less likely to be vulnerable to injury or illness) can provide a *gross estimation* of intelligence; tests of basic knowledge or vocabulary skills, for example, may provide scores that allow for estimation of intellect. An assessor should remember that the value of such tests as accurate estimations of intellect depends on the history of the client being assessed, with factors such as English fluency, presence of preexisting learning disability, poor education, and/or presence of acquired illness/injury that directly affect language skills potentially rendering such subtests inaccurate as estimates for any individual client.

For example, the Wechsler Test of Adult Reading (WTAR; Wechsler, 2001) was designed to provide an estimate of intellectual functioning prior to injury or illness that may have affected cognitive ability. It was normed for individuals ages 18–89. The measure is based on the reading of atypically pronounced English words, based on research showing that reading recognition tends to be a cognitive skill that "holds" across a wide variety of neurological changes (including normal aging). Of course, as noted above, the assumption is that the individual being assessed had normal English reading skills prior to the injury or illness and that the injury or illness did not affect reading or language skills directly. Scoring of the measure takes into account demographic factors (e.g., education level) that might be associated with achieved scores and that should be considered when interpreting the overall score. It is important to note that the WTAR, as with other measures of word-reading skills, has a wide range of error around the estimated score, and thus is appropriate only as a gross estimate of intellectual abilities.

However, estimating an individual's premorbid intellectual or other cognitive abilities is a task larger than a score on any one instrument. As in all assessment decisions, estimation of premorbid intellect should involve thoughtful consideration of other nontest data, such as a client's typical grades in school prior to the injury/illness, performance on nationally normed standardized tests (annual proficiency tests, ACT, SAT) during the school years (and predating the injury/illness), the client's overall level of education, and overall preinjury employment status. It should be noted that some of these factors still encompass individuals with a wide range of intellectual capacities. For example, although, on average, individuals with a college education have higher intellectual levels than those with a high school education and those with less than a high school education, there is still wide variability in the general intellectual level of individuals with college degrees. Similarly, whereas the cognitive complexity of one's occupation is generally correlated with intellect, there is still a wide range of levels of intellect among individuals in different professions. An assessor cannot assume that, just because a client is a doctor or lawyer, he or she has a high-average to superior level of premorbid intellect (although it is a safe bet that the individual had at least an average intellect). An assessor will consider any and all of these variables, as well as scores on tests such as the WTAR or subtests on intelligence tests that measure crystallized skills, when estimating premorbid intellect.

For the remainder of the decision-making questions in this chapter, it is assumed that the purpose of the assessment is to administer a comprehensive measure of intelligence to the client in question, not to estimate either current or premorbid intellect.

DOES THE WAIS-IV VALIDLY ASSESS THE CONSTRUCT OF INTELLIGENCE, GIVEN THE PURPOSE IN A SPECIFIC ASSESSMENT?

In order to determine whether a particular intelligence measure is appropriate for a given case, the assessor should carefully examine the evidence base for the construct validity of the instrument under consideration as a first step. Content validity for the WAIS-IV was addressed above; the organization that follows focuses on reliability, internal/structural validity, and external/diagnostic validity.

Reliability

The WAIS-IV

Every subtest of the WAIS-IV has an internal consistency of .8 or greater (note that the speeded tests do not have internal consistency calculations), and index scores (except Processing Speed) all have an internal consistency of .9 or greater. Test–retest (over an average of 22 days) was strong for most subtests (an exception was the Cancellation subtest). Interrater reliability for subtests requiring clinical judgment is also strong (Wechsler, 2008a).

The WJCOG

The internal consistency reliability was at .8 or greater for 94% of the subtests, and all but three of the cluster scores showed internal consistency reliabilities at .9 or above. Test–retest reliability was assessed only after a single day, and only 44% of the scores showed test–retest reliabilities of .8 or greater. Although 1-year stabilities were also reported, the results were not adequately documented to understand their validity (Wasserman, 2013; Woodcock, McGrew, Schrank, et al., 2007). Thus, overall, the WJCOG's reliability appears weaker than that of the WAIS-IV.

The SB5

The internal consistency reliabilities were generally .8 and above for the subtests and .9 and above for composite scores. Test–retest reliability (over an average of 7 days) across four age cohorts was generally .8 and above for subtests and index scores (Roid, 2003) and is generally comparable to that of the WAIS-IV.

Practice Effects

An important psychometric factor for an assessor to consider when using intelligence and other cognitive measures in repeated administrations is practice effects. All three instruments show some practice effects that can vary by subtest/index. Practice effects can also vary based on the general cognitive ability of the individual being assessed. An assessor who may be reassessing a client using an instrument the client has recently completed in another evaluation should be conscious of the potential for practice effects to affect the client's scores on the second administration.

Internal Validity

The WAIS-IV

The technical manual (Wechsler, 2008a) reported the results of a confirmatory factor analysis that generally supported the four-factor structure of the WAIS-IV. However, other researchers have used the WAIS-IV standardization sample to examine both exploratory factor analyses and confirmatory factor analysis of alternative models for the WAIS-IV structure. Some studies have shown support for only one- or two-factor models of the WAIS-IV (Canivez & Watkins, 2010), whereas others have argued that five-factor models (Benson, Hulac, & Kranzler, 2010) or modified four-factor models (Bowden, Saklofske, & Weiss, 2011; Ward, Bergman, & Hebert, 2012) best explain the variance in WAIS-IV subtests. Recently, Weiss, Keith, Zhu, and Chen (2013) showed that both four- and five-factor models fit the data in the standardization sample as well as in the clinical samples reported in the technical manual. The main discrepancy in four- and five-factor models is that the Perceptual Reasoning Index is actually comprised of two components, one associated with visual-spatial processing and the other associated with fluid reasoning (particularly notable when factor analyses include the supplemental subtests). An important question, however, with regard to consideration of internal structure to clinical interpretation, is how much variance any of the underlying factors account for, above and beyond the hierarchical factor of g. Data suggest that there is little incremental variance accounted for in the individual factors once the highest factor (g) has been taken into account.

The WJCOG

The confirmatory factor analysis reported in the technical manual (Woodcock, McGrew, Schrank, et al., 2007) shows at best only marginal support for the proposed seven-factor structure of the measure. This weakens conceptual arguments for interpretations of various factors and profiles on the WJCOG, as based on CHC theory or when interpreting cognitive profiles for clinical purposes. In fact, given that (as is true for the other intellectual measures) a high proportion of the variance in the scores is accounted for by g, with little left for any specific factors (Floyd, Shands, Rafael, Bergeron, & McGrew, 2009), interpretation of composite and subtest scores must be considered as less than pure measures of any particular factor or specific cognitive ability.

The SB5

Although intercorrelation tables show that the g loading for each subtest is high, which supports an overall hierarchical structure to the instrument, there was minimal support for the confirmatory factor analysis of the hypothesized five-factor model, as reported in the technical manual (Roid, 2003). Furthermore, other studies have not shown good support for the proposed five-factor structure (Canivez, 2008; Distefano & Dombrowksi, 2006; Williams, McIntosh, Dixon, Newton, & Youman, 2010). Thus, empirical data suggest that the SB5 should be interpreted only at the level of the composite score.

External Validity

The WAIS-IV

Data from the technical manual (Wechsler, 2008a) show strong and expected relationships between WAIS-IV and its predecessor, the WAIS-III, both for individuals in the standardization sample who took both instruments and for individuals with intellectual disability who completed both instruments. Similarly, in a sample of 16-year-olds who took both the WAIS-IV and WISC-IV, the data showed expected strong relationships. The WAIS-IV also showed strong relationships with achievement test scores, with some data suggesting differential relationships of specific WAIS indices to specific areas of academic achievement. The WAIS-IV also showed significant, though less strong (as expected), relationships with measures of other cognitive constructs, such as memory, executive functioning, and other neuropsychological instruments. Thus, good convergent and divergent concurrent validity is available for the WAIS-IV. Drozdick and Cullum (2011) also reported reasonable relationships of WAIS-IV with a measure of activities of daily living.

Given that the WAIS-IV includes measures meant to tap both crystallized and fluid aspects of intelligence, examination of changes to more crystallized and more fluid WAIS indices across age and in clinical disorders also provides evidence of its construct validity. In fact, the results of several special group studies generally support that the WAIS-IV's ability to identify the types of specific cognitive weaknesses associated with several clinical conditions (Wechsler, 2008a). In addition, Salthouse (2010) and Baxendale (2011) used the cross-sectional age data from the standardization sample to demonstrate that much greater age changes are associated, as expected, with more fluid measures, including the Processing Speed Index (PSI), Perceptual Reasoning Index (PRI), and Working Memory

Index (WMI), relative to the more crystallized tasks that are part of the Verbal Comprehension Index (VCI), even when statistically controlling for education as a confounding cohort. However, cross-sectional analyses are limited and vulnerable to potential cohort confounds when examining any age-related question.

The WJCOG

Data from the technical manual (Woodcock, McGrew, Schrank, et al., 2007) showed strong correlations of the WJCOG with other measures of intelligence, including earlier versions of both the Stanford–Binet and WAIS measures. The technical manual also reported strong associations between WJCOG scores and achievement test scores, consistent with expectations for a measure of intellect. In addition, given that the WJCOG is meant to be administered across the full developmental range, cross-sectional growth curves data reported in the technical manual are consistent with known cognitive changes across development and aging for the intellectual factors assessed within SB5 (as noted above, these analyses are limited by confounds associated with cross-sectional approaches to analyzing age changes). Although data from clinical samples are reported in the technical manual to provide further evidence of diagnostic validity, the demographic and diagnostic data for these samples are poorly documented, limiting their value. In addition, although the technical and interpretation manuals suggest many assessment–intervention linkages, these interpretations are conceptual at best and are not empirically based.

The SB5

As with the other two measures, there is evidence of strong correlations of the SB5 with composite scores from earlier versions of the WAIS and the WJCOG (concurrent validity), and the SB5 correlates strongly with achievement test data (Roid 2003). As with the WJCOG, the SB5 is designed to test across the full developmental range, and the technical manual provides good evidence of developmental changes in the cognitive factors assessed on the SB5 consistent with known age-related changes in specific cognitive skills (as noted above, these data are cross-sectional in nature and thus are limited in their ability to address age-related changes in intellect). The technical manual (Roid, 2003) also reports the results of several clinical studies, but given that most data suggest the SB5 can be interpreted only as a composite score, the value of these data for finding specific diagnostic patterns is limited.

IS THE WAIS-IV APPROPRIATE FOR USE WITH A SPECIFIC CLIENT?

As noted in Chapter 6, information on the overall validity of an instrument is necessary, but not sufficient, when considering whether to use that measure for a specific client. An assessor must also consider whether there is evidence that the measure is valid for individuals similar to the client in ways important to the construct under consideration (in this case, cognitive skills). Of course, there is some debate about which factors would be considered germane to the construct under consideration. Certainly age is a factor associated with cognitive and intellectual abilities, and, as noted above, with change in those abilities (particularly in the domain of fluid intelligence) over time. Thus, information on age invariance of internal and external validity data would be important to consider. There is also some evidence of reliable gender differences in specific cognitive skills, some of which might be assessed on subtests or indices of the intellectual measures being reviewed; thus, information on gender invariance might be useful to consider.

With regard to race/ethnicity differences, this is an area of particular importance, particularly given the social consequences often associated with intelligence assessment and the major public controversies about the use of intelligence tests with diverse individuals (Phelps, 2009). In this light, it is important to note that most empirical data on intelligence testing do not support the presence of any racial/ethnic bias in such instruments show (i.e., do not suggest that the measures show differential construct validity in diverse racial/ethnic groups), despite there still being evidence of reliable mean differences in intelligence in some diverse groups (Reynolds & Suzuki, 2013). It is also important to note that the most important confound to race/ethnic group differences on intellectual measures is SES; given that low SES likely reflects the lack of opportunity for a developing brain to reach its full potential (due to higher risk of teratogenic exposure, poorer nutrition, less intellectual stimulation, poorer schooling, as well as other neurobiological factors), group differences likely reflect actual differences in intellect (but not related to racial/ethnic group status per se), rather than representing a confound or test bias. As noted in Chapter 5, another extremely important variable to consider when individuals being assessed come from cultural backgrounds other than the dominant culture in which an assessment is taking place is each individual's degree of acculturation—which, in the case of intellectual tests, is most important with regard to language fluency and years of education in the cultural environment in which the specific intellectual test was developed. Thus, it is important to consider how each specific instrument has attempted to address concerns related to its use with diverse groups.

The WAIS-IV

The WAIS-IV is normed for individuals ages 16–90. These norms are representative for age, sex, race/ethnicity, self/parent education, and geographical region relative to the 2005 U.S. Census. Thus the norms include a relatively comprehensive and representative sample of the U.S. population, although there is underrepresentation of individuals from the lowest educational groups (Wechsler, 2008b). The Advanced Clinical Solutions array (Pearson, 2009a), whose purpose is to expand and enhance the clinical utility of the WAIS-IV, provides demographically adjusted scores for both subtests and index scores; scores can be adjusted on the basis of gender, race/ethnicity (European American, African American, Hispanic, Asian), and years of education. It should be noted, however, that there is significant controversy over the use of demographically corrected norms, given that any differences in scores might reflect real differences (see above and Chapters 5 and 12), and that use of such norms might diminish the predictive validity of the test scores (see Chapter 12).

When revising the instrument, WAIS-IV developers tried to minimize test-taking confounds related to hearing limitations, visual limitations, and motor limitations by changing test stimuli and decreasing time demands, which should make the measure more appropriate for use with individuals who have such limitations. In addition, there are more sample and practice items on the subtests, to decrease the confound of misunderstanding task demands and to increase the fair use of the instrument with diverse groups (Wechsler, 2008a).

With regard to potential item bias, the WAIS-IV developers conducted formal expert review of the items three times, using experts in cross-cultural work and in intelligence testing. The first review occurred at initial development, the second review during a tryout stage, and the third review occurred during the final standardization. Experts were asked to judge whether the items were culturally obsolete and whether the content was relevant to the domain being assessed and not confounded by construct-irrelevant (but perhaps culturally unfair) content. In addition to these content analyses, the WAIS-IV developers also conducted statistical bias analyses during the tryout stage of development, oversampling 73 African American and 93 Hispanic American participants to conduct item response theory and Mantel–Haenszel bias analyses (Wechsler, 2008a).

With regard to invariance of the WAIS-IV among diverse groups, there are few data available. Although the WAIS-IV developers used a diverse sample to examine both test–retest reliability and internal consistency, they did not provide data on whether these values were different in diverse subgroups. However, they did provide internal consistency estimates for the clinical subsamples described above, providing evidence of invariance of reliability within each subtest for clinical groups (Wechsler, 2008a). Similarly, although the WAIS-IV developers used a diverse sample to examine the internal validity of the instrument, there are no data available on whether the overall factor structure is invariant across different racial/ethnic groups or for males/females. However, the model was shown to be generally invariant across age groups (Wechsler, 2008a). In addition, Bowden and colleagues (2011) showed that the general factor structure is relatively invariant across U.S. and Canadian samples; Reynolds, Ingram, Seeley, and Newby (2013) showed general invariance in factor structure in individuals with intellectual disability; and Nelson, Canivez, and Watkins (2013) showed general invariance in factor structure in diverse clinical samples.

With regard to mean differences in diverse subgroups, Salthouse and Saklofske (2010), using the standardization sample data, found only very small gender differences on index scores, no larger than 0.2 SD, with higher PSI scores in females and higher PRI scores in males. Weiss, Chen, Harris Holdnack, and Saklofske (2010) also used the standardization sample data and found about 1 SD difference between African Americans and European Americans on the full-scale score. With regard to index scores, PRI showed the largest difference between these two groups, followed by VCI, then WMI, and then PSI. The researchers also examined the differences between these two groups based on birth cohort (age). The youngest birth cohort showed only a 10-point difference on the full-scale score, whereas in the oldest birth cohort, the difference was 17 points, suggesting that intellectual differences between these two groups are overall growing smaller in younger generations. In addition, the 1 SD difference was reduced to only 11 points when controlling for demographic factors. Weiss and colleagues also found an 11-point difference between Hispanic and European American samples on the full-scale score, with the biggest score difference on VCI, followed by WMI, then PRI, and then PSI. As with their analysis of African American and European American group differences, the full-scale difference was only 9 points in the youngest birth cohort, but 18 in the oldest birth cohort, again suggesting that the differences between racial/ethnic groups are shrinking across generations. In addition, the overall full-scale difference of 11 points was reduced to 6.5 points when controlling for demographics. As noted above and in previous chapters, the fact that there are group differences on the WAIS-IV is not, in and of itself, indicative of bias, if indeed the group differences reflect actual differences in the construct being assessed.

With regard to external validity, although the WAIS-IV developers used a diverse sample to test for external correlates, the samples were not big enough to examine whether the external correlates vary for diverse subgroups. Finally, although some of the clinical populations used to examine diagnostic validity of the WAIS-IV included diverse participants, there are no studies examining whether the patterns of performance within particular diagnostic groups were similar in majority or minority samples.

The WJCOG

The WJCOG standardization sample was collected from 1996 to 1999, based on 1996 census projections for the year 2000, and included 8,782 individuals ages 2 to 90-plus. However, in 2007, a normative update was published, using a newly stratified sample drawn from this original standardization sample, based on actual year 2000 census findings (Woodcock, McGrew, Schrank, et al., 2007). This restratification led to dramatic changes in some scores, which is a bit concerning for interpretation of scores on the instrument (Wasserman, 2013).

With regard to potential item bias, item development of the WJCOG was informed by expert review of items for potential item bias and sensitivity, which led to elimination or modification of items (Woodcock, McGrew, Schrank, et al., 2007). The WJCOG manual provides no data on whether there were empirical analyses for item bias during test development.

With regard to invariance of internal structure, data from the technical manual suggested that the factor structure was similar in fit in European American and non-European-American samples. The factor structure also seemed generally invariant across age (Taub & McGrew, 2004). Edwards and Oakland (2006) examined only the structure of General Intellectual Ability (GIA) across the 1,978 European American and 401 African American students in grades K–12 who were part of the original normative sample for the WJCOG. The g loadings for the subtests were generally similar across the two groups. As with the WAIS-IV, there were consistent mean score differences across the subtests, with the pattern generally consistent with general findings in the literature. Edwards and Oakland also found that correlations between the GIA and achievement test scores were similar in the two groups. Aside from these studies, there are few data available on the invariance of internal or external validity across diverse groups for the WJCOG.

The SB5

The SB5 can be administered to individuals from ages 2 to 96. The standardization sample consisted of 4,800 individuals stratified on age, geographic region, sex, race/ethnicity, and SES/education, based on the 2001 U.S. Census (Roid, 2003).

During the development of the SB5, tests and reviews for potential item bias occurred in three different rounds. The content of items was examined by expert reviewers on three occasions; reviewers were measurement experts and also members of diverse groups/researchers of diverse groups across gender, race/ethnicity, religion, and disability status. Empirical item bias analyses using item response theory (IRT) and differential item functioning (DIF) were also conducted across the three phases of development (Roid, 2003).

With regard to invariance of internal validity data, internal consistency of the scores was shown to be invariant across widely diverse groups in the standardization sample, as were the intercorrelation matrices across diverse groups. With regard to evidence for invariance of external validity data, scores on the SB5 correlated equally well with achievement scores across different gender and race/ethnicity groups (Roid, 2003).

$N = 1$ RELIABILITY AND VALIDITY

An important note with regard to the administration of individual intelligence tests is that they require a great deal of supervised training to administer correctly. Proper administration of any assessment tool (including structured interviews and self-report measures, in addition to cognitive measures) is always important, but for measures that involve reading of verbatim instructions, manipulation of stimuli, demonstration of items, accurate timing, start-and-stop rules, and sometimes complicated coding/scoring rules. Thus, extensive supervised administration practice and the double-checking of scoring are central to the reliability of intelligence test scores in an $N = 1$ format. It is my experience from decades of training students to administer cognitive and intellectual tests that students either focus too much on test administration, to the detriment of the assessment skills and processes being discussed in the present text, or they consider the correct administration of these instruments to be "beneath them," focusing instead on developing their higher-order assessment skills, to the detriment of collecting $N = 1$ test data in a standardized fashion. All assessors should be reminded of the absolute importance of ensuring that data collected during assessment have minimal error; examiner error is under the assessor's control.

Another important note with regard to $N = 1$ reliability is that accurate interpretation of intelligence tests requires that the client is giving forth full effort on the tasks being administered to him or her. Noncredible behavior is a problem for cognitive and intellectual/achievement tests, as the subtests typically grow more difficult as they proceed, with the potential for anxiety, frustration, and fatigue to contribute to poor/diminished effort. The assessor must be conscious of the client's mental status throughout the exam and recognize when there is a need for a break from what can be lengthy and anxiety-provoking procedures. In addition, noncognitive factors such as personality traits or test-taking styles can affect test performance. For example, some individuals are careful and deliberate when marking items on WAIS-IV Coding or Symbol Search, due to a desire to be neat and tidy, which might result in lower scores that do not actually reflect weaknesses in psychomotor processing speed per se. An assessor needs to remember to continue behavioral observations throughout the administration of tests (I encourage my students to write behavioral observations in the margins of the test protocols being administered, including nonverbal behaviors as well as direct quotes from the individuals being assessed).

Furthermore, a client can be motivated to deliberately behave in a noncredible manner on intelligence tests (or on components of intelligence tests) in order to attempt to behave in a way that is consistent with the identified behaviors of a particular disorder (e.g., intellectual disability) or to suggest that one has a specific type of cognitive impairment (e.g., slowed processing speed, poor working memory) to receive some external gain (see Chapter 4). Unfortunately, this possibility is not typically assessed within intelligence tests. However, studies have developed cutoff scores consistent with noncredible responding for some WAIS subtests and index scores (such as Digit Span and the PSI) (Larrabee, 2007), and the Advanced Clinical Solutions for the WAIS-IV and Wechsler Memory Scale—Fourth Edition (WMS-IV) (Pearson, 2009a) include subtests specifically developed to assess for noncredible behavior in cognitive testing.

An individual focused on assessment rather than testing will use data from an entire assessment battery to help interpret scores that, on their surface, might indicate impairment in a particular cognitive domain but instead are reflective of noncredible performance. For example, I have seen many assessment reports in which the assessor argued that the client requires extended time in an academic setting due to slowed information processing speed, as indicated by extremely low scores on psychomotor processing speed measures (e.g., WAIS-IV Coding and Symbol Search subtests, which comprise the PSI) or on measures of academic fluency (see below). However, often in such cases, examining the overall results of the assessment reveals that the client's performance on other administered subtests and tests that also require information-processing speed (in the form of time limits for providing answers) are well above average. In addition, the scores on the PSI are often so low in such cases that one would presume the individual would have difficulty carrying out tasks of everyday living that require psychomotor processing speed, such as driving a car, but extratest evidence suggests that this is not the case. Furthermore, it is often true in such cases that the individual in question has scored in the normal range (and sometimes well above normal) in timed high-stakes standardized testing during his or her school years, which is also inconsistent with the scores described above, *and* is inconsistent with a recommendation that the individual be granted extended time on tests because of slowed informa- tion processing speed. Thus, the assessor in such cases has made the fatal assessment error of focusing on only one isolated test score in a currently administered battery, without integrating that information with other con- current and historical evidence relevant to the referral question.

DECISION-MAKING ISSUES RELEVANT TO INTERPRETATION OF SCORES FROM INTELLECTUAL TEST BATTERIES

For measures as complex as intelligence measures are, it should not sur- prise an assessor that there are myriad interpretive guidebooks and com- puter programs designed to calculate the "clinical value" of every possible subtest score, every possible index/composite/cluster score, and every pos- sible discrepancy score that is available in the overall test profile. However, an assessor must be cautious about overinterpretation of all of these test scores and remember that assessment requires an examination of these test scores in the context of extratest data, as well as a consideration of psychometric issues associated with interpretation of more than one score concurrently within a battery.

Measures of Cognition Are Complex

Even though all of the intelligence measures reviewed above have subscales that are purported to measure more specific cognitive abilities beyond that represented by general intelligence, all of their subscales and subtests are interrelated, all of them have high g loading, and all involve more than one cognitive skill to accomplish them. Thus an assessor must remember that a poor score on one "specific" cognitive measure does not mean that the client lacks the ability to accomplish that one "specific" cognitive skill the measure purports to assess. Instead, a poor score on a specific cognitive measure should be weighted together with data from other measures within the battery, other scores from other tests, and other nontest data, before interpreting the score as indicative of impairment in a specific cognitive skill. The example of processing speed given earlier in this chapter illus- trates this point well. It is this cognitive complexity that makes intellectual measures strong in ecological validity (i.e., predicting real-world functioning), but that makes it difficult to interpret specific patterns of performance within the intellectual test battery with any degree of confidence.

Measures of Cognition Are Associated with Error

It is also important for an assessor to remember that there is error associated with each and every score on an intellectual measure. Given the internal consistency data reported above, although there is reasonable reliability for some of the higher-order factor/cluster/index scores on each of these measures, most of them do not have adequate reliability at the subtest level. It has been strongly recommended (American Educational Research Association, American Psychological Association, & National Council on Measurement in Education, 1999) that assessors always report confidence intervals around the scores obtained during assessment and consider them when interpreting the assessment data. Crawford and Garthwaite (2009) argue that expressing the end points of confidence intervals as percentile ranks may help both assessors and those who read assessment reports understand the interpretation of scores obtained during an assessment. Crawford, Garthwaite, Longman, and Batty (2012) provide a free program for obtaining this information for the WAIS-IV.

Discrepancy Scores Are Not Reliable for Clinical Decision Making

The manuals for all of the intelligence measures reviewed above provide guidance for calculating and interpreting various discrepancy scores within their test batteries, and supplemental interpretive guidebooks have also been published for these tests. As noted above, such an undertaking is somewhat suspect, given that none of the subtests (or indices) are pure measures of any particular cognitive construct. In addition, the reliability of the discrepancy scores should be sufficiently high so as to suggest that the discrepancy score can be trusted. Discrepancy score reliabilities (the consistency of the difference between two test scores) can be calculated from the internal consistency reliabilities of the two test scores in question and the correlation between those two tests. In order to feel confident in interpreting a discrepancy score, an assessor should consider only discrepancy scores with .9 or above reliability. In order to consider the discrepancy score as a means of generating a hypothesis that would require support from additional sources of data, the discrepancy score reliability should be at least .8.

Glass, Ryan, and Charter (2010) used the WAIS-IV data to calculate the discrepancy score reliabilities and showed that many subtest discrepancy scores were too low even for hypothesis generation; all *index* discrepancy scores (of note, no discrepancies utilizing PRI were examined because internal consistency reliability data were not available for those subtests) could be used to generate hypotheses for further exploration, and some of them (depending on the age group under consideration) were above .9 and thus might be useful for clinical decision making. Thus, at best, index discrepancy scores could be used as tentative hypotheses that, together with data from other test and nontest sources, may suggest differential patterns of cognitive strengths and weaknesses that are clinically meaningful. Although this issue has not been formally assessed with the WJCOG and the SB5, given the internal consistency data for their subtests and composite scores and the correlations among the various scores on these instruments, it is reasonable to expect similar findings with regard to concerns about subtest discrepancy analysis, and the need for an assessor to be very careful to consider even cluster/index discrepancy analyses as mere hypotheses requiring further support from other sources of data.

Base Rates for "Abnormal" Scores

As noted above, although intelligence tests tend to have strong psychometric properties and large and representative standardization samples, they also generate a high number of scores for interpretation. Information on the "abnormality" of such scores is key to interpreting their results. When scoring these tests (either via manuals or computerized printouts), an assessor will find the percentage of people in the standardization sample that scored below a certain score on an isolated subtest, which can give the assessor a sense of how rare such a low score is in isolation. However, in an assessment, the assessor is not considering any one score in isolation, but is considering multiple scores concurrently. Thus, the relevant base rates to consider (which are *not* provided by manuals or computer programs for these tests) are comprised of the "normal" number of "abnormal" scores, given the number of scores under consideration. When assessors consider that having at least one (or even sometimes quite a few more than one) "low" score would be expected, given the number of scores generated, they can decrease their likelihood of misdiagnosing cognitive impairment on the basis of an isolated low score.

In addition to considering this base-rate issue at the subtest/index score level, an assessor should consider this issue at the level of discrepancy analysis. Just as each of the tests reviewed above have many subtest and index scores, they also provide ways to calculate discrepancies among various scores/indices. For example, within the WAIS-IV standard battery, there are 10 standard subtests and four indices that generate 51 possible pairwise subtest/index discrepancy comparisons.

As a first step, the assessor can determine whether the difference obtained in any one of these comparisons is statistically significant (i.e., reliable), although such a determination only indicates that the difference is unlikely to have arisen due to measurement error. Due to good internal consistency, which makes for small confidence intervals, it is easy for an individual to have statistically reliable differences when subtest/index scores are compared to one another. Thus, a statistically reliable difference between two subtests or two indices is not a good indicator of cognitive impairment.

As a second step, the assessor can then determine (based on data provided in the test manuals) whether the difference between two scores is unusual (i.e., of low base rate). However, the manuals provide the base rates of such differences based on consideration of each discrepancy in isolation, not considering the number of concurrent comparisons being calculated. Thus, what is needed (and not provided in the test manuals or computerized scoring for the three instruments reviewed) is the "normal" number of "unusual" discrepancy scores, considering the number of comparisons being made.

Independent researchers have provided some data relevant to these base-rate issues for the WAIS-IV. For example, Brooks, Holdnack, and Iverson (2011) used the data from 900 people ages 16–69 from the WAIS-IV and the WMS-IV standardization sample, examining 20 subtests and 10 index scores. They used an "abnormality cutoff" of 1 SD below the mean (less than the 16th percentile). Of course, for each score considered in isolation, that means that 16% of the standardization sample scored the same or lower on that subtest/index. However, when considering the 10 index scores concurrently, almost half of the standardization sample had one or more index scores falling at or below that cutoff. The percentage of the standardization sample with "abnormal" scores varied by education; almost 88% of those with less than 8 years of education had at least one abnormal index score, but so did 56.5% of those with high school education, 45% of those with some college education, and 20.5% of those with college or more education. When considering the 20 subtests, 77% of the standardization sample showed at least one abnormal score. Even when using a more extreme score (5th percentile) to judge abnormality, 44.4% of the standardization sample showed at least one abnormal score when all 20 subtests were considered concurrently. The researchers concluded that, for people with average intelligence, having three or four WAIS/WMS index scores and subtest scores at or below 1 SD is common and not likely indicative of cognitive impairment.

With regard to discrepancy analyses, Binder and Binder (2011) examined the frequency of having abnormal scores on the WAIS-IV based on the highest subtest score. Although it was true that individuals with lower peak subtest scores more frequently had other scores that fell 1 *SD* below the mean, it was still the case that 18.8% of individuals whose peak highest subtest score was 2 *SD* or more above the mean still had at least one other subtest that fell 1 *SD* below the mean. Thus, the researchers were able to demonstrate that subtest variability/discrepancies are also common and thus not necessarily indicative of impairment. Crawford, Garthwaite, Longman, and colleagues (2012) provide a free computer program that takes into account the number of discrepancy comparisons on the WAIS-IV to help assessors consider this important issue when interpreting discrepancies. For example, they calculated pairwise differences between WAIS-IV index scores that, in isolation, occurred in < 5% of the standardization sample. When considering all pairwise comparisons together, however, about 20% of the standardization sample showed at least one such "rare" pairwise difference. When using a more liberal cutoff for "abnormal" pairwise comparisons (< 10% in isolation), 35.1% of the standardization sample showed at least one "abnormal" discrepancy when all pairwise comparisons were considered concurrently. Although there have been no similar calculations conducted for the WJCOG or the SB, there is no question that such a concern is relevant to these instruments as well, given the number of potential subtests, index scores, and discrepancy scores available for an assessor to interpret on these measures.

A RECOMMENDATION FOR AN EMPIRICALLY GUIDED PROCESS TO INTERPRETING THE WAIS-IV

The following sections describe recommended steps to take when conducting an empirically guided interpretation of findings from the WAIS-IV (which could be generalized and adapted to other intellectual measures as well). Of note, it is recommended that an assessor go through this process as part of reaching a "final conclusion" about how to interpret the instrument; as can be seen in Chapter 14, it is recommended that an assessor write only the final conclusion in the actual report.

Step 1

The assessor should first consider the administration of the test. Were there any examiner, examinee, or test environment variables that affected the reliability/validity of any of the subtests? If so, were supplemental subtests administered that could replace the invalid score, or will the scores be unreportable?

Step 2

The assessor should then record data on the various index scores (see Figure 11.1). Information to record includes (a) the actual index score, (b) the 95% confidence interval range for the score, (c) the percentile rank (recorded for the full confidence interval, not just the index score), and (d) a clinical description for the range of scores, considering the confidence interval (see the clinical manual for descriptive terms; Wechsler, 2008b).

Step 3

Next, the assessor should determine the level of interpretation of the overall scores. Starting with the Full Scale IQ, the assessor should determine whether there are differences among the index scores that would render the Full Scale IQ uninterpretable. To do so, the assessor can follow the next two substeps.

3a

Subtract the lowest index score from the highest index score. If the resulting figure is < 23 points (about 1.5 SD; cutoff recommended by Lichtenberger & Kaufman, 2013), then the Full Scale IQ might be interpretable.

3b

Subtract the lowest subscale score from the highest subscale score (of the 10 standard subscales that comprise the Full Scale IQ). If the resulting figure is < 10, there is no unusual scatter (base rate for 9 or less is 16% of the standardization sample). The assessor should remember that having too much scatter simply means that the index *likely* cannot be interpreted as a whole, not that it is indicative of impairment (Binder & Binder, 2011). In fact, if there is scatter among the subtests, *but* all the subtest scores fall above the mean (12 or higher is a recommendation of Lichtenberger & Kaufman, 2013) or below the mean (8 or lower), then this is likely not unusual scatter, and the Full Scale IQ can still be interpreted (assuming that 3a was true).

If both 3a and 3b suggest the Full Scale IQ can be reliably interpreted, then the assessor can describe the client's at the highest level (i.e., g) and proceed to Clinical Interpretation, below. If either 3a or 3b is violated, the assessor should move to Step 4.

Step 4

The assessor should determine whether the General Ability Index (GAI) or the Cognitive Proficiency Index (CPI) is interpretable, using the following steps.

4a

If the VCI and PRI differ by 23 or more, then the GAI is uninterpretable and the assessor should move to Step 5 to consider VCI and PRI separately. If the WMI and PSI differ by 23 or more, then the CPI is uninterpretable, and the assessor should move to Step 5 to consider WMI and PSI.

4b

The assessor should determine whether there is too much scatter within either GAI or CPI to interpret these indices, using Lichtenberger and Kaufman's (2013) recommendation of a "less than 5" (approximately 1.5 SD) point difference between the highest and lowest subtest score on either of these indices. If there is too much scatter on either the GAI or the CPI, then the assessor should move to Step 5 to consider the index scores separately.

If both the GAI and CPI are deemed reliable by these two standards, then the assessor can proceed to Clinical Interpretation (below), interpreting the profile at the level of GAI and CPI. If only one of them is reliable, the assessor can move to Clinical Interpretation for that index, and continue to Step 5 to further interpret the other one. If both GAI and CPI are not reliable, then the assessor should move to Step 5 for further interpretation of the full profile.

Step 5

The final step for the assessor is to consider the indices themselves, guided by the following substeps.

5a

The assessor should consider the internal consistency of each index, which involves examination of the scatter within the index. As noted above, Lichtenberger and Kaufman (2013) recommend using a rule of thumb of a "less than 5" (approximately 1.5 *SD*) point difference to consider the index scores as internally consistent. It should be noted, however, that such a difference is much more common for the PRI than for the other three indices, occurring in about 24% of the standardization sample, possibly reflecting the fact that the PRI has been shown to perhaps reflect more than one factor (as reviewed above). As noted above, if there is high scatter, it simply means that index cannot be interpreted as a whole, not that the individual has impairment, per se. However, the nature of the scatter can be used to generate hypotheses, as is noted in Clinical Interpretation.

5b

For the indices that are internally consistent, the assessor can compare them to one another, using the < 23 cutoff described above, comparing them in a pairwise fashion. Other authors (Glass et al., 2010) suggest using a method that minimizes the number of comparisons by comparing each individual index score to the mean of the index scores; however, Crawford, Garthwaite, Longman, and colleagues (2012) show that a large percent of the standardization sample will have at least one index score that is reliably different from the mean index score, again suggesting caution before interpreting this as clinically meaningful.

Clinical Interpretation

If on Step 3, the Full Scale IQ was judged to be interpretable, the assessor can focus the final clinical interpretation of the profile (and the subsequent write-up of the results) on reporting this highest-level score for the client. The various other indices can be reported in a descriptive fashion, but should not be described as unusual relative strengths/weaknesses because there were no reliable (or unusual) differences in the subtests/indices that comprised the overall Full Scale IQ score. The level of interpretation, then, for this type of profile is primarily at the normative level (i.e., how the scores compare relative to same-age peers).

If on Step 4, the GAI and/or the CPI were judged to be interpretable, the assessor can focus the final report on either (or both) at this level. Data on indices/subtests comprising either or both the GAI and CPI would be discussed in a descriptive fashion, but not as relative strengths or weaknesses. If both the GAI and CPI are interpretable, then they can be compared to one another; a difference of 23 points suggests an unusual and interpretable relative difference between the two indices, and thus they can be described as relatively unusual strengths/weaknesses; however, such interpretations must also consider the normative interpretation of the

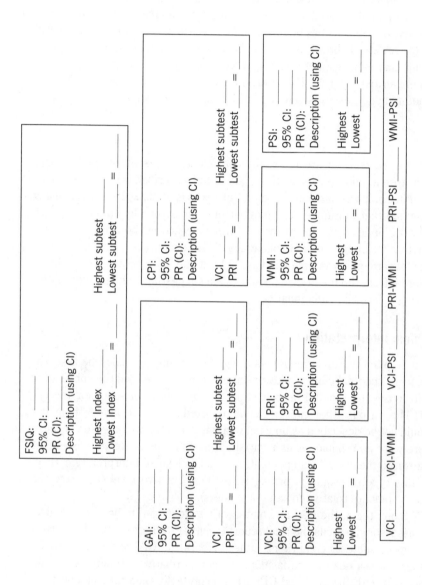

FIGURE 11.1. Worksheet for use in empirically guided interpretation of WAIS-IV protocols.

indices. In other words, if one of the indices is very superior and the other is simply average to high average, this relatively unusual ipsative difference is actually not clinically meaningful, in that both are normal to above normal in relation to the client's same-age peers.

If on Step 5 it was concluded that some of the indices could be interpreted, then clinical interpretation should focus on considering whether there are unusual differences between the indices that do not have too much scatter. The assessor should keep in mind the number of index comparisons that are being conducted when making this interpretation. Although a difference of 23 points on any one set of pairwise comparisons considered in isolation is relatively rare in the standardization sample, if all four indices are being compared to one another, data from Crawford, Garthwaite, Longman, and colleagues (2012) suggest that finding at least one "unusual" difference is not uncommon. The assessor should also remember that, because the PSI has lower reliability and a larger *SEM*, it is more likely to be discrepant from the other indices. Further, the assessor needs to remember that, at extreme scores, the likelihood of large differences increases. As noted above, the normative interpretation must also always be considered (i.e., the comparison of that client's data with the same-age peers) when considering a personal strength/weakness and before interpreting an unusual difference in indices as evidence of impairment.

If Step 5 indicated that an index simply had too much variability to be interpreted, then the assessor can focus at the subtest level for that index, providing descriptive normative data about the subtests. The data can be used to generate only very tentative hypotheses (to be followed by additional testing and/or considered in the context of other already available test and nontest data) about reasons for the variability; the assessor needs to also remember, as summarized above, that variability is not uncommon even in the standardization sample, and thus this variability is not necessarily indicative of impairment. For example, variability within the PRI may simply indicate that the client's pattern of performance is more consistent with the five-factor model for the WAIS-IV (described earlier in this chapter), and an assessor could consider follow-up testing with additional measures (not limited to the WAIS-IV supplemental measures) relevant to the separable factors to address whether that is a valid consideration for interpretation of the WAIS-IV data for that client.

A FEW WORDS ABOUT ACHIEVEMENT TESTS

Individually administered achievement tests are often used when a client presents with concerns about academic performance. Because this text is focused primarily on adult assessment, discussion of these tests is more limited, as they are used much more frequently in the assessment of children. However, a developmentally oriented assessor knows to ask about prior testing and knows to review results of any prior testing, which might include results from individually administered achievement tests. Furthermore, an assessor may still administer achievement tests to an adult client, if achievement tests are appropriate for the purpose of the referral question. The following brief discussion focuses on important decision-making issues relevant to the use of achievement tests in the assessment of adults.

Construct Validity

Achievement tests are meant to quantify an individual's achievement in basic academic domains and often focus on the academic domains that are part of federal guidelines relevant to identification of learning disabilities, including reading skills and reading comprehension, math skills and math applications, written expression (including spelling), and oral expression and listening comprehension. Some achievement tests cover these domains rather comprehensively (e.g., Wechsler Individual Achievement Test–III; Pearson, 2009b); others provide a screening for the most basic of these domains (e.g., Wide Range Achievement Test–IV; Wilkinson & Robertson, 2006), and still others have attempted to tie their achievement measures to overarching theories of cognitive/intellectual functioning (e.g., Woodcock–Johnson Tests of Achievement; Woodcock, McGrew, & Mather, 2007). Although educational achievement tests typically measure what has been learned within specific academic content domains, the context is often determined by the test developers and is not guided by federal or state guidelines regarding which aspects of academic content should be mastered by certain grades within the U.S. academic system. Some achievement tests also have parallel forms equated in difficulty level. Validity data are often tied specifically to, and limited to, content validity.

Other Psychometric Considerations

As with other cognitive measures, it is important to consider the internal consistency of achievement tests and the effect this has on confidence intervals and test interpretation. For example, some achievement tests have lower internal consistency than measures of intellectual ability, and thus have larger SEM and less precise confidence intervals. Another factor to consider is that often achievement tests allow for the reporting of age- or grade-equivalent scores, which are misleading and may be misinterpreted by many individuals.

As an example, a 20-year-old with a grade equivalent of eighth grade on a math task simply obtained a raw score that fell at the 50th percentile for individuals who completed eighth grade. This does not mean that the 20-year-old did not learn any math skills that are typically covered in more advanced grades. Similarly, an 8-year-old with a grade equivalent of 11th grade on a reading comprehension task simply obtained a raw score that fell at the 50th percentile for individuals who had completed the 11th grade; this does not mean that the 8-year-old should be moved to a high school level reading class.

As noted above, the most common use of achievement tests in psychological assessment is to identify individuals with learning disabilities. One way in which achievement tests are used is to document that an individual is "impaired" in a particular academic domain. However, the cutoffs that are used to determine whether a score is "impaired" vary greatly by test (and by state guidelines). It is often recommended that scores below the 16th percentile be interpreted as evidence of impairment. However, one must consider the base-rates issue raised above. Considering a score below the 16th percentile as impaired means that 16% of the normal standardization sample would be "impaired" on any isolated achievement subtest. Furthermore, given that most achievement tests also provide multiple subtests within specific academic domains, an assessor needs to consider the base rates of such a "low" score concurrently with all of the other tests in consideration. Given the studies cited above, it is likely extremely common for individuals to score in this range on at least one achievement test, when many achievement test scores are considered concurrently.

The Individuals with Disabilities Education Improvement Act (2004) also allows for the comparison of ability to achievement (i.e., discrepancy analyses) as a way to document the presence of a learning disability, although it is not required. Many interpretive manuals for achievement tests suggest comparing scores on ability and achievement tests by considering the expected score on an achievement test, given the score obtained on an ability test. Such a method makes several assumptions: (1) that this ipsitaive comparison is clinically meaningful (i.e., will indicate impairment in some way, which it might not; (2) that both measures assess the full range of scores in the same way—and this might not be true for achievement tests, which may not extend into the high-average/superior range for certain ages; and (3) that the discrepancy is somehow unusual.

First, such a relative discrepancy may not be indicative of impairment in any way. An individual with superior intellect and average to high-average achievement in a particular academic domain is not impaired or disabled in that academic achievement domain and should not receive any academic accommodations, given that there is no evidence of impairment from a normative standpoint, despite the relative difference in scores (and given this discrepancy, may not be unusual; see below).

Second, the distribution of some achievement test scores are skewed, with individuals at higher ages/grades reaching a ceiling on the tasks; thus, very high scores cannot be obtained in some cases. This is especially important to consider for someone whose ability test scores may indicate superior functioning; if the achievement test cannot measure superior achievement, then lack of a "superior" achievement score should not be misinterpreted as evidence of a relative weakness in achievement relative to ability.

Finally, having an ability–achievement discrepancy (or even multiple such discrepancies) may not be unusual. As noted above, when considering intra-ability discrepancies, multiple discrepancy comparisons could be calculated when an assessor has administered both ability and achievement tests. The base rates with which individuals might be expected to show a discrepancy or discrepancies, given the number of comparisons conducted, have not been systematically evaluated, but it is likely that the more unusual pattern is for a normal individual to show *no* variation in his or her performance across so many cognitive and academic domains.

Other manuals and researchers suggest using patterns of strengths/weaknesses on ability and achievement tests rather than ability–achievement discrepancies to determine whether an individual has a learning disorder (Flanagan, Alfonso, & Ortiz, 2012; Woodcock, McGrew, & Mather, 2007); this method typically results in even *more* discrepancy analyses because discrepancies among specific subtests, both across and within batteries, would also be considered "evidence" of impairment. For example, if an assessor administered the full WJCOG plus the Woodcock–Johnson Tests of Achievement, there would be intra-ability, intra-achievement, and ability–achievement discrepancies that could be calculated, resulting in a plethora of potential discrepancy comparisons. Any one of these discrepancies, considered in isolation, may appear to be rare in the standardization sample, but the real decision-making question is whether it is normal to have any discrepancies when so many of them are calculated concurrently. Although Flanagan and colleagues (2012) do caution individuals using this approach to corroborate test findings with other assessment evidence, there is no acknowledgment of the fact that discrepancies identified with such a method may be just normal variability in cognitive and academic performance among humans.

Finally, there is little to no control for, or consideration of, the potential for noncredible performance to affect achievement test scores, and yet there is ample evidence that this can and does occur when questions about academic failure or need for academic accommodations arise in psychoeducational testing (Alfano & Boone, 2007; Harrsion, Green, & Flaro, 2012).

12

Neuropsychological Screening and Assessment

Like all other arts, the Science of Deduction and Analysis is one which can only be acquired by long and patient study, nor is life long enough to allow any mortal to attain the highest possible perfection in it.
—SHERLOCK HOLMES, in *A Study in Scarlet*

Cognitive complaints are very common, and neuropsychological complaints with and without actual evidence of impairment are associated with myriad psychological, medical, and neurological disorders. In addition, cognitive concerns are seen in normal aging, as well as a host of personality styles, and thus occur in high base rates in the general population. Emotional distress also tends to be highly related to cognitive complaints. On the other hand, in some cases, individuals are unaware of their cognitive and neuropsychological impairments and thus do not report them accurately during interview or on questionnaires. Overall, such data indicate that one cannot measure cognitive dysfunction accurately by mere self-report. Individuals who either complain about cognitive concerns or who are known to be at risk of having cognitive impairment despite their lack of concerns should be considered candidates for neuropsychological evaluation.

Consistent with a developmentally oriented biopsychosocial model (see Chapter 3), a core competency of any psychologist conducting psychological assessment should be the ability to screen for neuropsychological impairment and to consider the possibility of a neurological contribution to a client's presenting concerns. However, the ability to conduct comprehensive neuropsychological assessment requires training well beyond that of a typical psychologist (or other professional trained to conduct psychological assessment). Clinical neuropsychology is a specialty area of training recognized by both the American Psychological Association and the Canadian Psychological Association. Minimal criteria for the specialty include obtaining a doctoral degree in psychology (from an accredited training program), completing a predoctoral internship (ideally with focus in clinical neuropsychology), and completing at least 2 years of supervised clinical experience by a clinical neuropsychologist (typically at the postdoctoral level, but which could include the predoctoral year and 1 year at the postdoctoral level). Various definitions of clinical neuropsychology exist, but all generally emphasize that the area of specialized knowledge, beyond that explicated in the rest of this text, is advanced knowledge of neuroscience and neurological bases of behavior.

This chapter presents a brief introduction to neuropsychological assessment, including discussion of neuropsychological screening. Decision-making issues unique to neuropsychological assessment are discussed, as these issues are relevant for any assessor who conducts neuropsychological screening or reviews neuropsychological reports as part of his or her evaluations of clients who have been previously assessed. These issues are equally relevant for individuals in training to conduct full neuropsychological evaluations.

INTRODUCTION TO NEUROPSYCHOLOGICAL ASSESSMENT

A neuropsychological evaluation can aid in the diagnosis of many conditions. For example, neuropsychological assessment can help to distinguish normal from abnormal performance (e.g., whether cognitive changes are consistent with normal aging or reflective of a pathological process) and can differentiate when presenting symptoms are reflective of a potential neurological dysfunction or not likely to be related to neurological issues. Although the advent of neuroimaging has greatly minimized the role of neuropsychological assessment in localizing areas of brain damage/dysfunction, there are still many conditions in which there may be no clear brain changes on structural or even functional imaging, but for which there is a pattern or profile of neuropsychological dysfunction suggestive of specific brain involvement (e.g., neurotoxicities, cardiovascular conditions, neuroendocrine conditions, neurodevelopmental disorders, neuropsychiatric disorders, early dementia, mild traumatic brain injuries) and for which neuropsychological evaluation can play a role in diagnosis.

In addition, even in conditions for which there is clear neuroimaging evidence of neurological damage, the extent to which that damage has affected functioning is not known without further evaluation; thus, neuropsychological assessment also plays a role in prognosis, disability determination, and making recommendations for interventions and/or accommodations to facilitate optimal functioning. There is a fair amount of evidence for the ability of various neuropsychological instruments to predict real-world functioning (depending on the condition and the tests under consideration) (Demakis, 2012; Marcotte & Grant, 2010). Neuropsychological assessment is also useful in tracking change, from identifying individuals at risk for future decline (e.g., early detection of dementia) to tracking that decline through the course of a dementing condition, to documenting response to various interventions or in the process of recovery from an injury or illness.

Two crucial components of a neuropsychological evaluation can be seen in the word "neuropsychological." The "neuro" part of the term indicates that the assessor should have advanced knowledge of, and experience with, empirical findings in neuroscience in order to apply that "brain–behavior" knowledge to the client in question. A neuropsychologist is best equipped to integrate the knowledge from neuropsychological tests with nontest neurological data (e.g., findings from structural and functional imaging, medical records documenting severity of injury, known neuropsychological effects of medications). However, the "psychological" part of the term should remind neuropsychologists that the dependent variable of focus in the evaluation is the *behavior* of the person. A psychological perspective is just as crucial to good neuropsychological assessment as a neurological perspective is. Training in clinical neuropsychology is highly consistent with the overall training for advanced assessment outlined throughout this text, with the addition of extra training in functional and clinical neuroscience.

Full neuropsychological batteries are lengthy and comprehensive. A list of neuropsychological domains typically covered in neuropsychological evaluation appears in Table 12.1. Although neuropsychological texts often describe the differences between a fixed and flexible battery approach to neuropsychological evaluation, the reality is that few people use a fixed battery of tests (Sweet, Moberg, & Suchy, 2000); even individuals who predominantly use one of the most common fixed batteries (i.e., the Halstead–Reitan Battery; Reitan & Wolfson, 1997) often augment the battery by including additional measures (e.g., memory measures).

What a flexible battery approach to assessment means, however, is that there are decision-making processes (including the selection of which constructs to measure, which measures of those constructs to administer, and how many measures of each of the constructs to administer) that become important potential sources of error in the assessment process. As noted in Chapter 1, although individual tests have reliability and validity

TABLE 12.1. Domains Typically Assessed in Neuropsychological Assessment

Domain	Description
Perception	Visual perception and auditory perception are most commonly assessed, but neuropsychologists might also assess tactile/somatosensory perception and/or gustatory/olfactory perception, depending on the referral question.
Motor functioning	Motor strength, fine and gross motor movements, apraxia
Orientation and attention	Orientation to time, place, personal information, basic attentional processes
Learning and memory	Immediate memory, learning efficiency, delayed memory in both verbal and nonverbal modalities (i.e., declarative memory), potentially also retrograde memory (autobiographical memory) or nondeclarative memory processes depending on referral question
Language skills	Both receptive (comprehension, both aurally and in reading) and expressive language (speaking and writing) skills; expressive skills including fluency, presence/absence of paraphasias
Visuospatial and visuoconstructional skills	Visuospatial orientation, mental rotation, ability to construct two- and three-dimensional stimuli, drawing tasks
Executive functioning skills	Working memory, decision making, abstract reasoning, inhibition, cognitive flexibility
Emotional functioning	Could include assessment for affect, emotion, motivation changes directly related to neurological conditions, or assessment for emotional reaction to illness/impairment; should also include assessment for premorbid personality and emotional issues that may impact current presentation.
Measures of noncredible behavior	Assessment for noncredible self-report and performance is necessary to any neuropsychological evaluation.

data, there is little evidence for the validity of the process of selecting, administering, and interpreting a collective of neuropsychological tests in the process of assessment.

In a flexible battery approach, the first decision being made by the assessor is which of these many constructs is most important to assess, given the referral question. For many flexible battery neuropsychologists, the goal is to select a battery of tests that will at least briefly screen most, if not all, of the areas listed in Table 12.1, with more elaborate testing of neu-ropsychological domains that are germane to the referral question or that become important as the neuropsychological evaluation unfolds (e.g., due to client responses to the interview, behavioral observations, performance on preliminary tests). The second decision being made is, of course, which of the many neuropsychological measures of the relevant constructs should be administered in any given case. Making this decision requires review of the construct validity of each instrument chosen to be part of the battery, as well as review of whether those measures are valid to use for the client in question (see Chapters 5 and 6).

CONSTRUCT VALIDITY OF NEUROPSYCHOLOGICAL ASSESSMENT

In a chapter meant only to introduce neuropsychological assessment, there is simply not space to examine the construct validity of every neuropsy-chological instrument available. However, the process by which these tests have been validated is briefly discussed, and an assessor should use this information to consider the relevant data for any specific neuropsychologi-cal test of a specific neuropsychological construct, to aid him or her in mak-ing decisions about which measures to administer to a particular client.

As in previous chapters discussing the construct validity of various tests, it is first important to consider the construct itself and (1) whether that construct is internally consistent or relatively heterogeneous; (2) whether that construct is stable over time or likely to be subject to state variability; (3) how that construct should behave in response to changes with age or any other relevant demographic variables; and (4) what kind of real-world data are related to the construct (diagnostic, neuroimaging, pre-diction of functioning). Such a construct review would then determine what evidence should be considered when examining the psychometric proper-ties of any specific measure of that construct.

For example, consider a test of verbal learning and memory ability. Such a measure may be somewhat more vulnerable to state-like changes in attention and arousal than a measure of vocabulary skill. Therefore, a valid measure of memory would likely show lower test–retest stability than would be expected for a valid measure of a more stable construct such as vocabulary. Because there are well-documented age-related changes in learning and memory skill, a valid measure of learning and memory should show declines in scores of individuals of different ages, or in older individu-als tracked over a reasonable time period. Declarative memory is related to intact functioning of the mesial temporal lobes, specifically the hippo-campus and surround, and thus functional imaging data showing activation of this brain region while healthy individuals complete the learning and memory task would provide evidence of construct validity, whereas individuals who have known damage to this region would be expected to show impairment in a valid measure of learning and memory. In fact, although some individuals have predicted that structural and functional imaging would eventually replace neuropsychological testing, imaging data have only provided good construct validity for many neuropsychological tests. Given that many neurological disorders are known to be associated with impairments in learning and memory ability, a valid measure of learning and memory should show sensitivity/specificity in the differential diagnoses of those disorders. Finally, if individuals with impaired learning and memory skills cannot function independently in some aspects of real-world functioning, a valid measure of learning and memory should be related to those skills as well.

For an assessor to comprehensively examine the construct validity of any neuropsychological measure for use with a particular client, the administration and technical manuals available for the test can be a good start, but as demonstrated in Chapters 9, 10, and 11, the assessor should also go further and look into the broader and more updated research literature for all measures under consideration. In addition, many neuropsychological tests are not copyrighted or are part of large test batteries for which publishing companies have gathered extensive psychometric and normative data in a manual. However, compendiums of neuropsychological tests, such as those by Lezak, Howieson, Bigler, and Tranel (2012) and Strauss, Sherman, and Spreen (2006), provide brief reviews of major psychometric properties for many neuropsychological tests and serve as a good starting point for considering which neuropsychological measures to administer to assess the relevant constructs in a particular assessment situation.

Because the main focus of this chapter is on neuropsychological screening, the Repeatable Battery for the Assessment of Neuropsychological Status (RBANS; Randolph, 2008) is used to illustrate construct validity issues.

SCREENING NEUROPSYCHOLOGICAL FUNCTIONING

As mentioned above, most psychologists lack competencies essential to conducting full neuropsychological evaluations. However, psychologists should be able to screen for neuropsychological concerns, in order to make informed decisions about the need to refer a client for more thorough neuropsychological evaluation. Although a screening evaluation should assess for relevant areas of cognition given the client's complaints or the referral question, most screens tend to assess only a narrow range of cognitive abilities. In addition, many screens are so easy that they assess for only gross levels of impairment and miss mild or subtler forms of impairment. Furthermore, like most cognitive and neuropsychological tests, brief screeners such as the Mini-Mental State Examination (MMSE; Folstein et al., 1975) are vulnerable to demographic factors such as age and educational level—factors that are not typically kept in mind when scores are interpreted.

RBANS (Randolph, 2008) is a neuropsychological screen that takes about 30 minutes to administer. It provides screening of attention, language, visuospatial/visuoconstructional skills, and verbal and nonverbal memory for ages 12–89. Although it was initially developed to serve as a core battery for the detection of dementia in older adults, it has been shown to be useful in many settings in which a neuropsychological screener can provide useful initial information about a client's cognitive status. There are four parallel forms to the test, allowing for serial testing using different items but with subtests equated in difficulty level. It serves as a good "bridge" between very short and gross measures of cognitive status (e.g., the MMSE) and a full comprehensive neuropsychological test battery.

CONSTRUCT VALIDITY OF THE RBANS
Internal Validity

Whereas the initial structure for the RBANS was developed based on theoretical relationships between tests of specific cognitive domains and the four overarching indices, studies have begun to examine the overall factor structure of the measure. Duff and colleagues (2006) found that two factors (verbal memory and visual processing) best fit the RBANS data in a sample of over 800 healthy older adults, with several subtests not fitting the two-factor solution. In an acute stroke sample, Wilde (2006) also identified two factors, although these were much broader than those identified by Duff and colleagues, with all verbally mediated subtests loading on a language/verbal memory factor and all visually mediated subtests loading on a visuospatial/visual memory factor. Garcia, Leahy, Corradi, and Forchetti (2008) found a three-factor solution (one factor specific to memory, one verbal factor, and one visuomotor factor) in a memory-impaired sample. Carlozzi, Horner, Yan, and Tilley (2008) analyzed data from a relatively small sample of veterans and identified a two-factor structure that generally represented a memory factor and a visuospatial factor. In a sample of over 600 patients referred for evaluation of dementia, Schmitt and colleagues (2010) identified a two-factor solution, with the first factor most strongly representing memory, and the second factor most strongly representing visuospatial and attention measures. The semantic fluency measure loaded on both factors. King, Bailie, Kinney, and Nitch (2012) examined the factor structure of use of the RBANS with 167 inpatients with schizophrenia and schizoaffective disorders and also identified the two factors of memory and visuomotor functioning; a higher-order factor of general neurocognitive functioning accounted for the most variance. Overall, the results of these various factor analyses suggest that there is little support for the proposed structure of the RBANS, but there is strong support for an overall memory factor and an overall visuospatial/visuomotor factor, particularly in samples of individuals for whom there is evidence of memory impairment.

External Validity

With regard to external validity, the RBANS has shown strong convergent and divergent validity relative to other, more comprehensive neuropsychological measures in a wide range of samples, including patients with acute stroke (Larson, Kirschner, Bode, Heinemann, & Goodman, 2005), individuals with severe traumatic brain injury (McKay, Casey, Wertheimer, & Fichtenberg, 2007; Pachet, 2007), and in mixed neurological patient samples (Gontkovsky, Hillary, & Scott, 2002). The RBANS has also shown strong correlations with measures of outcome, including return to work (Gold, Queern, Iannone, & Buchanan, 1999; Hobart, Goldberg, Bartko, & Gold, 1999), cognitive disability ratings (Larson et al., 2005), instrumental activities of daily living (IADL) ratings (Larson et al., 2005), and collateral reports of daily functioning (Freilich & Hyer, 2007; Hobson, Hall, Humphreys-Clark, Schrimsher, & O'Bryant, 2010) for patients with a wide variety of neurological and neurodegenerative conditions. Studies have also shown expected relationships of RBANS scores with functional and structural imaging findings in patients with Alzheimer's disease or stroke (Förster et al., 2010; Wilde, 2010).

The clinical utility of the RBANS has been demonstrated in the assessment of individuals with various neurological and neuropsychiatric conditions, including concussion and traumatic brain injury (Lippa, Hawes, Jokic, & Caroselli, 2013; McKay, Wertheimer, Fichtenberg, & Casey, 2008), psychotic disorders (Chianetta, Lefebvre, LeBlanc, & Grignon, 2008; Gogos, Joshua, & Rossell, 2010; Holzer et al., 2007; Iverson, Brooks, & Haley, 2009; Wilk et al., 2004), and diagnosis of mild cognitive impairment and dementia with varying etiologies (Beatty, Ryder, et al., 2003; Beglinger et al., 2010; Clark, Hobson, & O'Bryant, 2010; Duff, Beglinger, Theriault, Allison, & Paulsen, 2010; Duff, Hobson, Beglinger, & O'Bryant, 2010; Karantzoulis, Novitski, Gold, & Randolph, 2013; McDermott & DeFilippis, 2010; Morgan et al., 2010; Wagle et al., 2009, 2010).

The RBANS has also been shown to have utility in assessing change over time in response to treatment/surgical interventions/pharmacotherapy/rehabilitation in patients with cancer (Beglinger et al., 2007; Jansen, Cooper, Dodd, & Miaskowski, 2011), cardiovascular disease (Bauer et al., 2011; Takaiwa et al., 2009), psychosis (Bayless et al., 2010; Boggs et al., 2010), substance use and abuse (Green et al., 2010; Messinis et al., 2009; Schrimsher & Parker, 2008), obsessive–compulsive disorder (Csigo et al., 2010), general cognitive impairment (Smith et al., 2009), and Parkinson's disease (Rinehardt et al., 2010; Schoenberg et al., 2012), as well as in tracking recovery following stroke (Jorge, Acion, Moser, Adams, & Robinson, 2010) and delirium (Beglinger et al., 2011). Assessors interested in potentially using the RBANS with a specific clinical population or for a specific purpose can utilize these resources to examine the evidence for the value of the RBANS in those settings.

NEUROPSYCHOLOGICAL ASSESSMENT AND SCREENING IN DIVERSE GROUPS

As has been noted throughout this text, another important consideration for administration of any particular measure to a specific client is whether that measure is valid for use with that client. In the general realm of neuropsychological assessment, there has been mixed evidence for mean differences in diverse racial/ethnic groups on neuropsychological tests, with some researchers not finding any consistent differences (Manly & Jacobs, 2002) and other researchers documenting different mean scores on isolated tasks (e.g., Coffey, Marmol, Schock, & Adams, 2005; Fernandez & Marcopulos, 2008). However, as noted in previous chapters, finding mean differences between subgroups of people on tests is not, in itself, indicative of test bias. Some of these differences may reflect actual differences that are related to other factors (e.g., SES, educational level, physical and neurological health) that correlate with both race/ethnic status and with performance on neuropsychological tests (suggesting, in fact, that the mean score differences provide evidence for the construct validity of the test). What is necessary to determine whether neuropsychological tests are biased (i.e., inaccurate for some diverse groups) is to examine the literature on whether the measures show similar construct validity in those subgroups. For example, Siedlecki and colleagues (2010) identified an invariant factorial structure for a battery of neuropsychological tests that had been translated into Spanish and administered to Spanish speakers, relative to the factorial structure for the same battery administered in English to those fluent in English. Similarly, Mungas, Widamann, Reed, and Tomaszewski Farias (2011) found a common factorial structure for a battery of neuropsychological measures (both Spanish and English versions) administered to a large community-dwelling sample of African American, European American, English-speaking Hispanic, and Spanish-speaking Hispanic older adults. Data on the ability of neuropsychological measures to accurately diagnose neurological conditions, to be related to neuroimaging findings, and to predict real-world outcomes equally well in diverse groups are also important indicators for the lack of bias generally in neuropsychological instruments. Individuals interested in using specific neuropsychological tests in individuals from diverse backgrounds should carefully examine the empirical evidence for the validity of that test in individuals of similar backgrounds.

Of course, as with other tests reviewed in this text, one major issue in administration of neuropsychological tests to diverse clients is acculturation, particularly language fluency. However, as noted in Chapter 11, determining in which language it is appropriate to administer a test can be a very difficult task that requires careful thought. In addition, an assessor must be vigilant in determining the availability of good validity evidence for the translation of the test or tests prior to their use.

With regard to representativeness of neuropsychological normative data for particular clients, for any given neuropsychological test—especially for those that are not copyrighted or part of large copyrighted and published test batteries—there may be multiple independent samples of reasonable size that may or may not represent the client an assessor is evaluating and thus provide "normative" data. Books such as the previously mentioned compendiums (Lezak et al., 2012; Strauss et al., 2006), in addition to others (e.g., Mitrushina, Boone, Razani, & D'Ella, 2005), provide summaries of the normative data available for many neuropsychological tests. The assessor needs to make decisions about which set of normative data are most appropriate (along relevant cultural and demographic variables), given the client in question, as well as about the reliability (i.e., size) of the available sample.

Some researchers have provided race-specific norms for various neuropsychological measures (e.g., Lucas et al., 2005). However, it is extremely important that individuals act cautiously in the use of such norms, for many reasons (Gasquoine, 2009; Manly, 2005). First, as noted above and in previous chapters, simply finding mean differences between subgroups of people on tasks is not indicative of those scores being somehow inaccurate or biased; in fact, they may represent real group differences that have important implications for both diagnosis and prognosis. Second, with specific regard to prognosis, for many neuropsychological tests it may be best to use norms that are not corrected for any sociodemographic factor, if the assessment goal is to predict functioning on a universal task (Sherrill-Pattison, Donders, & Thompson, 2000; Silverberg & Millis, 2009). For example, research on predicting driving risk has shown that raw scores, without correction for age, are more related to driving outcomes than demographically corrected scores (Barrash et al., 2010).

Use of the RBANS with Diverse Groups

With regard to the RBANS specifically, the norms published in the manual were gathered from 690 12- to 89-year-olds in a stratified, nationally representative sample based on age, sex, race/ethnicity, educational level, and geographic region. The 20- to 89-year-old cohort included 90 people at each of six age groups, using the 1995 U.S. Census, and the 150 12- to 19-year-old members of the normative group were selected based on 2010 U.S. Census data (Randolph, 2008). A Spanish form available for the first two versions of the test has been validated only in the United States. There are also supplemental norms available for older adults (Beatty, Mold, & Gontkovsky, 2003; Duff et al., 2003) and for older African Americans specifically (Patton et al., 2003).

With regard to the use of the RBANS with diverse groups, Duff, Schoenberg, Mold, Scott, and Adams (2011) showed reliable gender effects in older adults on several of the subtests, consistent with known gender differences in cognitive abilities. The RBANS has also been examined for use in other countries, including China (Cheng et al., 2011; Lim, Collinson, Feng, & Ng, 2010), Spain (Muntal Encinas, Gramunt-Fombuena, Badenes Guia, Casas Harnanz, & Aguilar Barbera, 2012; Sanz, Vargas, & Marin, 2009); Australia (Green et al., 2008), Armenia (Azizian, Yeghiyan, Ishkhanyan, Manukyan, & Khandanyan, 2011), and in racial/ethnic subgroups within the United States (Johnson et al., 2011; O'Bryant, Falkowski, et al., 2011; O'Bryant, Hall, et al., 2011).

N = 1 VALIDITY ISSUES IN NEUROPSYCHOLOGICAL ASSESSMENT

An issue that arises more frequently with neuropsychological testing than with other types of psychological testing is the potential need to administer standardized tests in a nonstandardized fashion, due to testing individuals with various forms of sensory or motor impairment or disability or in less than optimal settings (e.g., at bedside). An assessor must make a conscious choice whether to administer no tests to individuals with such diverse presentations (and yet, it is likely decisions must still be made for this individual), or to administer the tests in a nonstandardized fashion and to consciously consider the effects of this nonstandardized administration on test interpretation and on overall conclusions drawn from the assessment. Given that an entire chapter of this text is devoted to the critical importance of assessing for noncredible reporting and behavior in all forms of assessment (see Chapter 4), here I only briefly review of some of the major domains of noncredible responding seen in neuropsychological referrals and mention some of the most validated procedures. In addition, a short discussion of the Effort Index in the RBANS is provided.

As noted in Chapter 4, malingered cognitive impairments occur with high base rates, and, as a consequence, researchers have attempted to outline specific diagnostic criteria for the malingering of neuropsychological impairment (Slick, Sherman, & Iverson, 1999), including evidence from formal tests of noncredible report and responding. Cutoffs and patterns of performance on existing neuropsychological tests have been identified as relatively specific to malingering/noncredible behavior in cognitive domains, including learning and memory, attention, visuospatial/visuoconstructional skills, motor speed, psychomotor processing, and abstract reasoning (Larrabee, 2007; Strauss et al., 2006). Of course, because neuropsychological assessment includes psychological assessment, noncredible symptom report is also highly relevant to neuropsychological evaluation (see Chapter 4). As indicated in consensus statements regarding the use of measures of noncredible responding in neuropsychological assessment (Heilbronner et al., 2009), consideration can also be given to inconsistencies between data obtained from formal tests and evidence from records and behavioral observation, as well as inconsistencies with what is known about the potential illness or injury that is alleged in the particular evaluation. Neuropsychologists also agree that it is best to use multiple validity measures covering multiple domains throughout an entire evaluation, with particular focus on validity measures that were developed to assess skills germane to the current evaluation (Heilbronner et al., 2009). As with any neuropsychological measures, an assessor should examine the evidence for the utility of specific measures of noncredible functioning prior to their use. The most important data will indicate the specificity of that measure in relation to noncredible functioning, given the diagnoses in question in a particular evaluation.

Assessment of Noncredible Responding on the RBANS

With regard to the RBANS, Silverberg, Wertheimer, and Fichtenberg (2007) created an Effort Index for the RBANS based on unusually low scores on two of the subtests (Digit Span, List Recognition) across a large outpatient clinical sample. Their initial data showed good accuracy in discriminating individuals likely malingering cognitive impairment from individuals with documented traumatic brain injury. Novitski, Steele, Karantzoulis, and Randolph (2012) created a variation of the scale and showed better specificity of their variant scale relative to a comparison group of individuals with amnesia, but no further analyses have been conducted with this variation. Young, Baughman, and Roper (2012) found that the original Effort Index had strong specificity but more limited sensitivity in a nongeriatric veteran sample. Duff, Spering, and colleagues (2011) showed good specificity of the original Effort Index in older adults who were cognitively intact or who had only mild cognitive impairment, but high false-positive rates for nursing home patients and older adults with more severe Alzheimer's disease, consistent with findings from Hook, Marquine, and Hoelzle (2009). Interestingly, with regard to use of the Effort Index as a prognostic rather than diagnostic tool, Moore and colleagues (2013) showed that the original Effort Index was related to the attendance of patients with schizophrenia in group therapy.

DECISION-MAKING ISSUES IN NEUROPSYCHOLOGICAL ASSESSMENT

While the assessment decisions that plague all testing certainly apply in neuropsychological testing, some are more unique to the neuropsychological setting. The following sections review important decision-making issues relevant to neuropsychological assessment, including issues discussed more comprehensively in previous chapters (including cognitive complexity of tests, definitions of impairment, and base rates of abnormal scores and discrepancies; see Chapters 10 and 11), but also issues more unique to neuropsychological assessment (including psychometric skew and its effects on score interpretation, lack of co-normed data, serial testing and reliable change, and the faulty logic sometimes seen by assessors who are examining brain–behavior relationships).

Complexity of Measures

Many neuropsychologists use the subtests of intellectual tests (see Chapter 11) as measures of neuropsychological skills. An important point to make is that the subtests selected as part of most intelligence tests are those that show the strongest relationship to general intelligence (i.e., *g*) and thus are naturally cognitively complex, often assessing more than one cognitive construct. Although this is a good trait for a test designed to capture variance in intelligence, it is not such a good trait for the purpose of creating more specific and focused cognitive and neuropsychological measures. In addition, as pointed out in the previous chapter, the internal consistencies of various subtests on intelligence tests are not high enough for clinical decision making, although many of them are high enough for hypothesis generation. Therefore, particularly in a case where a client shows unexpected and unusual variability on subtests of an intelligence test, in a pattern consistent with a known neuropsychological condition or disorder (or known area of brain dysfunction) and consistent with other test and nontest data, the subtests of the intelligence test may be informative in that particular neuropsychological assessment.

It is also true that, although neuropsychological measures that are specifically designed to assess focal cognitive domains are less likely to be cognitively complex, they nonetheless often involve several cognitive abilities and also tend to show moderate relationships with general intelligence; therefore, measures of intelligence (including premorbid intelligence; see Chapter 11) remain important cores to comprehensive neuropsychological assessment to aid in the interpretation of neuropsychological test findings. In addition, because neuropsychological measures are cognitively complex, an assessor needs to measure each important area of neuropsychological functioning with more than one instrument and needs to consider the overall pattern of test performances (and integrate these date together with nontest data) before interpreting any one neuropsychological test score as indicative of a specific cognitive impairment.

What Is Impairment?

Lezak and colleagues (2012) suggest that an assessor can use two methods of determining impairment on neuropsychological tests. One method is by looking at normative scores (i.e., comparing a client to an appropriate comparison group); as noted in previous chapters, cutoffs for determining that a score is impaired vary greatly in assessment, from cutoffs that still include a relatively large percent of a normative sample (such as a 1 *SD* cutoff, which falls at the 16th percentile) to much more conservative cutoffs for impairment (such as 1.5 or even 2 *SD* from the mean).

Another method advocated by Lezak and colleagues (2012) is less direct and involves comparing a client's scores to what the assessor would expect, given the client's premorbid abilities. Not only is such a determination problematic due to difficulties in estimating premorbid abilities and in identifying, with precision, what scores should be in specific cognitive domains based on estimated premorbid abilities (see Chapter 11), but this method also does not account for natural variability in scores that are of high base rate in the general population. Furthermore, it does not consider the issue of test skew, which is also very common in neuropsychological assessment.

Estimating Premorbid Abilities

As noted in Chapter 11, estimating premorbid intellect is a complex and difficult assessment task, and cannot be done by using merely the highest subscale score obtained by an individual. As an example, consider the following case: A 25-year-old male was being seen for a reevaluation because he was seeking extended time accommodations on the GRE, which were denied to him on the basis of a prior evaluation that was conducted during his senior year of college. At that time, he had sought an evaluation through his college counseling center and was granted extended time accommodations during his senior year due to a "processing speed disability secondary to a mild head injury" (note that the head injury in question was a concussion that reportedly occurred during his 10th-grade year in high school). Review of the prior evaluation showed that his WAIS-IV index scores all fell in the average to high-average range. The broad range of his WAIS-IV subtests scores included scores that mostly fell in the average to high-average range, but with one score (Vocabulary) falling in the superior range, and one score (Coding) falling in the low-average range. The prior examiner interpreted the vocabulary score as indicating that the young man had "superior" intellect, whereas the one low-average score was interpreted as "significantly discrepant from" his "superior" intellect and indicative of impairment on this basis. In addition, his "superior" intellect was used as the interpretive point for all other neuropsychological measures administered (some of which, due to their psychometric properties, did not assess the above-average range in performance; see below). All other data about this young man—including his performance on yearly proficiency tests, high-stakes testing during his postinjury high school years (ACT, SAT), his performance on neuropsychological tasks, and his high school and college grades—were consistent with the average to high-average intellect suggested by his overall WAIS-IV protocol and inconsistent with any impairment associated with his concussion in 10th grade. This case illustrates many decision-making errors on the part of the prior evaluator, in addition to mistakes in trying to estimate the young man's general level of functioning prior to the mild head injury.

Base Rates Revisited

Base Rates for Impaired Scores

Chapter 11 provided extensive coverage of the issue of base rates for "impaired scores" or for discrepant scores when considering the number of scores that have been generated within any particular test battery. Binder, Iverson, and Brooks (2009) provide a review of various factors that have been shown to be related to the likely number of "impaired" scores that might appear in a neuropsychological assessment. One factor, of course, is the mere number of tests given/discrepancies calculated. Another factor (as noted above) is the definition of "impairment" used by the assessor (i.e., what percentile is considered an impaired score). For example, Brooks, Iverson, Holdnack, and Feldman (2008) examined data from the Wechsler Memory Scale–III (Wechsler, 1997) battery in 550 healthy adults ages 55–87 years old. The scores compared included eight subscale scores and four index scores. In this sample, it was very common for healthy older adults to have up to three scores that fell less than or equal to 1 *SD* below the mean (the 16th percentile cutoff mentioned above), and was also very common for individuals to have at least one score that fell at 1.5 *SD* below the mean. With regard to score variability and discrepancies, Donnell and colleagues (2011) found that 67% of a sample of over 4,000 healthy participants showed discrepancies of 3 or more *SD* between their highest and lowest test scores in a battery of 21 neuropsychological measures.

On the RBANS, it is recommended that assessors use 80 as the cutoff for "normal" scores, which falls at the 16th percentile, with subtest scores of 7 or lower considered abnormal. Crawford, Garthwaite, Morrice, and Duff (2012) provided data on the number of abnormally low index scores that might be expected based on the normative data for the RBANS; these data should be useful to assessors who are carefully considering how to interpret an isolated "low" score on this measure.

As previously discussed, the reliabilities of the test scores themselves are also important factors in determining the likely number of impaired scores or "significant" score discrepancies in any given battery. Binder and colleagues (2009) provided the example of subtests from the Delis–Kaplan Executive Functioning System (DKEFS; Delis, Kaplan, & Kramer, 2001), which have lower reliabilities relative to many other neuropsychological measures. With over 100 possible scores to be calculated and many discrepancy scores to compare on this battery of tests, these lower reliabilities are particularly problematic.

Other factors to consider with regard to the base rates for impaired scores or "unusual" discrepancies in neuropsychological assessment are potential effects of the general ability of the person (i.e., his or her general intellect) and of sociodemographic factors (e.g., education). Some researchers have documented that individuals with extreme levels of intellect and education are more likely to have high variability in overall test scores and thus show more discrepancies when test scores are compared to one another (Brooks et al., 2008, 2011). Donnell and colleagues (2011) showed that this high variability is true of neuropsychological measures as well, as they are even less correlated with general intelligence (as compared to subtests of intelligence tests); scores on tests that are less correlated with intellect will show larger regression to the mean in comparison to intellectual disability for individuals with extremely high or extremely low IQ scores.

With regard to the RBANS, Randolph (1998) published base rates for index discrepancies (when considered in isolation). In addition, Patton and colleagues (2006) published base rates for index discrepancies in a large sample of community-dwelling older adults. Duff, Patton, and colleagues (2011) recently provided base-rate data for the 14 pairwise discrepancies among the RBANS subtests, based on data from over 700 community-dwelling older adults. These base rates were organized by general level of cognitive ability (based on RBANS total score). However, these data do not account for the number of comparisons (i.e., the percentages provided are based on each discrepancy considered in isolation). Crawford, Garthwaite, Morrice, and colleagues (2012) also published base rates of discrepancy scores on the RBANS, taking into account the number of comparisons being made.

The bottom line is that performance in the normal range on all measures in a large test battery is not necessary for an assessor to consider the overall test results as normal. In fact, what these studies show is that the likelihood of a cognitively healthy individual performing in the *normal* range on all cognitive and neuropsychological tests administered in a comprehensive battery is actually quite low! All of the factors above (as well as consideration of any "statistically abnormal" scores in the context of the rest of the assessment data) need to be considered when an assessor integrates all test and nontest data in the final stages of assessment (see Chapter 13).

Base Rates for Neurological Disorders

An assessor also needs to consider the base rates of the disorder in question when interpreting test scores. In the general population, base rates for neurological conditions are low, so most positive scores on a battery of tests will be false positives. If an assessor is working in a neurological setting, the rates of the disorder in question *may* be higher, meaning that it is less likely that a positive score in a battery of tests is a false positive. However, an assessor still needs to consider the individual case in making that determination. Given that individuals are more likely to refer themselves for "diagnosis" for some conditions, they may well present to specialty clinics where the base rates of the disorder in that setting should not necessarily be applied to that individual.

Psychometric Properties of Neuropsychological Tests

When tests are designed so that most people succeed on most items, then test scores are compressed into just a few values at the upper extent of the score range, leaving little variability of scores in the normal and high normal range. As noted in Chapter 11, this low level of variability can occur on achievement tests, depending on the area of academic achievement and the age or grade level of the individual being assessed. In the neuropsychological realm, list learning and recall tests, confrontational naming tests, and tasks assessing psychomotor speed are great examples of tests that are highly skewed in their score distributions.

There are several implications of a truncated range of scores. First, scores with a small amount of variability will have lower reliabilities and thus require larger confidence intervals for their valid interpretation. Second, when a client receives well above-average scores on a measure of intelligence (which has a normal distribution), but does not score above average on other neuropsychological measures for which it is *impossible* to score higher than just "average," due to the skewed distribution, this discrepancy in scores does not indicate a "relative impairment" in the client but is a natural consequence of the test score distribution. Finally, when a test generally has a tight range of scores but a "tail" of more extreme scores, the weight of those extreme scores becomes exaggerated by the small standard deviation of the distribution of scores. This exaggerated weight can make slightly abnormal scores seem very abnormal (Donnell et al., 2011), which also has implications for comparing scores across different tests.

Availability of Co-Normed Data

There are some neuropsychological tests and test batteries that have co-normed scores across measures of a wide variety of constructs (e.g., the Neuropsychological Assessment Battery; Stern & White, 2003). However, when neuropsychologists use a flexible battery and select tests that have norms from different samples, it can be more difficult to compare scores across the different tests, due to potential differences in the normative samples of the tests being used and differences in the types of standard scores being reported for the various tests. Some researchers have suggested converting all scores to z-scores in order to compare them to one another, but this "solution" does not adequately address the problem. Of course, even in the case of co-normed data, the problem of skewed distributions of scores (as discussed above) can lead to inaccurate standard scores being compared to one another. Donnell and colleagues (2011) suggest using percentile ranks to compare scores across tests, but an assessor must also continue to consider the normative sample(s) being used to interpret clients' performances on each individual test across a flexible battery.

Assessing for Reliable Change

A common issue to address in neuropsychology is whether there is evidence of change over time. Evidence of decline over time might be diagnostic (e.g., in a degenerative dementia); evidence of improvement over time might help to document treatment response or natural recovery from an acute injury or illness. When a neuropsychologist reevaluates a client who has undergone prior testing, he or she must remember that, even in tests that show relative test–retest reliability over time, there is still error in the score due to measurement error in the test and transient variability in patient functioning over time (due to factors such as fatigue, arousal, alertness, orientation, mood, effort).

To know whether differences in scores across two administrations reflect real change over time, an assessor needs to access data that reflect what the likely retest score would be if there were no real change in functioning. This process includes examining the internal consistency of the measure being administered, the test–retest reliability data (with consideration of the time interval for those data), and evidence of practice effects. For example, a learning and memory test that does not have a parallel form is likely to show very large practice effects over a short duration of time in intact individuals. McCaffrey, Duff, and Westervelt (2000) provide data from various papers on control samples and patients diagnosed with various conditions as result of repeated testing at different time intervals.

Unfortunately, there is no clear evidence that there is a lack of a practice effect after some time period, meaning that there may still be a need to consider practice effects even if the reevaluation occurs several months later (well past the known practice effects findings for the test). As an example, I once overheard an older couple on their way up a stairway "practicing" verbal fluency and also rehearsing the story from Form A of the RBANS; this couple had participated in a dementia screening study about 18 months prior and were returning to participate in a rescreening. While they were likely surprised when Form B was administered, meaning that their practice of Form A's story did them no good, clearly there was test sophistication (practicing fluency tasks, knowing they would need to recall a story at an immediate and delayed time period) that might have led to changes in performance due to practice effects. There is also some suggestion that practice effects may stabilize over many repeated administrations in a brief time period (Falleti, Maruff, Collie, & Barby, 2006). I am reminded of a training rotation on a liver transplant unit where the nursing staff apparently administered the Trail Making Test every time they conducted a mental status exam (about every hour of the day), resulting in patients' practically drawing of the proper dot connection patterns with their eyes closed.

In addition, the assessor needs to consider whether the measure has floor or ceiling effects (i.e., can change even be seen on the measure?) and whether premorbid functioning level or even current level of cognitive impairment might impact the ability of the test to show real change. Regression to the mean (extreme scores tend to revert toward the mean at readministration) is a statistical artifact, but will affect the ability to determine real change over time in individuals with extreme scores at Time 1. In addition, tests with more measurement error generally (i.e., less reliability) have more regression to the mean. There is also no clear evidence that any particular type of neuropsychological impairment would lead to a lack of a practice effect. For example, would individuals with severe memory problems not show an expected practice effect on a learning and memory test? As noted by Heilbronner and colleagues (2010), it is possible that seeing no change between Time 1 and Time 2 testing obscures real evidence of decline, due to practice effect, and it is also possible that lack of a practice effect when you would expect to see one could indicate memory impairment.

Furthermore, the assessor needs to consider base rates for change. If the assessor is comparing a huge battery of repeated tests and finds reliable changes on only one of these comparisons, this may well be in the likelihood of a "normal" finding. It would be more powerful to see the same pattern of change across multiple test scores of the same construct before an assessor could conclude with confidence that a client's ability in a certain domain had either improved or declined.

With regard to the RBANS, there are four parallel forms of the test, making it potentially valuable for use in serial evaluation (or when a client has been seen recently by someone else using the same instrument and the assessor wishes to minimize practice effects). The internal consistency reliabilities for the indices are mostly .8, which is good for hypothesis testing, whereas reliability of the subtests tends to be a bit lower (and it should be noted that several subtests actually use test–retest reliability data, as internal consistency data are not available, given the nature of the measures). Test–retest reliability data for adolescents (with a 14- to 31-day delay between testing) were .63–.85, and reliability data from adults (tested with a 33- to 43-week delay between testing) were .55–.88, with practice effects on index scores ranging from increases of 1.4 to 8.1 points (with the exception of the Language Index, which showed a decline of almost 2 points); as would be expected, there were higher practice effects on memory measures (Randolph, 1998). In addition, Duff and colleagues (2005) examined test–retest reliability for slightly over a year, on average, in a large community-dwelling older-adult sample. The reliability data were quite similar to that reported over a much shorter time interval in the RBANS manual (ranging from .58 to .83). Practice effects were generally not seen over this longer delay, although the Language Index also showed a decline consistent with that reported in the RBANS manual over a shorter time period. In general, Immediate and Delayed Memory Indices were the only ones to show some practice effect in a small percent of their sample. Patton and colleagues (2005) provide base rates for changes over time in RBANS scores over both 1-year and 2-year intervals for almost 300 community-dwelling older adults.

Faulty Logic

One of the largest contributors to diagnostic error when individuals administer neuropsychological tests but do not conduct appropriate assessment is the faulty logic of applying what is known about brain–behavior relationships to a sample of behavior when there are no other findings suggesting a brain implication. Miller (1983) noted that, because there is ample empirical evidence that damage to certain brain regions will cause specific types of neuropsychological impairment, it can be tempting for assessors who see low performance on a neuropsychological measure of that particular construct to conclude that the client being assessed has damage to that particular area of the brain. For example, as noted early in this chapter, it is known that mesial temporal damage (particularly to the hippocampus) leads to impaired learning and recall of new information (anterograde declarative memory impairment). However, just because a client performs poorly on a measure of learning and recall does not mean that he or she has dysfunction of the hippocampus. There are myriad reasons that an individual may perform poorly on a learning and memory task, including, but not limited to, poor attention, poor hearing, lack of fluency in the language of the task (all leading to poor input), or noncredible behavior or aphasia (all leading to poor output). Neuropsychological tasks are cognitively complex and can be affected by many non-neurological factors. Interpreting neuropsychological tests correctly does require additional neuroscientific knowledge about brain–behavior relationships, but also requires the psychological skills and good decision-making needed in assessment generally.

13

Putting the Data Together
Empirically Guided Integration
of Assessment Information

It is of the highest importance in the art of detection to be able to recognize, out of a number of facts, which are incidental and which vital. Otherwise your energy and attention must be dissipated instead of being concentrated.
—SHERLOCK HOLMES, in *The Reigate Squires*

The process of putting all the information together to reach decisions is the most difficult part of an assessment, and one that combines the science outlined in all previous chapters with the "art" of the assessor. This chapter reviews statistical versus clinical approaches to decision making in assessment (first discussed in Chapter 2). Then an empirically informed approach to integration of assessment data is presented, with a case example to illustrate the various stages of the approach.

STATISTICAL APPROACHES TO DECISION MAKING

In a statistical approach to decision making, information is combined using mechanical processes that (in theory) require little, if any, subjective interpretation, with great reliability across decision makers. Ideally the process and the formulas used arise from the empirical literature (e.g., the known sensitivity and specificity of particular test scores for the decision being made). In a statistically guided decision-making approach (Bell & Mellor, 2009; Millis, 2009), an assessor starts with the base rate that a particular client has disorder X (the pretest odds). Knowing no other information about the client, the base rate of a disorder can be used to generate the odds that a client has the disorder: odds = probability/(1 − probability). For example, if disorder X occurred with 50% base rate, then the odds of the client having the disorder are .50/(1 − .50) = 1. The assessor can then determine whether the client falls above the cutoff score from a measure with known sensitivity/specificity for disorder X to calculate a likelihood ratio, using the formula sensitivity/(1 − specificity). For example, perhaps the assessor has a screening measure for disorder X with 80% specificity and 60% specificity. Using the above formula, this generates a likelihood ratio of 2. The posttest odds that this client has disorder X is calculated as (pretest odds) × (posttest odds); in this case, 1 × 2 = 2. To convert the posttest odds to a posttest probability, the assessor can use the following calculation: probability = odds/(1 + odds). In this case, the probability is 2/(1 + 2), which is about 67%. Thus, because the client was positive on the screener, the odds that the client has disorder X have moved from 50 to 67%. What if the available test score had lower specificity (as many screening tests do)? Assuming the screening test had only 40% specificity, using the calculations above, the posttest probability that the client had disorder X would only be 57%, with little improvement over the pretest prediction. If there are more known predictors available, these steps can be repeated, with the posttest probabilities converted back into the posttest odds to be used in the next set of calculations.

Although this method sounds reassuringly clear-cut and highly appealing to the empirically minded assessor, there are many difficulties in using even this simple statistical method to aid decision making in assessment. First, to calculate the pretest odds, the assessor needs to know the base rate of disorder X for the client in question. Any individual-level data about a person (age, gender, racial/ethnic status, education) and data about the specific setting in which the assessment is taking place (inpatient clinic, outpatient clinic, forensic evaluation) may affect the prior probability of a certain disorder, making it more or less likely than the overall population prevalence. So determining the pretest odds can be difficult and even in the best of circumstances requires some subjective judgment.

In addition, when there are multiple tests that could be used to determine posttest probabilities, decisions must be made about which test or tests to use. In order to increase accuracy in judgment, the tests need to be conditionally independent (i.e., not correlated with one another once the disease status is taken into account). Frequently, data from psychological tests are not conditionally independent because they measure similar things. It is highly unlikely, given the lack of specificity of many symptoms and complaints (and test scores) in psychological assessment and the high overlap in psychological constructs, that such conditional independence could occur.

Third, even a decision to use only one available test score can be difficult, given currently available data on accuracy of diagnostic prediction for psychological tests. As Bell and Mellor (2009) emphasized, suitable statistical formulae or actuarial tables do not exist or are not sufficiently developed in many fields of psychological judgment. A particular problem is lack of specificity data in differential diagnosis; most available data distinguish presence/absence of certain disorders rather than different disorders from one another. Therefore, it is rare to have findings from even one potential predictor to enter into this statistical decision-making method.

A related problem is that use of statistical decision making requires that the decision is a binary one ("Does the client have disorder X or not?"). In the realities of clinical practice, there are usually multiple decisions an assessor is making, multiple hypotheses that must be compared and contrasted to one another. In addition, those multiple hypotheses are often not mutually exclusive; that is, a client may have more than one condition or have more than one contributing factor to his or her presenting concerns.

Yet another problem occurs even when a statistical formula can be developed to assist an assessor in making a decision. There are always individuals who fall "close" to the cutoffs on the scale (or scales) used in such procedures. What about a client who is 1 point from the cutoff of being called "positive" or "negative" on a scale? A categorical approach (that doesn't account for confidence intervals) can lead to error for individuals near the cut point. Although there has been more emphasis on publishing odds ratios across a series of cut points for measures, to allow assessors to weight the confidence with which conclusions can be drawn, it is still rare to find those data in the literature.

A final problem for many statistical formulae is that they do not take into account nontest data (beyond perhaps that represented by demographics and clinical setting to determine pretest odds). In order to truly integrate assessment data, an assessor should look for convergence across *all* sources of data, not just test scores, and with consideration of the validity of both the test and nontest data. In the real world of assessment, the available data may be not only somewhat invalid but also inconsistent or incomplete. As yet, there are no clear no evidence-based guidelines on how to integrate all assessment data in this manner. For this reason it is pretty safe to predict that computers will not replace human assessors just yet in making decisions about clinical data.

CLINICAL APPROACHES TO DECISION MAKING

As Bell and Mellor (2009) noted, clinical and statistical approaches do not differ in the types of data gathered, the setting in which clinical decisions are made, or the methods by which data are collected (interview, tests, records review, collateral report). The main distinction between a clinical and statistical decision-making approach is in how the data are integrated. Clinical approaches may be more appropriate when the explicit prediction rules are not available or when relevant data in a particular case are not part of the existing statistical models (Bell & Mellor, 2009). Although some argue that assessors cannot use both approaches simultaneously, because they may lead to contradictory conclusions (Grove et al., 2000), use of both (when available) may help clarify uncertainty. Spengler (2013) summarized data from two meta-analyses that showed that, although the effect sizes for mechanical/statistical decision making were reliably stronger than those of clinical decision making, the effect was small at best when looking across a range of decisions (Grove et al., 2000) and even smaller when looking specifically at psychological prediction (effect sizes ranged from -0.12 to -0.16; Aegisdottir et al., 2006).

Clinical judgments involve idiographic multifaceted multidimensional conceptualizations of unique individuals. The assessor is needed to determine which information about the individual is relevant in considering the prior probabilities for each of the many hypotheses generated during the evaluation. The assessor is needed to determine what data to gather, and whether that data are valid for interpretation, to assist in determining the postevaluation odds that a client does or does not have a disorder in question (and whether other nondiagnostic factors are relevant to the presenting problem). During this integration, the assessor needs to remember that no single finding from one test (or one other source of data) should be given as much weight as the results that emphasize consistency across test and nontest data. These various judgments are dependent on the assessor's knowledge of the underlying science of psychopathology (see Chapter 3), on his or her knowledge of the assessment literature on the psychometrics of various instruments (see Chapters 5, 6, and 9–12), as well as on his or her clinical skills in gathering both test and nontest data (see Chapters 7 and 8) and judging their validity for integration in the $N = 1$ case (Chapter 4). However, the clinical decision-making approach can be empirically informed and subject to conscious and deliberate deductive reasoning processes (see Chapter 2). As noted in Chapter 7, if an assessor holds him- or herself accountable for the decision-making procedures he or she uses, decision-making accuracy can be improved (Brtek & Motavildo, 2002). The following sections provide an outline of a recommended, empirically informed approach to the integration of assessment information.

A RECOMMENDED METHOD FOR EMPIRICALLY INFORMED INTEGRATION OF ASSESSMENT DATA

Step 1: Restate All Hypotheses

The assessor should start with a conscious process of restating all the major problems and concerns the client presented with and all the potential contributory factors (diagnoses and/or explanatory factors that may not lead to diagnoses), which should serve as the list of potential hypotheses. Doing so will help the assessor resist representativeness bias and availability bias (see Chapter 2), and force him or her to review what is known from developmental biopsychosocial research to potentially explain the symptoms and problems the client is experiencing (see Chapter 3). The assessor should always remember to include the hypotheses of "no diagnosis" and "noncredible presentation," given their high base rates. Of course at this point in an evaluation, an assessor may have already "ruled out" certain hypotheses or already feel that the weight of the evidence "rules in" certain other hypotheses, but, as these decisions were likely based primarily on unconscious reasoning processes (see Chapter 2), it is in the assessor's best interest to deliberately and consciously review each hypothesis that was under consideration at any point during the assessment.

For example, consider a typical referral question that I see in my practice: young adults in their first years of college who are convinced that they have ADHD. The typical behavioral problem encountered by these students is that they are (or perceive themselves to be) receiving poor grades in college, or that they have to work too hard to receive the grades they expect to receive. Some of the many known contributing factors to poor grades include:

1. ADHD.
2. Learning disability (LD).
3. General cognitive ability that would predict increasing academic struggles as courses get harder.
4. Poor study habits.
5. Lack of readiness for college level work (i.e., poor preparation in high school).
6. Contributions from substance misuse.

7. Poor daily habits related to sleeping and eating that might contribute to less than adequate cognitive functioning.
8. Psychological adjustment to college or psychological disorders in which a primary symptom is "poor attention."
9. Undiagnosed neurological condition that might be related to the primary symptoms and complaints.
10. Noncredible presentation, often for the purpose of obtaining stimulant medications and/or academic accommodations.

So there are at least 10 (nonmutually exclusive) hypotheses for the assessor to consider as potential contributors to this common, young-adult complaint.

Step 2: Consider Baseline Likelihood of Each Hypothesis

The assessor should take each hypothesis generated in Step 1 and consider the likelihood that each is true (keeping in mind that more than one hypothesis may be true; in the real world decisions are not orthogonal). It may be difficult to generate actual base rates for some hypotheses, but there should still be enough available data to determine whether each hypothesis is more or less likely to be true.

Base rates of ADHD vary in college students, but are certainly less than 4% (American Psychiatric Association, 2013). Similarly, base rates for learning disorders (particularly if never diagnosed before) are very low in this population. Base rates for general cognitive ability that might make college difficult are hard to pinpoint, but certainly given the wide range of cognitive abilities in the general population and the increasing number of students who at least start college, it is plausible that a student may not have the cognitive skills necessary to easily succeed in the college environment. The likelihood of this hypothesis may also depend on the admission policies of the university in question. Hypothesis 4 (poor study habits) does occur with high base rates in college students (Babcock & Marks, 2011). Recent data also suggest that lack of readiness for college-level work is a high base-rate hypothesis. Estimates suggest that fewer than half of students who graduate from high school have the bare minimum qualifications to even apply to college (Greene & Foster, 2003). Data from the ACT suggest that only 25% of students taking the ACT score in a way suggesting readiness for entry-level college courses (ACT, Inc., 2007). Again, the likelihood for this to be a supported hypothesis may depend on the admission requirements of the school in question.

Another high base-rate hypothesis is substance misuse. Rates of substance misuse on college campuses are extremely high (U.S. Department of Health and Human Services, 2013). Similarly, rates of poor daily habits that might contribute to academic failure are also high (e.g., poor sleep) (Gaultney, 2010). Rates of psychological adjustment/disorders (Hypothesis 8) are high in college samples (Hunt & Eisenberg, 2010; Gallagher, 2010). On the other hand, rates of undiagnosed neurological conditions (Hypothesis 9) are likely low in a healthy young sample. Finally, rates of noncredible performance (Hypothesis 10) in college students presenting with concerns about ADHD are high, ranging from 10 to over 40% (Harrison & Edwards, 2010; Marshall et al., 2010; Pella, Hill, Shelton, Elliott, & Gouvier, 2012; Sullivan, May, & Galbally, 2007; Suhr, Hammers, Dobbin-Buckland, Zimak, & Hughes, 2008). Thus, there are many more likely hypotheses to consider than that the individual in question has ADHD.

	Base rate
ADHD:	Low
LD:	Low
Low cog.:	Low
Study skills:	High
College readiness:	Medium to high
Substance use:	High
Daily habits:	High
Psych. issues:	Medium to high
Neuro. condition:	Low
Noncredible:	Medium

Step 3: Consider the Constructs Underlying Each Hypothesis

The assessor should step back and consciously and deliberately review what evidence is actually needed to support each and every hypothesis. For example, evidence for a diagnosis of ADHD would include clear evidence of a developmental course, clear evidence of impairment in multiple settings (not just academic), and a clear set of symptoms, together with ruling out many other explanatory factors (which are some of the alternative hypotheses listed above). Similarly, evidence for a learning disorder diagnosis should show clear evidence of developmental impairment in an area of academic functioning (not just poor college grades) and rule out many other explanatory factors.

Step 4: Consider Evidence for/against Each Hypothesis

The assessor should then work to consider and build the evidence to both confirm and disconfirm each hypothesis. This deductive reasoning step involves the conscious and deliberate consideration of the weight of evidence with regard to all hypotheses under consideration (see Chapter 2). For each piece of evidence, the assessor needs to decide:

1. How well it fits each hypothesis under consideration.
2. Validity of the piece of evidence in the $N = 1$ setting.
3. Its use in disconfirming (or confirming) other hypotheses.

The assessor needs to remember that there will be much overlap, in that pieces of evidence may support or disconfirm many of the hypotheses. Not only must the assessor keep in mind all potential data that represent the construct(s) underlying each hypothesis, but also that data may represent more than one construct. The assessor also needs to remember that absent findings may well constitute disconfirming evidence for some hypotheses.

Evidence from Self-Report

In the interview, "hypothetical student" (HS) reported difficulty with paying attention in class lectures or when studying, and indicated that he can't concentrate for more than an hour at a time on readings for his courses. He described having this difficulty "all his life." Upon further questioning, he endorsed an adequate number of symptoms to meet (symptom) criteria for ADHD, predominantly inattentive type. In terms of the consequences of his reported symptoms, he stated that he is currently on academic probation due to getting a couple of F grades in the past two semesters (both math classes). He recalled that he "sometimes" got in trouble in elementary and middle school for talking out of turn in class and he reported "terrible" grades in high school because he "didn't try" and "didn't care." He denied taking any honors or AP courses and reported his ACT score as 19. He denied any history of or current behavioral problems but called himself a "space cadet" who forgets everything unless others remind him. He also reported that he waits until "the last minute" to do his homework, complete readings for his courses, write papers, or study for tests. By his report, he crams the night before exams, starting the evening before and studying up to the test time (missing other classes if necessary). He blamed his "ADHD" for his study habits. He estimated that he misses about 40% of his morning classes due to these study habits (as well as his general habit of staying up until 2:00 or 3:00 in the morning to play videogames and sleeping until at least 11:00 A.M.). He reported that he "knows" he has ADHD because he took a couple of stimulants to help him stay up and study for really important exams and found that they helped him concentrate. In fact, he reported that his home physician diagnosed him with ADHD over the winter break and gave him samples of Ritalin so that he could have some to use; he indicated that he sought the evaluation because the local college health center would not renew his prescription without a thorough evaluation, despite his prior diagnosis. He denied psychological problems or any history of psychological treatment, although he acknowledged feeling a little worried and down about his academic probation and fearful that he would be dismissed from college. He denied health problems except for seasonal allergies and a concussion received in high school (during a football game, with a loss of consciousness for about 10 minutes, a negative computed tomography (CT) scan, headaches for a week, but no permanent consequences). He also noted having a lot more headaches recently, especially while reading, and wondered if he needs glasses. He reported that he started drinking in high school and drinks socially; when pressed, he indicated that he typically drinks three nights per week, and at least one of those nights he is likely to drink to black out. By his report, he usually does not rise before 1:00 or 2:00 P.M. on weekends due to being out very late drinking the night before.

HS was also administered some self-report questionnaires. He completed a self-report checklist, the Conners' Adult ADHD Rating Scale—Long Form (CAARS; Conners et al., 1998). Although he scored high on the CAARS DSM-IV ADHD scale for Inattentive Symptoms and Total ADHD symptoms, his T-scores were above 90, which the CAARS manual indicates should be considered potential symptom overreport. He also scored significantly above the cutoff on a new indictor of infrequently endorsed symptoms on the CAARS (Suhr et al., 2011). These responses call into question the validity of his self-report of symptoms during interview (as well as any interpretation of the data from this self-report questionnaire). HS was also administered the MMPI-2-RF (Ben-Porath & Tellegen, 2011). He scored high on RBS, NUC, COG, NFC, STW, and SUB. RBS has been shown to be related to failure on measures of noncredible performance (Gervais, Ben-Porath, Wygant, & Green, 2007), and NUC and COG are also both vulnerable to overreporting of symptoms (Bolinger, Reese, Suhr, & Larrabee, 2014). Therefore, his scores on the MMPI-2-RF also call into question the validity of his self-reported cognitive symptoms.

To summarize evidence from HS's self-report, although he reported symptoms consistent with the DSM description of ADHD, his self-report on the CAARS and the MMPI-2-RF raises some concerns about the validity of his self-reported symptoms, making this weak evidence for Hypothesis 1. He does not endorse a history of learning disorder and thus self-report data do not support Hypothesis 2. There is no self-report data to assist in making judgments about Hypothesis 3. There is clear self-report evidence of poor study habits (Hypothesis 4); the assessor should remember that these poor study habits are common in college students generally, not just seen in those with ADHD. With regard to Hypothesis 5, there are some indicators in his self-report (lack of honors or AP courses, lower ACT scores) that suggest this hypothesis remains plausible. Based on his self-report, there is definite support for Hypothesis 6. He also self-reported poor sleep habits, suggesting support for Hypothesis 7. Based on his self-report, there is no evidence of psychological adjustment to college or psychological disorders in which a primary symptom is poor attention. Although he does have a history of a mild head injury, the research literature on this type of injury does not support Hypothesis 9 as a cause of his current academic troubles. Finally, given the initial evidence of some invalid self-reporting, Hypothesis 10 has some support.

	Base rate	Self-report
ADHD:	Low	Weak
LD:	Low	None
Low cog.:	Low	None
Study skills:	High	Strong
College readiness:	Medium to high	Medium
Substance use:	High	Strong
Daily habits:	High	Medium
Psych. issues:	Medium to high	Weak
Neuro. condition:	Low	None
Noncredible:	Medium	Medium

Evidence from Behavioral Observations

HS was alert, oriented, cooperative, and attentive throughout testing. He asked minimal questions but answered questions quickly. His mood was euthymic and his affective expression was broad and appropriate. He made good eye contact. He showed no unusual motor movements and was able to sit still for long hours of testing without need for a break. He yawned frequently and indicated that he had gotten only 5 hours of sleep the night before the evaluation. The assessor noted that he had trouble reading some of the finer print on clinic forms, having to hold the paper closer to his eyes rather than reading it from the tabletop, prompting further discussion of the last time he'd had his eyes checked (several years prior). Overall, behavioral observations are not particularly supportive of any hypothesis, other than perhaps his need for more sleep, but do raise concerns about a potentially important but incidental finding regarding his eyesight.

	Base rate	Self-report	Behavioral observation
ADHD:	Low	Weak	None
LD:	Low	None	None
Low cog.:	Low	None	None
Study skills:	High	Strong	None
College readiness:	Medium to high	Medium	None
Substance use:	High	Strong	None
Daily habits:	High	Medium	Weak
Psych. issues:	Medium to high	Weak	None
Neuro. condition:	Low	None	None
Noncredible:	Medium	Medium	None

Evidence from Collateral Report

HS's mother provided some information in a phone interview. She reported that no teachers had ever raised any concerns about his behavior or academic performance. She reported trying to encourage him to take honors and AP courses but that he was so busy with athletics that he didn't want to. She described him as "disinterested" in school but denied that he had ever had any academic or behavioral problems. She reported that his "weakest" subject seemed to be math, although he did "just fine" through precalculus and had never required any special services when learning math in school. She reported that he reached developmental milestones normally and that he had been quite healthy; she also denied any psychological concerns. She indicated that she had been worried about his mild head injury at the time that it occurred, but that he seemed to recover fully within a few weeks, with no signs of any permanent damage. She was not aware of his current study habits, drinking habits, health habits, psychological symptoms, or health problems. Overall, evidence from his mother is not supportive of Hypothesis 1, and generally equivocal for other hypotheses.

	Base rate	Self-report	Behavioral observation	Collateral report
ADHD:	Low	Weak	None	None
LD:	Low	None	None	None
Low cog.:	Low	None	None	None
Study skills:	High	Strong	None	None
College readiness:	Medium to high	Medium	None	None
Substance use:	High	Strong	None	None
Daily habits:	High	Medium	Weak	None
Psych. issues:	Medium to high	Weak	None	None
Neuro. condition:	Low	None	None	None
Noncrebible:	Medium	Medium	None	None

Evidence from Prior Diagnoses Given

It is important for assessors to consider whether prior diagnoses that were given to clients were valid. Frances (2013) noted that most psychological diagnoses and prescriptions are made by primary care physicians who have received little training in psychological diagnosis (or in appropriate use of psychotropic medications). Frances also cites evidence that physicians (and others) may provide "updiagnoses" to help patients gain something valuable, such as school accommodations, and that this practice is a major cause of diagnostic inflation. In this case, HS recalled filling out an "ADHD" questionnaire and taking "a computer test" administered by the doctor's secretary in the waiting room. The assessor in this case could ask for the medical records pertaining to the diagnosis (see below), but based on the student's report of the background for that prior diagnosis, it is not strong support for Hypothesis 1.

	Base rate	Self-report	Behavioral observation	Collateral report	Prior diagnosis
ADHD:	Low	Weak	None	None	Weak
LD:	Low	None	None	None	None
Low cog.:	Low	None	None	None	None
Study skills:	High	Strong	None	None	None
College readiness:	Medium to high	Medium	None	None	None
Substance use:	High	Strong	None	None	None
Daily habits:	High	Medium	Weak	None	None

Psych. issues:	Medium to high	Weak	None	None	None
Neuro. condition:	Low	None	None	None	None
Noncredible:	Medium	Medium	None	None	None

Evidence from Prior Records

HS's school records indicated no academic concerns and noted no behavioral concerns. He performed in the proficient (never accelerated or advanced) range on annual proficiency exams. His high school grades were mostly B's, with a few C's, which stand in contrast with his self-report of his high school performance. As he noted during the interview, the academic records show that he took no honors or AP courses and in some cases appeared to have taken a basic level (particularly in math and sciences) rather than a college-prep level of the same course. This academic record helps to disconfirm Hypotheses 1, 2, and 3, as there is no evidence of academic impairment consistent with any of those developmental conditions. Furthermore, it calls into question the validity of his self-report of impairment earlier in his academic career because his report of "horrible" high school grades is not consistent with his record. It does provide some evidence for the "college readiness" hypothesis.

	Base rate	Self-report	Behavioral observation	Collateral report	Prior diagnosis	Academic records
ADHD:	Low	Weak	None	None	Weak	None
LD:	Low	None	None	None	None	None
Low cog.:	Low	None	None	None	None	None
Study skills:	High	Strong	None	None	None	None
College readiness:	Medium to high	Medium	None	None	None	Some
Substance use:	High	Strong	None	None	None	None
Daily habits:	High	Medium	Weak	None	None	None
Psych. issues:	Medium to high	Weak	None	None	None	None
Neuro. condition:	Low	None	None	None	None	None
Noncredible:	Medium	Medium	None	None	None	Some

Evidence from Screening Results

Records from HS's doctor show that the doctor administered an unknown self-report screen of ADHD-type symptoms with no known psychometric properties. However, given the nonspecificity of "ADHD" symptom report (Harrison et al., 2013), this scale is of limited value. The doctor's report also provided information on HS's performance on a computerized continuous performance test, on which there were 16 different possible standard scores to consider, only two of which fell out of the range of normal. Continuous performance tests are inappropriate in the diagnosis of ADHD, given their lack of specificity (i.e., they are vulnerable to too many other conditions, including several of the alternative hypotheses in HS's case) (Solanto, Etefia, & Marks, 2004), and also given the sheer number of scores generated, questioning the value of interpreting two of 16 possible scores as indicative of ADHD (see Chapters 11 and 12). Overall, although the screening results may be consistent with Hypothesis 1, they are also consistent with Hypotheses 6, 7, 8, 9, and 10.

	Base rate	Self-report	Behavioral observation	Collateral report	Prior diagnosis	Academic records	Med. screen results
ADHD:	Low	Weak	None	None	Weak	None	Weak
LD:	Low	None	None	None	None	None	Weak
Low cog.:	Low	None	None	None	None	None	None
Study skills:	High	Strong	None	None	None	None	None
College readiness:	Medium to high	Medium	None	None	None	None	None
Substance use:	High	Strong	None	None	None	None	Weak
Daily habits:	High	Medium	Weak	None	None	None	Weak
Psych. issues:	Medium to high	Weak	None	None	None	None	Weak
Neuro. condition:	Low	None	None	None	None	None	Weak
Noncredible:	Medium	Medium	None	None	None	Some	Weak

Evidence from Current Test Results

HS was administered the WAIS-IV. Overall, his scores fell in the average range, with variability completely within normal range, considering the evidence presented in Chapter 11. Although he had one "low" score

(7) on Mental Arithmetic, his other working memory scores were higher (10 and 11 on Digit Span and Letter Number Sequencing, respectively). The assessor noted as a potential explanation that the Mental Arithmetic subtest requires good math fluency, and that HS muttered that he wished he could "use a calculator" and tried to write the problems down with his finger on the desktop when completing the items. Therefore, it is possible that his performance on this task was lower because it measures other constructs (math fluency, math anxiety) in addition to working memory skills. In addition, as noted in Chapter 11, one "low" score in a battery such as the WAIS-IV is not unusual and thus unlikely to be clinically meaningful, in the absence of other evidence consistent with the low score (Binder et al., 2009; Brooks et al., 2008; Schretlen, Munro, Anthony, & Pearlson, 2003). Statistically normal performance on all measures in a large cognitive test battery is not necessary in order to classify the general results as normal (Brooks et al., 2008). HS was also administered an achievement test, on which his scores were consistent with average intellect and his status as a high school graduate. On a brief battery of neuropsychological measures, he performed in the normal range on all, with the exception of performance on a verbal learning and memory task, which was below expectations. However, his performance on a measure of noncredible behavior (the Word Memory Test; Green, 2005) was indicative of invalidity.

	Base rate	Self-report	Behavioral observation	Collateral report	Prior diagnosis	Academic records	Med. screen results	Cog. test results
ADHD:	Low	Weak	None	None	Weak	None	Weak	None
LD:	Low	None	None	None	None	None	Weak	None
Low cog.:	Low	None	None	None	None	None	None	None
Study skills:	High	Strong	None	None	None	None	None	None
College readiness:	Medium to high	Medium	None	None	None	None	None	None
Substance use:	High	Strong	None	None	None	None	Weak	None
Daily habits:	High	Medium	Weak	None	None	None	Weak	None
Psych. issues:	Medium to high	Weak	None	None	None	None	Weak	None
Neuro. condition:	Low	None	None	None	None	None	Weak	None
Non-credible:	Medium	Medium	None	None	None	Some	Weak	Some

Step 5: Final Integration

A review of the above table allows the assessor to quickly examine the evidence for and against each potential hypothesis to explain HS's current academic problems. With regard to the first hypothesis, there is at best only weak evidence in support of this low base-rate hypothesis. The weak self-report data should be considered in the context of other evidence questioning the validity of his self-reported symptoms and self-reported impairment. His prior diagnosis was made by a primary care physician on the basis of highly nonspecific screening results and little examination for alternative explanations of HS's symptoms. Otherwise there is no evidence in support of this hypothesis. There is no evidence for Hypotheses 2 and 3. Regarding Hypothesis 4, there is strong support in his self-report that his study skills are lacking, although no other source of evidence is available for this particular hypothesis; however, it is already a very high base-rate hypothesis. Hypothesis 5 is also reasonably supported by his own self-report, his mother's report, and his academic records. Hypothesis 6 is supported by HS's self-report and his MMPI-2-RF scores. However, an assessor wishing to consider whether a formal diagnosis is appropriate should gather additional data on whether HS does/does not meet criteria for a substance-related diagnosis. If, however, the assessor feels that there is enough evidence to raise the possibility that HS should consider cutting back on his alcohol use due to its potential contribution to his presenting problem, then further data may not be needed.

Similarly, although there is evidence from HS's self-report, behavioral observations, and potentially his screening test scores that chronic lack of sleep may be contributing to his presenting symptoms, an assessor who felt that it would be important to address whether HS met diagnostic criteria for a sleep disorder should either gather additional data about sleep and/or consider referring HS for a sleep evaluation. Overall, in HS's case, there is little evidence for a contribution of psychological issues to his presenting concerns. There is also little to no evidence that any neurological disorders are contributing to his concerns; his head injury history is not clinically meaningful in this case. Finally, there is support from multiple sources for the final high base-rate hypothesis of noncredible behavior, both in terms of self-report and performance on cognitive tests, all the more important given the potential for secondary gain (receipt of stimulant medication).

Final Step: Write Out the Story

The final step is for the assessor to "write it out." This step provides the first draft of the results and impressions section of the report and also helps an assessor prepare for the feedback session (see Chapter 14). In "writing it out," the assessor should make certain that the final integration of the evaluation findings covers the following issues:

1. *Explaining the presenting problem by answering the referral question, clarifying the diagnosis, and/or identifying causal and contributing factors.* In the case of HS, the focus should be on the self-reported concerns and the problems that they are related to (academic probation), rather than focus on only one hypothesis (ADHD).

2. *Providing consistent converging evidence, with consideration of possible explanations for inconsistent or diverging data or acknowledgment of the puzzling results that don't fit.* In this case, because HS specifically mentioned the diagnostic hypothesis of ADHD (and he had been given the diagnosis in the past), this particular hypothesis should be addressed comprehensively to show why it has been disconfirmed. In the case of HS, there is little in his history, behavioral presentation, or test results that support a diagnosis of ADHD. He lacks a history of any behavior or impairment consistent with this disorder. His behavior during testing was not consistent with ADHD. Although he self-reported symptoms that sound like ADHD, they are also consistent with several other hypotheses, and some of the data suggest that he overreported symptoms and impairment, raising some concerns about the validity of HS's self-report data. Overall, his cognitive and neuropsychological test scores do not support a diagnosis of ADHD, but instead are either well within the normal range and with normal variability seen in healthy young adults, or may be invalid for interpretation due to evidence for some low/poor effort on some select attention and memory tasks. Although he was given the diagnosis of ADHD in the past, this diagnosis was based on a short interview, screening tests that the research literature shows are not specific to ADHD, and without careful exclusion of other potential factors important to consider prior to making the diagnosis. Furthermore, his self-reported reaction to stimulant medication is not, in and of itself, diagnostic of ADHD, and in fact might be related to addressing issues with chronic fatigue and sleepiness. Finally, there is evidence for the contribution of several other factors to his current academic issues, including poor study habits, lack of readiness for college-level courses (particularly math), substance misuse, and fatigue related to poor sleep habits. Evidence for the importance of these factors to academic performance can be emphasized in both the report and during feedback. Ultimately a "no diagnosis" hypothesis is the final conclusion, together with evidence for the contribution of several addressable factors (plus some noncredible behavior) for his concerns.

3. *Dealing with incidental findings that are still important to providing the best care for the client.* In the case of HS, it would be important to indicate that poor eyesight may interfere with his ability to see the blackboard or projector in class or to read his textbooks, which could affect his academic work.

4. *Considering postevaluation recommendations for both the primary findings and the incidental findings, which might include treatment recommendations, referral for other nonpsychological care, and/or need for specialty evaluation by other experts.* In HS's case, referring him to available resources (study skills workshops, free tutoring or peer review sessions, supplemental instruction opportunities for some classes) to address his study skills and habits is important. Depending on his chosen major (e.g., if it involved a lot of math), consideration of career resources to help him determine whether there are other ways for him to achieve his career goals might be warranted. Based on the available data, the assessor should address sleep and drinking issues as relevant contributors to academic performance, but cannot reach diagnostic conclusions on these issues based on the existing evidence. The assessor could recommend that HS work to improve his sleep habits and cut down on his drinking and suggest that, should he find it difficult to meet these goals, he might consider further evaluation for either sleep or substance-related issues. Alternatively, if the assessor feels there is existing evidence that HS might not be able to address either concern without help, the assessor could make those referrals as part of the recommendations. The inappropriate use of other people's medications should be strongly discouraged. Given the potentially incidental but important finding about his vision, a recommendation for an eye exam would be appropriate.

14

Feedback and Report Writing

Nothing clears up a case so much as stating it to another person.
—SHERLOCK HOLMES, in *Silver Blaze*

The American Psychological Association (2010) ethical code mandates the provision of assessment results to clients in most circumstances, which should be done in the form of a feedback session. Communication of assessment results is also typically conducted in the form of a formal report. This chapter discusses the potential therapeutic value of assessment feedback, with general suggestions for providing assessment feedback that is both beneficial to clients and remains true to assessment findings. In addition, a "scientist-detective" approach to report writing is described.

CLINICAL ISSUES IN PROVIDING CLIENTS WITH FEEDBACK

When providing a client with feedback, an assessor must be aware of the client's current mental state, including his or her capacity to understand (and/or later recall) the feedback and respond to it in a way that is beneficial to him or her. At times, the client's current psychological state can make it difficult for him or her to pay attention to and recall the feedback after the session; other times, the nature of a client's cognitive impairments make comprehension and/or recall of feedback less likely. In addition, when information is contradictory to clients' beliefs about "what is wrong" with them, it can be hard for them to retain the disconfirmatory information for later recall. In some cases, clients may need to have someone with them (with their permission) to hear the feedback, and in other cases, clients may need to review the feedback at another time after the initial feedback session.

The assessor also needs to remember that, although communication in the official report (see below) and communication to the client during the feedback may not be exactly the same, for good clinical reasons, it is possible that the client will read the report later. Thus, the assessor needs to balance the appropriateness of the feedback for that clinical moment with the information that is presented in the report, in order to prevent contradictory statements and misinterpretation.

FEEDBACK CAN BE THERAPEUTIC

In addition to the value of assessment for making treatment decisions, evidence shows that providing feedback about assessment results can, in and of itself, be therapeutic. Some studies have documented the benefits of assessment feedback on several important outcome variables, including decreased distress about symptoms (Finn & Tonsager, 1992; Newman & Greenway, 1997), improved self-esteem (Finn & Tonsager, 1992; Newman & Greenway, 1997), increased hope (Finn & Tonsager, 1992), improved therapeutic alliance (Ackerman, Hilsenroth, Baity, & Blagys, 2000; Hilsenroth, Peters, & Ackerman, 2004), more follow-through with treatment recommendations (Ackerman et al., 2000; Ougrin, Ng, & Low, 2008), and increased engagement in treatment (Michael, 2002), relative to attention controls. Feedback has even been shown to have positive effects when compared to traditional therapy. For example, Newman (2004) showed that one 2-hour feedback session about personality assessment results was as effective as five 1-hour traditional therapy sessions in improving symptom distress and self-esteem in adolescents.

In a recent meta-analysis of 17 studies examining the effects of receiving assessment feedback (Poston & Hanson, 2010), an overall effect size of 0.42 was found for therapeutic feedback on a host of outcome variables. It is important to note that this meta-analysis included studies that simply provided assessment feedback in a therapeutic manner as well as studies that used a formal therapeutic assessment approach advocated by Finn and Tonsager (1992); some assessment feedback sessions also utilized psychotherapeutic techniques, making the specific effect of assessment feedback difficult to isolate. In addition to these critiques of Poston and Hanson's conclusions, Lilienfeld, Garb, and Wood (2011) pointed out that some dependent variables were not analyzed in Poston and Hanson's meta-analysis and noted the lack of control for "assessment placebo" or "Barnum" effects (i.e., providing people with feedback, even if not necessarily unique or accurate, which has been shown to have powerful effects). Poston and Hanson (2011) reanalyzed their data, addressing concerns about assessment feedback studies that included therapy components as well as missing dependent variables, and their reanalysis still supported a small to medium effect of assessment feedback. However, it is clear that further study is necessary to isolate the specific benefits of assessment feedback to individuals undergoing evaluation.

Making Feedback Therapeutic

Although there are highly structured therapeutic assessment procedures (such as that presented by Finn & Tonsager, 1992), a more general therapeutic assessment process is one in which the assessor works hard to maintain empathy for the client and to work collaboratively with him or her to define the assessment goals and to share the assessment results in a feedback session. As noted in Chapter 1, when an assessor starts an assessment knowing that assessment feedback can be a therapeutic process, it will likely influence the assessor's approach to the entire evaluation in ways that make the process a true assessment rather than just diagnostic testing. In other words, to be truly therapeutic, an assessment needs to provide more than a diagnosis. Thus, the comprehensive assessment process discussed throughout this text is one that is the most likely to benefit the client at the time of feedback. Proponents of therapeutic assessment agree that the narrow focus of diagnostic assessment is typically insufficient for understanding treatment needs because it does not speak to severity and chronicity of symptoms and problems, presence or absence of comorbidities, presence of other strengths/weaknesses, the contribution of other factors to the presenting concern (e.g., environmental context), etc. With regard to the actual feedback session, however, when an assessor remembers that the ultimate goal is usually to benefit clients in some way, a natural structure to the feedback session can be identified. This structure is described below.

Framing the Feedback Session

First, the assessor can set the tone for the assessment feedback session as a time in which he or she will answer the client's initial question(s) as well as make recommendations for what the client should do next. If the client's initial question was about whether he or she had a specific diagnosis, such a question can be reframed in terms of what specific problems the client identified as most problematic, and the assessor can point out that the goal of the assessment was to identify all causes and contributors to that problem in order to make the best recommendations. This first step provides a "framework" for the feedback session, reminding the client of the reasons he or she sought an evaluation (or was referred for one) and the general structure of what is to come ("I will review results and conclusions with you, make some recommendations, and give you time to ask any questions you may have").

Integrative Discussion of the Impressions

Second, the assessor can provide conclusions about the assessment, emphasizing both the evidence base for those conclusions (i.e., the support from various aspects of the assessment data as well as disconfirmatory evidence) and the strength of those conclusions given the confirmatory and disconfirmatory evidence. It is often useful to couch this discussion within a psychoeducational framework (using a developmentally oriented biopsychosocial lens; see Chapter 3) to help the client understand those conclusions. Depending on the client, it might be helpful to start chronologically and restate the client's presenting concerns, integrating into that description the other causes/contributions/contexts to bring the "story" to the client's present situation; other times it may be helpful to start with the "bottom line" and then draw back on various pieces of the developmentally oriented biopsychosocial model to support the conclusion. Determining which approach to use is often a clinical decision (and may have been made by the assessor during integration of the data; see Chapter 13). This decision may also influence the structure of the final assessment report (see below).

Regardless of the general structure for the feedback, a recommended approach is to speak from the level of the constructs that were assessed, rather than from each individual and unique data point (or each individual score in a test battery). By following the integrative approach to considering the data recommended in Chapter 13, the assessor should be ready to guide the client through a discussion of the results at this macro-construct level of understanding. It is also recommended that the assessor tie that integration back to the client's real-life experience and real-world problems during the discussion.

WHEN FEEDBACK IS "NEGATIVE"

Sometimes the evaluation conclusions are contrary to what the client wants to hear. However, thinking of these occasions as "negative feedback" does not incline the assessor to think of these moments as equally beneficial and therapeutic to the client, even if they are uncomfortable at the time. Generally, clients tend to believe feedback that makes them seem similar to others (i.e., applies to everyone as accurate, e.g., the Barnum effect), confirms what they already think about themselves, and bolsters self-esteem or makes them think that others will think well of them. Thus, Finn (2007) suggests that an assessor start with feedback that verifies clients' usual thinking about themselves, then give feedback that might slightly modify clients' thinking about themselves, and then move to findings that are discrepant from clients' usual ways of thinking about themselves, while continuing to point out where those findings are still consistent with clients' real-world experiences and concerns.

For example, consider the case of a college student who was in an abnormal psychology course and used information from his textbook to "diagnose" himself with ADHD, which he needed to have "confirmed" in an evaluation so that he could get access to stimulant medications. His presentation during the first interview suggested that he was acutely uncomfortable; he could not make eye contact with the assessor and had an odd and eccentric way of speaking. At the second interview, he admitted to experiencing some "maybe atypical" thought processes at times when he was "inattentive and distracted" in his courses, which included some mildly paranoid thoughts about classmates and beliefs that "somehow" professors were lecturing about things that had specific and special relevance to him, which then caused him alarm and made him question whether the professors could read his mind. He indicated that he had already "run through" three roommates, who all moved out rather quickly after moving in, and he was currently living alone, with no friends or social support and little contact with family (which he preferred). He asked highly unusual questions about the psychological and cognitive tests that he was administered, often appearing to miss the point entirely, despite directions or items being repeated for him. Ultimately, after a thorough assessment, it was clear that the client met criteria for schizotypal personality disorder. During feedback, the assessor took the approach of focusing specifically on the client's presenting concerns (rather than his presenting "diagnosis"); pointed out all of the symptoms, experiences, behaviors, and observations that were made and formally assessed, confirming with the client that these all "made sense" and "rang true" for him; and then began to explain how together they really painted a different picture than one typically seen in individuals with ADHD. After further discussion, during which the client actually (almost) seemed to warm up to the assessor as he began to understand the conclusions, he made the following observation: "Gee, I guess I was looking in the wrong part of the DSM!"

Assessors can also find it difficult to give "bad news" to clients (i.e., when assessors' own value judgments, anxieties, and personal reactions to the diagnosis make them personally uncomfortable and they project this discomfort onto clients). Many psychologists have seen this when they work in a consultative role, particularly with other health care providers who are not trained in assessing or addressing psychological issues; the psychologist becomes the "go-to" person when suicidal ideation, abuse, sexual issues, substance misuse, and other "hard" diagnoses come to the forefront and need to be discussed with clients. Psychologists tend to become worried about feedback when they anticipate that the feedback will make the client angry, hostile, or overly emotional. (A short list of such anticipated situations would include diagnoses such as a degenerative dementia with no known treatment, psychotic disorder of some sort, lack of diagnosis in someone convinced that he or she has a diagnosis, implications of psychological contributions to physical presentation in someone convinced that he or she only has a physical illness, and when someone has behaved noncredibly during the evaluation.) For example, in the case just presented above, the student assessor was very nervous about having to talk with a client about his unusual beliefs and implying that they were perhaps not reality based, particularly given how adamant the client was that he needed stimulant medications and had ADHD. The assessor was worried that the client would become hostile and angry. After role-playing the feedback several times, the assessor was able to make the feedback therapeutic for the client and successfully encouraged him to enter therapy as well as complete a psychiatric consultation.

Another illustrative case is that of a severely depressed and actively suicidal university student in her second year of college who was also referred for evaluation due to her academic probation status. She reported that ever since she had begun college, she had felt like she "didn't belong" and that she was a "total failure." Although she indicated that she had been valedictorian of her high school class, she felt that she didn't seem to be able to comprehend anything in most of her class lectures; she thought this might be due to the large lecture format as compared to her small high school, but also reported that college lecture information was covered "overwhelmingly fast" and that she couldn't comprehend most of her textbooks either. As a result of her difficulty, she was on continued academic probation and was in danger of being expelled. She had been actively utilizing every available resource on campus to help her with study and academic skills, although they had not been successful. She also reported that she even had difficulty following regular conversations with her dorm mates over lunch or dinner, which made her feel like an "idiot."

Her school records showed that she had attended a magnet school in which her entire class consisted of 12 students; although she had been given A and B grades, she'd had to take the state's graduation test five times before she was able to pass, and her ACT scores were in the single digits. She recognized that this information somehow might have indicated that she would struggle in college, but that her high school guidance counselor had not seem concerned and actively encouraged her to go to college; because she had been admitted to college, she didn't think this history was necessarily relevant. However, she knew "something" was wrong; she just wasn't sure what was wrong and why she was doing so poorly in school.

Intellectual testing showed that she was performing in the borderline range of intellect, and her scores on achievement testing were quite consistent with this level of intelligence. No clear cognitive impairments or strengths were seen in any additional neuropsychological testing, but rather her overall pattern of scores was generally consistent with borderline intellectual functioning. Psychological testing confirmed her severe depressive symptoms and her active suicidal ideation, as well as overwhelming anxiety and distress over her current life situation, but with otherwise healthy psychological history, good coping skills, and high levels of family and peer support.

The student in training who conducted the evaluation was extremely worried about giving "bad news" to the client about her borderline cognitive abilities. I reminded the student that the client "already knew" how poorly she was functioning academically, and that the assessment would help her better understand the cognitive contributions to her poor academic performance, despite her best efforts. A therapeutic approach to feedback was taken, couched in terms of both the client's weaknesses (of which she was well aware at the level of consequences, but had never understood in terms of her own cognitive abilities), and her strengths, with recommendations to work with career services to identify careers that were inviting to her as well as educational approaches that might get her to those careers without a 4-year college degree and/or with a more "hands-on" approach to learning and training. In addition, given her psychological status, a recommendation for therapy was made and a suicide prevention contract was initiated. The feedback session was highly successful, and the client indicated that she left the feedback with more hope for her future than she had experienced in a long time. The client attended a couple of therapy sessions, but indicated that simply having someone confirm her weaknesses while emphasizing her strengths and helping her to identify a way to "find another path" to her career goals (i.e., the feedback session) had provided her with positive motivation to move on to a community college near her hometown and thus she discontinued therapy.

PROVISION OF FEEDBACK WHEN THE CLIENT BEHAVED NONCREDIBLY

The most difficult feedback session to prepare for is one in which the data suggest that the client responded in a noncredible way during the assessment, either by reporting symptoms noncredibly or by behaving noncredibly on performance measures. As noted in Chapter 4, such data simply indicate that the results for some tests are invalid and cannot be interpreted. It is always important for an assessor to explain the basis of his or her opinions or conclusions, as noted above, but in the case of a client behaving noncredibly, it is also important to be careful to avoid providing specific information about ways in which the noncredible behavior was determined, so that the assessor doesn't preclude the validity of such measures for future use with either the same client (i.e., coaching the client to be a more sophisticated malingerer in future evaluations) or with other clients (by violating test security).

As noted in Chapter 4, identifying noncredible responding does not indicate a particular reason for the noncredible responding, and thus the assessor can focus the feedback on the behavior exhibited by the client, pointing out that this unfortunately made certain tests difficult to interpret (or invalid). It is important for an assessor to remember that there still might be some test data that can be interpreted in feedback to the client (e.g., as noted in Chapter 4, if some test results are still in the normal range, suggesting no impairment). It is also important for an assessor to remember all the other nontest data that may still be relevant to interpret and discuss with the client. Reviewing components of "invalidity shock," as presented in Chapter 4, can help the assessor increase the likelihood that feedback about noncredible responding goes as well as it can (although, given that sometimes the motivation for behaving noncredibly is one of external gain, the assessor also needs to be ready for the feedback to not go well, despite his or her best efforts).

Implications of the Conclusions

Another important aspect of providing therapeutic feedback is to tie the conclusions and impressions to the recommendations being made. Helping clients to understand and accept the assessment conclusions is a first step to explaining what should "come next" and what might benefit clients in regard to addressing their presenting concerns. Just as clients may not be ready to hear what an assessor has to say, what clients define as "help" may not match what the evaluation indicates are the most beneficial recommendations. Using a psychoeducational approach that is grounded in empirical evidence (e.g., "Research shows that X can be very effective for people with concerns like yours") can help, as well as providing specific information about where the client can follow through with any recommendations that are made.

WHEN CONCLUSIONS ARE MIXED

Sometimes an evaluation ends up raising more questions than it might answer. There may be some clear conclusions, whereas others are merely tentative and require further procedures (often referral to others) prior to reaching conclusions. In addition, some presenting problems cannot be addressed until some of the other clearer conclusions (and recommendations) have been successfully addressed. It is important for an assessor to be clear on the status of all of a client's presenting concerns and how they interconnect with the recommendations being made.

Consider the following case: A 19-year-old male college student was referred for an evaluation for ADHD. He reported that he was having trouble focusing on schoolwork outside of the classroom and in class lectures. At the initial appointment he was quite insistent that his problems could be addressed with stimulant medication. His grade point was near a 2.0 (his high school GPA had been 3.0). He indicated that, since middle school, teachers had commented that he often seemed "out of it" and inattentive (school records confirmed these qualitative comments), but he had never been referred for any sort of evaluation. Both he and his parents self-reported symptoms consistent with ADHD, both currently and in childhood, and the pattern of testing in a neuropsychological battery was supportive of mild problems with sustained attention, vigilance, working memory, and psychomotor speed (and no evidence of noncredible responding). Although he reported that he had always been healthy and had no history of injuries, illnesses, or hospitalizations, a thorough examination of his daily routine revealed that he slept 12–16 hours in a 24-hour period, but that he never felt rested. He reported that he could fall asleep "on a dime" and that this had been true through his middle and high school years (in fact, he admitted to sleeping through many of his high school classes). He mentioned that in middle school, during a physical for sports, the physician had recommended that he consider having a sleep evaluation, but he and his parents had never followed through. With further questioning, he indicated that his roommates could "barely stand" his snoring and gasping at night, and that he often awoke with a severe headache. He also admitted to buying stimulant medications from other students in order to force himself to stay awake in college classes.

The feedback session focused on his major sleep concerns and the fact that they strongly suggested he was experiencing obstructive sleep apnea; conclusions about whether he had ADHD were delayed pending the follow-through on a sleep evaluation recommendation. At the feedback session he was angry because he was "convinced" that he had ADHD, and he insisted that any continued evaluation after the sleep study "finds nothing" would need to be provided to him for free, since he had already paid for the evaluation but wasn't "hearing what I wanted to hear" in the feedback session. However, when he showed his parents the evaluation report, they insisted he follow up with the sleep evaluation. He was diagnosed with obstructive sleep apnea and began using a continuous positive airway pressure (CPAP) mask, which successfully alleviated all of his symptoms. He called back 2 months later and asked the front desk staff to "apologize on my behalf" to his assessor because he realized now how important that feedback and the recommendation were to providing him with appropriate treatment for his concerns.

Recording Response to Feedback

Finally, the assessor should allow time for and assess the client's response to the feedback (and record that response; see below). The focus when assessing the client's response should include accuracy of understanding (seeing if the client can repeat/paraphrase the main conclusions and recommendations), how relevant the client feels the conclusions are to his or her situation, and the client's affective reaction. And questions raised by the client should be answered. The most likely questions will arise when the information provided does not align with the client's expectations regarding the diagnosis and/or recommendations for treatment.

REPORT WRITING

The approach to report writing described below is the culmination of the scientist-detective perspective of assessment that has been the theme of this text. While reports are meant to communicate to others (and thus are like feedback), they are also used to document the assessment and often are part of a patient's medical or psychological record. As such, one way to view a report is like a research report. The report includes a number of components: (1) a restatement of the referral question (the hypothesis); (2) the procedure used to examine the question (measures administered, methods used, e.g., collateral interviews, review of records); (3) the nature of the data collected and the validity and strength of those data (the results); (4) the final impressions (a discussion of the convergence of data across sources, with consideration of discrepant results, leading to an answer to the referral question); and (5) recommendations for follow-up and/or treatment (implications).

Because the report is also a communication to the person who made the referral, the assessor must view the report as an important communication tool, with specific consideration of the primary reader of the report when writing. However, although the assessor must consider the most likely audience for the report when writing it, he or she must also remember the potential for other individuals to read the report in the future. A report should reflect a balance between the use of readable/accessible language and the use of jargon/scientific terms. Most importantly, opinions, impressions, and judgments should be surrounded with the evidence that supports them, and limitations to those opinions, impressions, and judgments should also be clearly stated. The following material describes common elements of a psychological report that is written from a scientific-detective perspective. A sample report is provided in Appendix 14.1 at the end of the chapter.

Identifying Information

Identifying information about the person at the time of the assessment should be given at the very top of the report. This can include demographic information, but should also include who made the referral, the dates the client was seen, the date of the final report, and a list of everyone involved in conducting the assessment and writing the report.

Reason for Referral

The first section of text in the report should clearly state the reason for referral. In a sense, this is the question or questions the report will answer (i.e., the initial hypotheses to be considered). It can be helpful here to clarify the source of these questions; for example, the referring physician may have had a specific diagnostic question to answer, but the client may have added other concerns and questions to be addressed in the evaluation. In order to remind the reader (and the assessor!) that the assessment focus is not merely to identify a diagnosis, even when a referral question refers specifically to a diagnosis, it is a good habit to follow such a statement with a brief summary of the most primary problems the client (or referral source) is reporting (particularly when they are relevant to the impressions and recommendations).

Assessment Procedure

The next section of the report lists the various assessment procedures that were followed and should include names of anyone who was interviewed (including their relationship with the client), what other records were gathered and evaluated as part of the evaluation, and all tests that were administered. It is important to note that inclusion of *all* procedures helps to emphasize the significance of nontest data to the final opinions and impressions in the report. A complete list of measures administered to the client can comprise a subsection of this section of the report, or could be placed immediately subsequent to this section. This is also a good place to provide the acronyms for all tests (in parentheses following their full names) in case an examiner decides to refer to them further in the body of the report.

History/Background Information

The next section of the report addresses the history and/or background information. This is where the assessor builds the client's story, at this point based on interview information (client, collaterals) as well as records that were reviewed. In a sense, this section provides a summary of the "results" from the nontest sources of data that were part of the assessment process. Thus, it is important to reflect accurately the source of the data within this section and their likely accuracy.

There is no "right" way to tell a client's story. Sometimes it makes the most sense to take a developmental approach and start with a chronological history of the first onset of the symptoms/problems forward to the current presentation, whereas other times it can make more sense to start with the client's current presentation, followed by a chronological history. In either case, the assessor should keep in mind a developmentally informed bio-psychosocial model when writing to ensure a comprehensive report of the client's current presentation in the context of all potential past and current contributing and consequential factors.

It is important for the assessor to be clear about the source of "factual" information that is reported. In addition, to the extent possible, judgments and opinions in this section should be substantiated with supportive evidence. For example, it is far too common to see reports in which a statement by a client is presented as fact, such as "The client performed very poorly on her PSAT exam in ninth grade." In this case, if the data were gathered only by self-report, the assessor should say, "The client *reported* that she performed very poorly on her PSAT exam in ninth grade" (and hopefully, followed by the actual PSAT exam results in a records review). This is true for any data gathered from the client, including medical history ("the client *indicated* that he had never been hospitalized" rather than "there is no history of hospitalization"), symptoms ("the client *denied* experiencing prior psychological symptoms or seeking psychological treatment in the past" rather than "the client has no psychological history"), to provide just a few examples.

When there are extensive records and a detailed self-report, it might be useful to have two summary subsections in the background portion of the report: one based on self-reported history and one based on records review. In other cases, it is better to integrate information from self-report with other sources of data (records, collateral interviews) in order to point out the consistencies and inconsistencies in history across different sources of data. Either approach can be appropriate, depending on the case at hand, and is an important clinical judgment for an assessor to make.

The information included in the background section should be relevant to answering the referral questions; thus, it is not necessarily a detailed summary of every single bit of historical detail that happened to be gathered along the way, when the assessor was still using inductive reasoning and exploring any and all possibilities and hypotheses at hand. Several factors are important in helping the assessor determine whether the information is relevant to include. One factor is, of course, whether the information is, in fact, relevant to the final conclusions that are being drawn. The assessor needs to keep in mind that absence of a fact is also sometimes relevant information (e.g., the absence of any actual traumatic event that would meet Criterion A for PTSD is important factual information). In addition, the assessor should still make a conscious effort to include information that is potentially contrary to the conclusion being drawn; in later sections, the assessor should then discuss both the converging and diverging information in the integration of all available data. A second factor is whether the person who is most likely to receive the report might need to have the information under consideration. The assessor should try to anticipate the reader's questions and provide answers while writing. A third factor is to consider whether a known piece of information gathered during the assessment process that seems irrelevant to the specific issues at hand has the potential to harm the client. If it is not in the best interest of the client to include a certain piece of information and it is truly irrelevant to answer the questions raised, it should not be included.

Behavioral Observations

This section should include a summary of behavioral observations taken throughout the entire evaluation, from each visit if there is more than one, and across the different contexts of interview and test completion. As noted in Chapter 7, these data provide information relevant to the evaluation itself (i.e., may provide examples of symptoms, behaviors, coping strategies, etc., that have either diagnostic or intervention value), and can also speak to the $N = 1$ validity of data that were gathered from the client (interview, self-report measures, and cognitive testing).

Results

There are many different styles of reporting results that appear in psychological testing books. In my opinion, many of these approaches serve to overemphasize the scores on tests, resulting in (1) minimal consideration of data from other sources and (2) no integration of test data across different tests or with other nontest sources of information. For example, many assessors take a test-by-test approach in which each test is first described in great detail, including a statement about what the test is supposedly measuring, followed by a description of how the client actually does on each and every component of the test (sometimes even down to the item level!). Not only does this approach result in an overly lengthy report, but it also tends to create an "isolationist" view of each test as its own entity. In order to place tests in their proper context, as well as to keep reports as brief as possible, this approach should be discouraged.

I advocate an approach to reporting results that is meant to (1) place tests in their proper context, as just part of the data that should be used to form impressions and opinions; (2) keep the focus on the constructs being assessed, rather than each individual assessment data point from each test administered; and (3) emphasize the person being assessed, not the tests themselves. Table 14.1 provides some general dos and don'ts for report writing that I recommend.

In order to keep the results focused on the relevant constructs that were assessed, rather than on the individual tests, the assessor should organize test results by grouping tests of similar constructs together in the results section. When necessary, interpretive results from a prior subsection could be referred to again in the next section, particularly for complex measures known to tap more than one construct (which is most of them!).

With regard to provision of raw data (i.e., actual test scores), I am of mixed mind about including them in reports. Although the ethics code of the American Psychological Association (2010) makes it clear that clients can access their raw data and release them to anyone, there is an important balance to facilitate between clients' accessing of raw data and their ability to interpret the data correctly (misinterpretation could lead to client harm). In addition, there is the potential to violate test security when raw data (all the way down to the level of client verbatim response, which is what is indicated in the ethics code) are provided to others. I tend to adopt the strategy

TABLE 14.1. Dos and Don'ts in Writing Results from Formal Tests

Do	Don't
Test description	
Indicate that the client completed a certain test to assess a broad construct, listing either the test name or the acronym if provided earlier in the report.	Provide a lengthy description of the measure, the constructs it purportedly measures, and what the client actually had to do to perform the measure.
Test items	
Provide no discussion of test items (even critical items from measures such as MMPI-2-RF or PAI should be discussed as the construct they are assessing rather than stating the individual item content).	List responses to specific items and try to interpret the test in this manner.
Provision of scores	
Either provide only the level of the scores that can be interpreted (i.e., percentiles, descriptors for level of test performance) *or*, if actual test data are provided, put them in context.	List every single score without providing context (percentiles, standard scores, confidence intervals).
Report overall test results for multiscore tests/test batteries at the level of interpretation determined during steps described in Chapters 10, 11, and 12.	Interpret every single score for every single subtest in great detail.
Write about the performance of the person on the constructs that were assessed, being clear when you are speaking about a client's ipsative/relative strengths/weaknesses and when you are speaking about a client's performance relative to a comparison group.	Write about the tests, rather than the client's performance/behavior on the test.
Describing score variability	
When describing normal variability in a profile, be clear this is merely descriptive and not diagnostic; place emphasis only on scores and discrepancies that actually may have clinical meaning (when integrated with other nontest data).	Refer to scores or score discrepancies as abnormal, clinically meaningful, unusual, or impaired when the data show they are not.
Invalid scores	
Clearly indicate that certain scores are not reported or interpreted because of evidence of invalidity.	Report invalid scores, but then explain that they may not be interpretable.

of creating an appendix for a report (often not attached when sent to potential readers, but available upon request, as required by the ethics code), in which various valid test scores are summarized, rather than including them in tables in the body of reports or embedded in the text of reports. Provision of every single data point in a report adds unnecessary length to it, invites misinterpretation by readers who lack a full understanding of statistics and psychometrics, and also gives undue weight to test scores over other sources of data. When data must be included in the report itself, the assessor should focus on provision of standard scores and percentiles for the valid test scores, surrounded by their confidence intervals, to put them in their appropriate context for later interpretation.

The astute reader will have noticed the reference to *valid* test scores. It is of absolute importance that an assessor *avoid reporting* invalid test scores in the report as if they could be validly interpreted. It is too easy for test scores (even if marked with some kind of asterisk or other footnote as invalid) to be transferred forward for other purposes without the invalidity disclaimer. In addition, reporting that scores on a specific instrument were at a certain level that indicates that they were invalid may well violate test security and make the client more likely to be able to avoid detection for his or her noncredible behavior in the future. It should be noted that in the sample report provided in Appendix 14.1, the scores even for invalid measures are given at the end of the report, so that the reader can see how test scores were incorporated into the sample report.

Finally, by taking a more integrative approach to the reporting of results, the assessor is better able to keep the focus on the person being assessed, rather than the minutiae of each test score. Talking about all tests in terms of their integrated constructs, from the standpoint of descriptive statements (and perhaps percentiles), and talking about them in terms of how the person performed, rather than the test itself, will help the reader stay focused on the person.

Impressions

Much like the discussion section of a research paper, the assessor should work to put all the data together to support the final conclusions being drawn, in specific answer to the referral question or questions. The assessor should start with the primary findings and then explain more incidental findings. Writing this section can help the assessor prepare for the feedback session (and is what I recommend that my students do prior to conducting a feedback session). If there is a clear diagnosis, it can be placed here together with the diagnostic code or codes (DSM, ICD) that are being given. The integrative process described in Chapter 13 is the mental exercise that, once completed, should result in the formulation of the "bottom line" in this section of the actual report.

Recommendations

Recommendations should refer back to the main conclusions and impressions to help the reader see why they are being made, and they should be specific, providing the client with particular referral sites, resources, individuals, and/or clinics that can assist the client in carrying out those recommendations.

Why Would a Report Need a Summary?

Because my approach to assessments is very focused, it doesn't make sense to write a summary section. If an assessor writes such a lengthy report that a summary is needed, the assessor should know that the only thing any reader is going to read is the summary section.

Feedback

I always include this section in my reports, due to clinical experience. In my experience, often clients have been evaluated elsewhere, and what they report they were told at feedback is not congruent with what reports from that evaluation seem to conclude. This makes it difficult to know if the client did not understand or recall the feedback correctly, or perhaps the prior assessor failed to provide accurate feedback to the client. Therefore, placing a comment about the client's understanding of the feedback and reaction to it allows future readers to know what was said to the client. This information also can facilitate appropriate follow-up care and a smoother transition for other health care providers who will work with the client and access the report because the specific recommendations, and the fact that they were communicated to the client, are clearly articulated in the report.

Report Caveat

I always conclude reports with the following statement: "This assessment was conducted to answer the specific referral question above and may not be complete for other purposes." Other assessors add caveats about the potential for the results to be outdated within a certain time period. These sorts of caveats help to remind future readers that any assessment, although valid at the time it was conducted and for the specific purpose for which it was conducted, may not be valid if the report is too old or was conducted for some other purpose. Such caveats serve as an overarching "limitation" statement that should remind individuals who wish to use the evaluation for a purpose other than what it was intended, or decades after it was written, that it would be inappropriate to do so.

Appendix 14.1. Sample Psychological Report

Confidential Report
Student, date of report
Page 1 of [total pages]

Name of Practice
Psychological Report

Name: Hypothetical Student   *Date(s) of evaluation*: [all dates given]
Date of report: [date report finalized]   *Age*: 22
Education: College sophomore   *Sex*: Male
Referred by: Self   *Examined by*: [list all involved in
                                                         examination]

Reason for Referral

Hypothetical Student referred himself to [Practice Name] for concerns about his attention and concentration skills. He reported that he was currently on academic probation at [College Name] due to his attention and concentration problems. He indicated that he sought the present evaluation because he could not get a renewed prescription for Ritalin from [College Health Center Name] without the evaluation. He reported being diagnosed with attention-deficit/hyperactivity disorder by his general physician when he was home for winter break a few months ago.

Evaluation Procedures

Phone interview with Mr. Student's mother
Academic records from [School Name]
Medical report dated [give date] from Dr. [Doctor Name]

Tests Administered

Conners' Adult ADHD Rating Scale—Long Form (CAARS)
Minnesota Multiphasic Personality Inventory–II—Restructured Format (MMPI-II-RF)
Wechsler Adult Intelligence Scale–IV (WAIS-IV)
Word Memory Test (WMT)
Wechsler Individualized Achievement Test–III (WIAT-III)
Auditory Verbal Learning Test (AVLT)
Stroop Color and Word Test (SCWT)
Trail Making Test (TMT)

History

Mr. Student reported that he has had "lifelong" difficulties with paying attention and concentrating. Specifically, he noted difficulties paying attention during class lectures and when studying for his courses, and he reported that he can't concentrate for more than an hour at a time when reading. Although these were his main concerns, upon direct questioning he also indicated that he tends to be messy and disorganized, has trouble finishing assignments on time (mostly because he procrastinates until the night before they are due), and finds himself easily distracted when he tries to read course material or study for exams. In addition, he reported that he makes a lot of careless mistakes when writing papers, such as leaving out words, misspelling words that he "knows" how to spell, and making grammatical errors that he easily identifies later when the papers have already been submitted. He described his general study style as waiting until "the last minute" to do homework, complete readings, write papers, and study for tests. By his report, he "crams" the night before tests, starting the evening before and studying up to the test time, missing other classes, if necessary, to continue studying. When asked, he estimated that he misses about 40% of his morning classes. He also described himself as a "space cadet" who forgets everything unless other people remind him.

Although Mr. Student reported that these concerns and problems were "lifelong," he indicated that he first noticed them during his middle school years. However, he reported that in elementary and middle school he "sometimes" got into trouble for talking out of turn in class. He denied any problems with motor restlessness, impulsivity, or conduct or other behavioral issues. He denied ever receiving discipline from his teachers for anything other than talking out of turn, and specifically denied ever being sent to the principal's office, having detention, or being suspended or expelled from school. Of note, his mother indicated that no teachers had ever raised any concerns with her about either his behavior at school or his academic performance. This report is consistent with his school records, which revealed no academic or behavioral concerns from elementary school through high school. He denied any behavioral difficulties in high school or since entering college.

Mr. Student indicated that his attention and concentration concerns have had a negative impact upon his academic functioning. Whereas he reported his grades through middle school as mostly A's and B's, he described his high school grades as "terrible." He attributed these "terrible" grades in part to his attitude; he indicated that he "didn't try" and "didn't care" about school at that time. Of note, although he characterized his high school grades as "terrible," school records showed that he received mostly B's, with just a few C grades (in high school math courses). Consistent with his self-report, his grades prior to high school were all A's and B's. Mr. Student reported that he did not take any honors or AP courses during his high school years; consistent with this report, his school records revealed that he took some college preparatory courses, but no honors or AP courses, and tended to take "basic-level" courses in math and sciences rather than the college preparatory level of the same courses. His mother indicated that she tried to encourage him to take harder courses to better prepare himself for college, but that he was "so busy" with athletics that he didn't want to; she described him as generally "uninterested" in school. She reported that, although he was relatively weak in math, he never had any problems learning math in school, never received any special services for math or for any other academic subject, was never held back, and never failed any proficiency tests. She also indicated that he passed the [State Name] graduation test on the first try. This report is consistent with the school records that were reviewed, which show that Mr. Student performed in the proficient range in every academic area on annual proficiency exams.

Mr. Student denied psychological problems or any history of psychological treatment; this was consistent with his mother's report. He acknowledged that he currently felt a bit "worried" and "down" about his academic probation and fearful that he would be dismissed from college, but indicated that he generally feels "good" and does not tend to ruminate on these thoughts or feel depressed by them. He reported that, although he typically gets 7 hours of sleep a night, he usually stays up until 2:00 or 3:00 A.M. playing videogames and then sleeps in, often until at least 11:00 A.M. According to Mr. Student's report, he started drinking alcohol while in high school. He described himself as a "social" drinker, indicating that since starting college he drinks three nights per week, typically Thursday through Saturday evenings. By his report, on at least one of those nights per week, he drinks to blackout stage, typically on Friday evening, and on the other nights he drinks four beers, at most. By his report, he has not engaged in any illegal or risky behavior during drinking episodes; when he blacks out, a roommate or friend usually helps him get back to his room. In addition, he denied ever experiencing hangovers and indicated that he feels his drinking is "pretty typical" for undergraduate students. He indicated that on weekends he often does not rise until 1:00 or 2:00 P.M. due to being out with friends drinking the night before. He denied the use of any other recreational substances.

Mr. Student's mother indicated that her son was born full term with no complications during pregnancy or delivery. She also reported that he met all developmental milestones on time. She described her son as generally healthy, with no major illnesses or injuries requiring hospitalization, with the exception of an emergency room visit his sophomore year of high school due to a concussion incurred during a football game. According to Mr. Student, he was unconscious for about 10 minutes at that time and was taken to a hospital, where a head CT scan showed "no damage." He was taken out of play for 2 weeks. Both Mr. Student and his mother noted that he experienced headaches for about a week after the concussion, but was he able to return to school 3 days after the injury and noticed no academic or cognitive problems as a result of it. Mr. Student denied having any current health problems or taking any medications, except taking over-the-counter medications for seasonal allergies. Mr. Student also observed that he has had more headaches frequently, especially when reading, and expressed the idea that he may need glasses.

Mr. Student noted that, over the recent winter break, he spoke with his general physician about his attention and concentration concerns. He also mentioned to the physician that he had "borrowed" some stimulant medications from another student to help him study for a really important exam and that he felt he had benefited from them. By his report, the physician "did a couple of tests" and diagnosed him with ADHD, providing him with "samples" of Ritalin to use during the spring semester. According to the medical records from Dr. [Doctor Name], Mr. Student was administered some sort of self-report questionnaire on ADHD symptoms, although the scale was not named and no actual scores were provided for interpretation. In addition, Mr. Student was administered some sort of continuous performance test that was not named; nevertheless, 16 different scores from that test were reported in tabular form. Two of those scores were interpreted as out of the range of normal (reaction time variability, omission errors). Mr. Student expressed frustration that [College Health Center Name] would not give him a prescription for Ritalin without the present evaluation because "I was already diagnosed."

Behavioral Observations

Mr. Student was seen on two occasions for a total of 5½ hours of assessment within a 2-week window of time. He arrived on time for both sessions. Mr. Student was alert, oriented, cooperative, and attentive throughout the interview and testing. He asked minimal questions of the examiner, but answered questions quickly and fluently; his speech was congruent with his level of education. His mood was euthymic and his affective expression was broad and appropriate. He made good eye contact. He showed no unusual motor movements and was able to sit still for long hours of testing without need for a break. He yawned frequently and indicated that he had gotten only 5 hours of sleep on the night before the first testing session; he slept a similar amount the night before the second session. It was noted that Mr. Student had difficulty reading some of the fine print on consent forms, holding the forms closer to his eyes rather than reading them from the tabletop. When asked, he indicated that he had not had his vision checked in several years. However, there were no other observed difficulties with vision, and repeated checks with Mr. Student throughout testing suggested he did not have difficulty seeing any test stimuli.

Test Results

Self-Report Instruments

Mr. Student completed the CAARS, a self-report measure of current ADHD symptoms for adults. His scores on all scales fell in the normal range, with the exception of the DSM-IV Inattentive Symptoms scale and the Total ADHD Symptoms scale. However, his scores on these two scales were so elevated that concerns must be raised about the potential for symptom overreport on these measures.

Mr. Student also completed the MMPI-2-RF to assess personality and psychological characteristics. Although his scores suggest that he answered the questions consistently, his score on at least one validity scale raised concerns about the validity of his self-report of cognitive symptomatology. Although his scores on other measures suggested that he endorsed a high number of neurological and cognitive complaints, these scores must be interpreted in light of his validity scale scores. He also reported a high degree of stress, worry, and concern, which are generally consistent with his presentation during the interview, about his own ability to address his current issues.

Performance Measures

Mr. Student's score on a measure of performance validity suggested that he was not performing credibly on this measure, raising concerns about the interpretability of other test scores assessing attention and memory constructs. Indeed, Mr. Student's performance on a measure of verbal learning and recall were well out of the range of normal and suggestive of noncredible responding; in the context of his invalid completion of another measure of performance validity, these scores cannot be interpreted.

Mr. Student was administered the WAIS-IV to assess his intellect and general cognitive functioning. His general intellect fell in the average range, with normal variability in his cognitive strengths and weaknesses (verbal reasoning average to high-average range, perceptual reasoning average range, working memory low-average to average range, psychomotor processing speed average to high-average range).

Of note, although Mr. Student's WAIS-IV Working Memory Index fell in the low-average to average range, this score is consistent with normal variation in cognitive performance and was primarily related to his relatively low score on a test of mental arithmetic (16th percentile), by which he was particularly frustrated and requested use of a calculator. His performance on the other subtest comprising the working memory index fell at the 50th percentile, and his performance on a supplemental working memory subtest fell at the 63rd percentile, relative to his same-age peers.

His performance on a task requiring psychomotor processing speed and cognitive flexibility was also normal for his age, consistent with his average to high-average scores on psychomotor processing speed measures of the WAIS-IV.

Mr. Student's performance on a measure of assessing response inhibition was normal for his age.

Mr. Student was also administered an achievement test, the WIAT-III. His performance in all academic domains was in the average range relative to his same-age peers, consistent with his academic history and level of intellect.

Impression

Mr. Student's history, behavioral presentation, and test scores are not consistent with a diagnosis of ADHD. His developmental and academic histories provide no evidence of impairing problems in attention, concentration, inhibition, or impulsiveness consistent with the diagnosis. Although he currently reports symptoms that could be consistent with ADHD, these symptoms are not specific to ADHD, and given his scores on validity measures, are likely related to symptom overreport. Similarly, his overall pattern of scores on cognitive tests provides no evidence of cognitive impairment consistent with ADHD.

Although Mr. Student is currently on academic probation, there are many other potential contributing factors to his academic difficulties. First, his reported study skills are inadequate for success in the college setting. Second, given his academic record, he was likely not prepared to be successful in college-level coursework. Other potential contributing factors include his sleep patterns, which have resulted in some sleep deprivation and a tendency to miss many of his morning classes, and his misuse of alcohol on a regular basis, including frequent blackouts.

Recommendations

Mr. Student should take advantage of the many academic resources available on campus, including [list of what is available; may include supplemental instruction courses, free tutoring, study skills and test-taking courses, special workshops for students on academic probation]. If he predicts he will struggle specifically with certain academic coursework (e.g., math courses, given his lack of college-level preparation in this academic area and his prior failing math grades), he is advised to start the semester by talking with the course instructor, identifying all available resources for that course, scheduling time to use them all semester, and scheduling extra study time for that course into his regular study schedule.

Mr. Student should also consider adjusting his sleep habits to better match his academic schedule or not sign up for morning courses. Lack of class attendance likely has a significant impact on his academic success. If Mr. Student struggles with adjusting his own sleep schedule, he might consider consulting with [College Health Center Name or Psychological Counseling Center Name, if sleep resources are available at one of those sites].

In addition, Mr. Student should strongly consider the potential impact of his alcohol use 3 days a week on both his time available for his academic work and on his cognitive abilities. We strongly recommend he cut down on his drinking; if he finds this difficult to do on his own, he might consider consulting with [College Health Center Name or Psychological Counseling Center Name, if substance use resources are available at one of those sites].

In addition, Mr. Student may need to have his vision checked (even though vision problems did not appear to affect the results of the present evaluation), as poor vision may be impacting his ability to see the blackboard/projector in class and/or to read his textbooks comfortably without straining.

Feedback

Feedback was given to Mr. Student on [date]. It was explained to him that his history and current presentation are not consistent with a diagnosis of ADHD. His test scores were explained to him, including the normal variability in his cognitive strengths and weaknesses and his overall average abilities, as well as their implications for success in college. The potential contributions of sleep, alcohol use, limited college preparedness, and poor study skills were explained to him. He was provided with a resource guide to study skills, and it was explained to him that study skills and habits, like all habits, can be hard to learn on his own and take time and active participation to implement correctly. He insisted that his poor study skills are a result of his ADHD and thus cannot be "fixed." He suggested that his reaction to stimulant medication in the past was diagnostic of ADHD, and the research evidence about this claim was discussed with him. He expressed his disappointment with the conclusions of the evaluation, but acknowledged that his parents also informed him that his sleeping habits and lack of class attendance were important factors contributing to his current academic standing; he also indicated that he had recently been trying to cut back on his alcohol use and noticed that he was able to get more homework done on weekends as a result.

_____   _____

[Names, degrees, signatures of all involved in the evaluation]

Note: This assessment was conducted to answer the specific referral question above and may not be complete for other purposes.

Test Scores

Note: All scores are provided in this sample report for the reader's benefit. In an actual report, I would not include scores that were invalid, but would mark them as invalid for interpretation. In addition, all *italicized comments* below the tables would not be included if the actual test data were in the report.

CAARS T Scores

A	B	C	D	E	F	G	H
54	55	49	44	90+	59	90+	58

As noted in Chapter 13, according to the CAARS manual, scores this high on E and G are possibly related to symptom overreport.

MMPI-2-RF T Scores

CNS	VRIN-r	TRIN-r	F-r	Fp-r	Fs	FBS-r	RBS	L-r	K-r	EID	THD	BXD	RCd
0	58	50	51	51	58	62	97	47	42	64	57	60	62
RC1	RC2	RC3	RC4	RC6	RC7	RC8	RC9	MLS	GIC	HPC	NUC	COG	SUI
56	61	54	59	42	57	59	51	52	46	59	70	97	45
HLP	SFD	NFC	STW	AXY	ANP	BRF	MSF	JCP	SUB	AGG	ACT	FML	IPP
39	51	68	65	59	39	43	42	50	69	51	48	49	51
SAV	SHY	DSF	AES	MEC	AGGR-r	PSYC-r	DISC-r	NEGE-r	INTR-r				
55	50	57	36	65	41	47	47	56	49				

WAIS-IV

Index/subtest	Scaled/index score	95% confidence interval (CI)	Percentile (95% CI)	Interpretation
Verbal Comprehension	108	102–113	55–81	Average to high average
Similarities	13			
Vocabulary	12			
Information	10			
Comprehension	10			
Perceptual Reasoning	100	94–106	34–66	Average
Block Design	10			
Matrix Reasoning	9			
Visual Puzzles	11			
Figure Weights	9			
Working Memory	92	86–99	18–47	Low average to average
Digit Span	10			
Arithmetic	7			
Letter Number Sequencing	11			
Processing Speed	105	96–113	39–81	Average to high average
Symbol Search	11			
Coding	11			
Full Scale IQ	102	98–106	45–66	Average

WMT

For the sake of protecting test security, these data not provided in the sample report.

WIAT-III

Subtest	Standard score	95% CI	Percentile
Reading Comprehension	100	89–111	50
Word Reading	91	84–98	27
Pseudoword Decoding	108	103–113	70
Spelling	112	106–118	79
Numerical Operations	113	108–118	81

The 95% CI percentiles are not available in the computerized scoring system for this test.

AVLT

Subtest	Raw score	Comparison data (ages 20–29) mean (*SD*)
Trials 1–5 total	25	56.7 (7.3)
Immediate Recall	5	11.5 (2.3)
Delayed Recall	4	11.3 (2.5)
Delayed Recognition	9	14.3 (1.1)

Stroop Color and Word Test Scores

Word	Color	Color Word	Interference
44	46	40	44

The manual for the test does not provide confidence intervals.

TMT

Subtest	Percentile (college student norms)
Part A Time	30–40
Part B Time	50–60

References

Achenbach, T. M., Krukowski, R. A., Dumenci, L., & Ivanova, M. Y. (2005). Assessment of adult psychopathology: Meta-analyses and implications of cross-informant correlations. *Psychological Bulletin, 131,* 361–382.

Ackerman, S. J., Hilsenroth, M. J., Baity, M. R., & Blagys, M. D. (2000). Interaction of therapeutic process and alliance during psychological assessment. *Journal of Personality Assessment, 75,* 82–109.

Acklin, M. W. (2002). How to select personality tests for a test battery. In J. N. Butcher (Ed.), *Clinical personality assessment: Practical approaches* (2nd ed., pp. 13–22). New York: Oxford University Press.

ACT, Inc. (2007). Rigor at risk: Reaffirming quality in the high school core curriculum. Retrieved from *www.act.org/research/policymakers/pdf/rigor_report.pdf*.

Aegisdottir, S., White, M. J., Spengler, P. M., Maugherman, A. S., Anderson, L. A., Cook, R. S., et al. (2006). The meta-analysis of clinical judgment project: Fifty-six years of accumulated research on clinical versus statistical prediction. *The Counseling Psychologist, 34,* 341–382.

Alfano, K., & Boone, K. B. (2007). The use of effort tests in the context of actual versus feigned attention-deficit/hyperactivity disorder and learning disability. In K. B. Boone (Ed.), *Assessment of feigned cognitive impairment: A neuropsychological perspective* (pp. 366–383). New York: Guilford Press.

Alloy, L. B., Abramson, L. Y., Urosevic, S., Walshaw, P. D., Nusslock R., & Neeren, A. M. (2005). The psychosocial context of bipolar disorder: Environmental, cognitive, and developmental risk factors. *Clinical Psychology Review, 25,* 1043–1075.

Alloy, L. B., Abramson, L. Y., Whitehouse, W. G., Hogan, M. E., Tashman, N. A., Steinberg, D. L., et al. (2000). The Temple–Wisconsin cognitive vulnerability to depression project: Lifetime history of Axis I psychopathology in individuals at high and low cognitive risk for depression. *Journal of Abnormal Psychology, 109,* 403–418.

American Academy of Pediatrics. (2000). Clinical practice guideline: Diagnosis and evaluation of the child with attention-deficit/hyperactivity disorder. *Pediatrics, 105,* 1158–1170.

American Educational Research Association, American Psychological Association, & National Council on Measurement in Education. (1999). *Standards for educational and psychological testing.* Washington, DC: Author.

American Psychiatric Association. (2013). *Diagnostic and statistical manual of mental disorders* (5th ed.). Arlington, VA: Author.

American Psychological Association. (2000). *Report of the Task Force on Test User Qualifications.* Washington, DC: Author.

American Psychological Association. (2002). Ethical principles of psychologists and code of conduct. *American Psychologist, 57,* 1060–1073.

American Psychological Association. (2010). *Ethical principles of psychologists and code of conduct.* Washington, DC: Author.

Anderson, J. L., Bellbom, M., Bagby, R. M., Quilty, L. C., Veltri, C. O. C., Markon, K. E., et al. (2013). On the convergence between PSY-5 domains and PID-5 domains and facets: Implications for assessment of DSM-5 personality traits. *Assessment, 20,* 286–294.

Ansell, E. B., Kurtz, J. E., DeMoor, R. M., & Markey, P. M. (2011). Validity of the PAI Interpersonal Scales for measuring the dimensions of the interpersonal circumplex. *Journal of Personality Assessment, 93,* 33–39.

Antony, M. M., & Barlow, D. H. (Eds.). (2010). *Handbook of assessment and treatment planning for psychological disorders* (2nd ed.). New York: Guilford Press.

Arango-Munoz, S. (2011). Two levels of metacognition. *Philosophia, 39,* 71–82.

Archer, R. P., Buffington-Vollum, J. K., Stredny, R. V., & Handel, R. W. (2006). A survey of test use patterns among forensic psychologists. *Journal of Personality Assessment, 87,* 64–94.

Arnoult, L. H., & Anderson, C. A. (1988). Identifying and reducing causal reasoning biases in clinical practice. In D. Turk & P. Salovey (Eds.), *Reasoning, inference, and judgment in clinical psychology* (pp. 209–232). New York: Free Press.

Avdeyeva, T. V., Tellegen, A., & Ben-Porath, Y. S. (2012). Empirical correlates of low scores on MMPI-2/MMPI-2-RF restructured clinical scales in a sample of university students. *Assessment, 19,* 388–393.

Ayearst, L. E., & Bagby, R. M. (2010). Evaluating the psychometric properties of psychological measures. In M. M. Antony & D. H. Barlow (Eds.), *Handbook of assessment and treatment planning for psychological disorders* (2nd ed., pp. 23–61). New York: Guilford Press.

Azizian, A., Yeghiyan, M., Ishkhanyan G., Manukyan, Y., & Khandanyan, L. (2011). Clinical validity of the Repeatable Battery for the Assessment of Neuropsychological Status among patients with schizophrenia in the Republic of Armenia. *Archives of Clinical Neuropsychology, 26,* 89–97.

Babcock, P., & Marks, M. (2011). The falling time cost of college: Evidence from half a century of time use data. *Review of Economics and Statistics, 93,* 468–478.

Barlow, D. H. (2005). What's new about evidence-based assessment? *Psychological Assessment, 17,* 308–311.

Barrash, J., Stillman, A., Anderson, S. W., Uc, E. Y., Dawson, J. D., & Rizzo, M. (2010). Prediction of driving ability with neuropsychological tests: Demographic adjustments diminish accuracy. *Journal of the International Neuropsychological Society, 16,* 679–686.

Bauer, L., Pozehl, B., Hertzog, M., Johnson, J., Zimmerman, L., & Filipi, M. (2011). A brief neuropsychological battery for use in the chronic heart failure population. *European Journal of Cardiovascular Nursing, 48,* 587–595.

Baxendale, S. (2011). IQ and ability across the adult life span. *Applied Neuropsychology, 18*, 164–167.

Bayless, J. D., McCormick, J. M., Brumm, M. C., Espe-Pfeifer, P. B., Long, J. J., & Lewis, J. L. (2010). Pre- and post-electroconvulsive therapy multidomain cognitive assessment in psychotic depression: Relationship to premorbid abilities and symptom improvement. *Journal of ECT, 26*, 47–52.

Beatty, W. W., Mold, J. W., & Gontkovsky, S. T. (2003). RBANS performance: Influences of sex and education. *Journal of Clinical and Experimental Neuropsychology, 25*, 1065–1069.

Beatty, W. W., Ryder, K. A., Gontkovsky, S. T., Scott, J. G., McSwan, K. L., & Bharucha, K. J. (2003). Analyzing the subcortical dementia syndrome of Parkinson's disease using the RBANS. *Archives of Clinical Neuropsychology, 18*, 509–520.

Beck, A. T., & Steer, R. A. (1988). *Beck Hopelessness Scale*. San Antonio, TX: Psychological Corporation.

Beck, A. T., & Steer, R. A. (1990). *Manual for the Beck Anxiety Inventory*. San Antonio, TX: Psychological Corporation.

Beck, A. T., & Steer, R. A. (1991). *Manual for the Beck Scale for Suicidal Ideation*. San Antonio, TX: Psychological Corporation.

Beck, A. T., Steer, R. A., & Brown, G. K. (1996). *Beck Depression Inventory manual* (2nd ed.). San Antonio, TX: Psychological Corporation.

Beglinger, L. J., Duff, K., Allison J., Theriault, D., O'Rourke, J. J. F., Leserman, A., et al. (2010). Cognitive change in patients with Huntington disease on the Repeatable Battery for the Assessment of Neuropsychological Status. *Journal of Clinical and Experimental Neuropsychology, 32*, 573–578.

Beglinger, L. J., Duff, K., van der Heiden, S., Moser, D. J., Bayless, J. D., Paulsen, J. S., et al. (2007). Neuropsychological and psychiatric functioning pre- and post-hematopoietic stem cell transplantation in adult cancer patients: A preliminary study. *Journal of the International Neuropsychological Society, 13*, 172–177.

Beglinger, L. J., Mills, J. A., Vik, S. M., Duff, K., Denberg, N. L.,Weckmann, M. T., et al. (2011). The neuropsychological course of acute delirium in adult hematopoietic stem cell transplantation patients. *Archives of Clinical Neuropsychology 26*, 98–109.

Belanger, H. G., Curtiss, G., Demery, J. A., Lebowitz, B. K., & Vanderploeg, R. D. (2005). Factors moderating neuropsychological outcomes following mild traumatic brain injury: A meta-analysis. *Journal of the International Neuropsychological Society, 11*, 215–227.

Belar, C. D. (2009). Advancing the culture of competence. *Training and Education in Professional Psychology, 3*, S63–S65.

Bell, I., & Mellor, D. (2009). Clinical judgments: Research and practice. *Australian Psychologist, 44*, 112–121.

Ben-Porath, Y. S. (2012). *Interpreting the MMPI-2-RF*. Minneapolis: University of Minnesota Press.

Ben-Porath, Y. S., & Tellegen, A. (2011). *Minnesota Multiphasic Personality Inventory–2 Restructured Form manual for administration, scoring, and interpretation*. Minneapolis: University of Minnesota Press.

Benson, N., Hulac, D. M., & Kranzler, J. H. (2010). Independent examination of the Wechsler Adult Intelligence Scale—Fourth Edition (WAIS-IV): What does the WAIS-IV measure? *Psychological Assessment, 22*, 121–130.

Berner, E. S., & Graber, M. L. (2008). Overconfidence as a cause of diagnostic error in medicine. *American Journal of Medicine, 121,* S2–S33.

Bickman, L., Wighton, L. G., Lambert, E. W., Karver, M. S., & Steding, L. (2012). Problems in using diagnosis in child and adolescent mental health services research. *Journal of Methods and Measurement in the Social Sciences, 3,* 1–26.

Binder, L. M., & Binder, A. L. (2011). Relative subtest scatter in the WAIS-IV standardization sample. *The Clinical Neuropsychologist, 25,* 62–71.

Binder, L. M., Iverson, G. L., & Brooks, B. L. (2009). To err is human: "Abnormal" neuropsychological scores and variability are common in healthy adults. *Archives of Clinical Neuropsychology, 24,* 31–46.

Binder, L. M., & Rohling, M. (1996). Money matters: A meta-analysis of the effect of financial incentives on recovery from closed-head injury. *American Journal of Psychiatry, 153,* 7–10.

Binder, L. M., Rohling, M., & Larrabee, G. (1997). A review of mild head trauma: Part 1. A meta-analytic review of neuropsychological studies. *Journal of Clinical and Experimental Neuropsychology, 19,* 421–431.

Blais, M. A., Baity, M. R., & Hopwood, C. J. (Eds.). (2011). *Clinical applications of the Personality Assessment Inventory.* New York: Taylor & Francis.

Boccaccini, M. T., Rufino, K. A., Jackson, R. L., & Murrie, D. C. (2013). Personality Assessment Inventory scores as predictors of misconduct among sex offenders civilly committed as sexually violent predators. *Psychological Assessment, 25,* 1390–1395.

Boggs, D. L., Kelly, D. L., McMahon, R. P., Gold, J. M., Gorelick, D. A., et al. (2012). Rimonabant for neurocognition in schizophrenia: A 16-week double blind randomized placebo controlled trial. *Schizophrenia Research, 134,* 207–210.

Bolinger, E., Reese, C., Suhr, J., & Larrabee, G. (2014). Susceptibility of the MMPI-2-RF Neurological Complaints and Cognitive Complaints Scales to over-reporting in simulated head injury. *Archives of Clinical Neuropsychology, 29,* 7–15.

Boone, K. B. (Ed.). (2007). *Assessment of feigned cognitive impairment: A neuropsychological perspective.* New York: Guilford Press.

Boone, K. B. (2012). *Clinical practice of forensic neuropsychology: An evidence-based approach.* New York: Guilford Press.

Bornovalova, M. A., Blazei, R., Malone, S. H., McGue, M., & Iacono, W. G. (2012). Disentangling the relative contribution of parental asociality and family discord to child disruptive disorders. *Personality Disorders: Theory, Research, and Treatment, 4,* 239–246.

Bornstein, B. H., & Emler, C. (2000). Rationality in medical decision making: A review of the literature on doctors' decision-making biases. *Journal of Evaluation in Clinical Practice, 7,* 97–107.

Borrell-Carrio, F., Suchman, A. L., & Epstein, R. M. (2004). The biopsychosocial model 25 years later: Principles, practice, and scientific inquiry. *Annals of Family Medicine, 2,* 576–582.

Bowden, S. C., Saklofske, D. H., & Weiss, L. G. (2011). Invariance of the measurement model underlying the Wechsler Adult Intelligence Scale–IV in the United States and Canada. *Educational and Psychological Measurement, 71,* 186–199.

Brooks, B. L., Holdnack, J. A., & Iverson, G. L. (2011). Advanced clinical interpretation of the WAIS-IV and WMS-IV: Prevalence of low scores varies by level of intelligence and years of education. *Assessment, 18,* 156–167.

Brooks, B. L., Iverson, G. L., Holdnack, J. A., & Feldman, H. H. (2008). Potential for misclassification of mild cognitive impairment: A study of memory scores on the Wechsler Memory Scale–III in healthy older adults. *Journal of the International Neuropsychological Society, 14,* 463–478.

Brown, T. A., Di Nardo, P. A., & Barlow, D. H. (1994). *Anxiety Disorders Interview Schedule for DSM-IV (ADIS-IV).* New York: Oxford University Press.

Brtek, M. D., & Motavildo, S. J. (2002). Effects of procedure and outcome accountability on interview validity. *Journal of Applied Psychology, 87,* 185–191.

Bruchmuller, K., Margraf, J., & Schneider, S. (2012). Is ADHD diagnosed in accord with diagnostic criteria?: Overdiagnosis and influence of client gender on diagnosis. *Journal of Consulting and Clinical Psychology, 80,* 128–138.

Bufka, L. F., & Camp, N. (2010). Brief measures for screening and measuring mental health outcomes. In M. M. Antony & D. H. Barlow (Eds.), *Handbook of assessment and treatment planning for psychological disorders* (2nd ed., pp. 61–94). New York: Guilford Press.

Bush, S. S. (2009). What to do after making a determination of malingering. In J. E. Morgan & J. J. Sweet (Eds.), *Neuropsychology of malingering casebook* (pp. 530–540). New York: Psychology Press.

Bush, S. S., Ruff, R.M., Troster, A. I., Barth, J. T., Koffler, S. P., Pliskin, N. H., et al. (2005). Symptom validity assessment: Practice issues and medical necessity: NAN Policy and Planning Committee. *Archives of Clinical Neuropsychology, 20,* 419–426.

Butcher, J. N. (2002). Clinical personality assessment: An overview. In J. N. Butcher (Ed.), *Clinical personality assessment: Practical approaches* (2nd ed., pp. 1–6). New York: Oxford University Press.

Butzlaff, R. L., & Hooley, J. M. (1998). Expressed emotion and psychiatric relapse: A meta analysis. *Archives of General Psychiatry, 50,* 551–564.

Byrne, B. M., & Campbell, T. L. (1999). Cross-cultural comparisons and the presumption of equivalent measurement and theoretical structure: A look beneath the surface. *Journal of Cross-Cultural Psychology, 30,* 555–574.

Byrne, B. M., Stewart, S. M., Kennard, B. D., & Lee, P. W. H. (2007). The Beck Depression Inventory–II: Testing for measurement equivalence and factor mean differences across Hong Kong and American adolescents. *International Journal of Testing, 7,* 293–309.

Byrne, B. M., Stewart, S. M., & Lee, P. W. H. (2004). Validating the Beck Depression Inventory–II for Hong Kong community adolescents. *International Journal of Testing, 4,* 199–216.

Cacioppo, J. T., Hawkley, L. C., & Thisted, R. A. (2010). Perceived social isolation makes one sad: 5-year cross-lagged analyses of loneliness and depressive symptomatology in the Chicago Health, Aging, and Social Relations Study. *Psychology and Aging, 25,* 453–463.

Cacioppo, J. T., Hughes, M. E., Waite, L. J., Hawkley, L. C., & Thisted, R. A. (2006). Loneliness is a specific risk factor for depressive symptoms: Cross-sectional and longitudinal analyses. *Psychology and Aging, 21,* 140–151.

Calhoun, P. S., Collie, C. F., Clancy, C. P., Braxton, L. E., & Beckham, J. C. (2011). Use of the PAI in assessment of posttraumatic stress disorder among help-seeking veterans. In M. A. Blais, M. R. Baity, & C. J. Hopwood (Eds.), *Clinical applications of the Personality Assessment Inventory* (pp. 93–112). New York: Taylor & Francis.

Camara, W. J., Nathan, J. S., & Puente, A. E. (2000). Psychological test usage: Implications in professional psychology. *Professional Psychology: Research and Practice, 31*, 141–154.

Camilli, G., & Shepard, L. A. (1994). *Methods for identifying biased test items.* Thousand Oaks, CA: Sage.

Campbell, D. T., & Fiske, D. W. (1959). Convergent and discriminant validation by the multitrait–multimethod matrix. *Psychological Bulletin, 56*, 81–105.

Canel-Cinarbas, D., Cui, Y., & Lauridsen, E. (2011). Cross-cultural validation of the Beck Depression Inventory–II across U.S. and Turkish samples. *Measurement and Evaluation in Counseling and Development, 44*, 77–91.

Canivez, G. L. (2008). Orthogonal higher-order factor structure of the Stanford–Binet Intelligence Scales—Fifth Edition for children and adolescents. *School Psychology Quarterly, 23*, 533–541.

Canivez, G. L., & Watkins, M. W. (2010). Investigation of the factor structure of the Wechsler Adult Intelligence Scale—Fourth Edition (WAIS-IV): Exploratory and higher-order factor analyses. *Psychological Assessment, 22*, 827–836.

Carroll, J. B. (1997). The three-stratum theory of cognitive abilities. In D. P. Flanagan, J. L. Genshaft, & P. L. Harrison (Eds.), *Contemporary intellectual assessment: Theories, tests, and issues* (pp. 122–130). New York: Guilford Press.

Carlozzi, N. E., Horner, M. D., Yan, C., & Tilley, B. C. (2008). Factor analysis of the Repeatable Battery for the Assessment of Neuropsychological Status. *Applied Neuropsychology, 15*, 274–279.

Charter, R. A., & Feldt, L. S. (2001). Meaning of reliability in terms of correct and incorrect clinical decisions: The art of decision making is still alive. *Journal of Clinical and Experimental Neuropsychology, 23*, 530–537.

Cheng, Y., Wu, W., Wang, J., Feng, W., Wu, X., & Li, C. (2011). Reliability and validity of the Repeatable Battery for the Assessment of Neuropsychological Status in community-dwelling elderly. *Archives of Medical Science, 7*, 850–857.

Chianetta, J. M., Lefebvre, M., LeBlanc, R., & Grignon, S. (2008). Comparative psychometric properties of the BACS and RBANS I patients with schizophrenia and schizoaffective disorder. *Schizophrenia Research, 105*, 86–94.

Chronbach, L. J., & Meehl, P. E. (1955). Construct validity in psychological tests. *Psychological Bulletin, 52*, 281–302.

Clark, J. H., Hobson, V. L., & O'Bryant, S. E. (2010). Diagnostic accuracy of percent retention scores on RBANS verbal memory subtests for the diagnosis of Alzheimer's disease and mild cognitive impairment. *Archives of Clinical Neuropsychology, 25*, 318–326.

Coffey, D. M., Marmol, L., Schock, L., & Adams, W. (2005). The influence of acculturation on the Wisconsin Card Sorting Test by Mexican Americans. *Archives of Clinical Neuropsychology, 20*, 795–803.

Conners, C. K., Erhardt, D., & Sparrow, E. P. (1998). *Conners' Adult ADHD Rating Scale—Self-Report: Long Version.* North Tonawanda, NY: Multi-Health Systems.

Conrad, P., & Potter, D. (2000). From hyperactive children to ADHD adults: Observations on the expansion of medical categories. *Social Problems, 47*, 559–582.

Cook, T. D., & Campbell, D. T. (1979). *Quasi-experimentation: Design and analysis issues for field settings.* Boston: Houghton Mifflin.

Craig, R. J. (2013). Assessing personality and psychopathology with interviews. In

J. R. Graham, J. A. Naglieri, & I. B. Weiner (Eds.), *Handbook of psychology: Vol. 10. Assessment psychology* (2nd ed., pp. 558–582). New York: Wiley.

Crawford, J. R., & Garthwaite, P. H. (2009). Percentiles please: The case for expressing neuropsychological test scores and accompanying confidence limits as percentile ranks. *The Clinical Neuropsychologist, 23*, 193–204.

Crawford, J. R., Garthwaite, P. H., Longman, R. S., & Batty, A. M. (2012). Some supplementary methods for the analysis of WAIS-IV index scores in neuropsychological assessment. *Journal of Neuropsychology, 6*, 192–211.

Crawford, J. R., Garthwaite, P. H., Morrice, N., & Duff, K. (2012). Some supplementary methods for the analysis of the RBANS. *Psychological Assessment, 24*, 365–374.

Cromer, K. R., Schmidt, N. B., & Murphy, D. L. (2007). An investigation of traumatic life events and obsessive–compulsive disorder. *Behaviour Research and Therapy, 45*, 1683–1691.

Cronbach, L. J., & Meehl, P. E. (1955). Construct validity in psychological tests. *Psychological Bulletin, 52*, 281–302.

Croskerry, P. (2009). A universal model of diagnostic reasoning. *Academic Medicine, 84*, 1022–1028.

Crupi, V., Tentori, K., & Lombardi, L. (2009). Pseudodiagnosticity revisited. *Psychological Review, 116*, 971–985.

Csigo, K., Harsanyi A., Demeter, G., Rajkai, C., Nemeth, A., & Racsmany, M. (2010). Long-term follow-up of patients with obsessive–compulsive disorder treated by anterior capsulotomy: A neuropsychological study. *Journal of Affective Disorders, 126*, 198–205.

Danzinger, P. R., & Welfel, E. R. (2001). The impact of managed care on mental health counselors: A survey of perceptions, practices, and compliance with ethical standards. *Journal of Mental Health Counseling, 23*, 137–150.

Dawson, N. V., & Arkes, H. R. (1987). Systematic errors in medical decision making: Judgment limitations. *Journal of General Internal Medicine, 2*, 183–187.

De Figueiredo, J. M. (2013). Distress, demoralization, and psychopathology: Diagnostic boundaries. *European Journal of Psychiatry, 27*, 61–73.

Delis, D. C., Kaplan, E., & Kramer, J. H. (2001). *Delis–Kaplan Executive Function System*. San Antonio, TX: Pearson.

Demakis, G. J. (Ed.). (2012). *Civil capacities in clinical neuropsychology: Research findings and practical applications*. New York: Oxford University Press.

Derogatis, L. R. (1994). *Symptom Checklist-90-R administration, scoring, and procedures manual* (3rd ed). Minneapolis, MN: National Computer Systems.

Di Nardo, P. A., Brown, T. A., & Barlow, D. H. (1994). *Anxiety Disorders Interview Schedule for DSM-IV: Lifetime Version*. New York: Oxford University Press.

Distefano, C., & Dombrowski, S. C. (2006). Investigating the theoretical structure of the Stanford–Binet—Fifth Edition. *Journal of Psychoeducational Assessment, 24*, 123–136.

Donnell, A., Belanger, H., & Vanderploeg, R. (2011). Implications of psychometric measurement for neuropsychological interpretation. *The Clinical Neuropsychologist, 25*, 1097–1118.

Dovidio, J. F., & Fiske, S. T. (2012). Under the radar: How unexamined biases in decision-making processes in clinical interactions can contribute to health care disparities. *American Journal of Public Health, 102*, 945–952.

Doyle, A. C. (1892/2011). *The adventures of Sherlock Holmes* (Project Gutenberg version). Retrieved from *www.gutenberg.org/files/1661/1661-h/1661-h.htm#1*.

Dozois, D. J. A., & Covin, R. (2004). The Beck Depression Inventory–II (BDI-II), Beck Hopelessness Scale (BHS), and Beck Scale for Suicide Ideation (BSS). In M. Hersen (Series Ed.), D. L. Segal & M. Hilsenroth (Vol. Eds.), *Comprehensive handbook of psychological assessment: Vol. 2. Personality assessment and psychopathology* (pp. 50–69). Hoboken, NJ: Wiley.

Dozois, D. J. A., & Dobson, K. S. (2010). Depression. In M. M. Antony & D. H. Barlow (Eds.), *Handbook of assessment and treatment planning for psychological disorders* (2nd ed., pp. 344–389). New York: Oxford University Press.

Drozdick, L. W., & Cullum, C. M. (2011). Expanding the ecological validity of WAIS-IV and WMS-IV with the Texas Functional Living Scale. *Assessment, 18,* 141–155.

Drozdick, L. W., Wahlstrom, D., Zhu, J., & Weiss, L. G. (2012). The Wechsler Adult Intelligence Scale—Fourth Edition and the Wechsler Memory Scale—Fourth Edition. In D. P. Flanagan & P. L. Harrison (Eds.), *Contemporary intellectual assessment: Theories, tests, and issues* (3rd ed., pp. 197–223). New York: Guilford Press.

Duff, K., Beglinger, L. J., Schoenberg, M. R., Patton, D. E., Mold, J., Scott, J. G., et al. (2005). Test–retest stability and practice effects of the RBANS in a community-dwelling elderly sample. *Journal of Clinical and Experimental Neuropsychology, 27,* 565–575.

Duff, K., Beglinger, L. J., Theriault, D., Allison, J., & Paulsen, J. S. (2010). Cognitive deficits in Huntington's disease on the Repeatable Battery for the Assessment of Neuropsychological Status. *Journal of Clinical and Experimental Neuropsychology, 32,* 231–238.

Duff, K., Hobson, V. L., Beglinger, L. J., & O'Bryant, S. E. (2010). Diagnostic accuracy of the RBANS in mild cognitive impairment: Limitations on assessing milder impairments. *Archives of Clinical Neuropsychology, 25,* 429–441.

Duff, K., Langbehn, D. R., Schoenberg, M. R., Moser, D. J., Baade, L. E., Mold, J., et al. (2006). Examining the Repeatable Battery for the Assessment of Neuropsychological Status: Factor analytic studies in an elderly sample. *American Journal of Geriatric Psychiatry, 14,* 976–979.

Duff, K., Patton, D., Schoenberg, M. R., Mold, J., Scott, J. G., & Adams, R. L. (2003). Age- and education-corrected independent normative data for the RBANS in a community-dwelling elderly sample. *The Clinical Neuropsychologist, 17,* 351–366.

Duff, K., Patton, D. E., Schoenberg, M. R., Mold, J., Scott, J. G., & Adams, R. L (2011). Intersubtest discrepancies on the RBANS: Results from the OKLAHOMA Study. *Applied Neuropsychology, 18,* 79–85.

Duff, K., Schoenberg, M. R., Mold, J. W., Scott, J. G., & Adams, R. L. (2011). Gender differences on the Repeatable Battery for the Assessment of Neuropsychological Status subtests in older adults: Baseline and retest data. *Journal of Clinical and Experimental Neuropsychology, 33,* 448–455.

Duff, K., Spering, C. C., O'Bryant, S. E., Beglinger, L. J., Moser, D. J., Mold, J., et al. (2011). The RBANS Effort Index: Base rates in geriatric samples. *Applied Neuropsychology, 18,* 11–17.

Eaton, W. W., Muntaner, C., Smith, C., Tien, A., & Ybarra, M. (2004). Center for Epidemiologic Studies Depression Scale: Review and revision (CESD and

CESDR). In M. E. Maruish (Ed.), *The use of psychological testing for treatment planning and outcome assessments: Vol. 3. Instruments for adults* (pp. 363–378). Mahwah, NJ: Erlbaum.

Edwards, O. W., & Oakland, T. D. (2006). Factorial invariance of Woodcock–Johnson III scores for African Americans and Caucasian Americans. *Journal of Psychoeducational Assessment, 24,* 358–366.

Elhai, J. D., Naifeh, J. A., Zucker, I. S., Gold, S. N., Deitsch, S. E., & Frueh, B. C. (2004). Discriminating malingered from genuine civilian posttraumatic stress disorder: A validation of three MMPI-2 Infrequency scales (F, Fp, and Fptsd). *Assessment, 11,* 139–144.

Elstein, A. S. (2009). Thinking about diagnostic thinking: A 30-year perspective. *Advances in Health Sciences Education, 14,* 7–18.

Elstein, A. S., Shulman, L. S., & Sprafka, S. A. (1978). *Medical problem solving: An analysis of clinical reasoning.* Cambridge, MA: Harvard University Press.

Endicott, J., & Spitzer, R. L. (1978). A diagnostic interview: The Schedule for Affective Disorders and Schizophrenia. *Archives of General Psychiatry, 35,* 837–844.

Engel, G. (1977). The need for a new medical model: A challenge for biomedicine. *Science, 196,* 129–136.

Exner J. E., & Erdberg, P. (2002). Why use personality tests?: A brief history and some comments. In J. N. Butcher (Ed.), *Clinical personality assessment: Practical approaches* (2nd ed., pp. 7–12). New York: Oxford University Press.

Falleti, M. G., Maruff, P., Collie, A., & Barby, D. G. (2006). Practice effects associated with the repeated assessment of cognitive function using the CogState Battery at 10-minute, one week and one month test–retest intervals. *Journal of Clinical and Experimental Neuropsychology, 28,* 1095–1112.

Faust, D., Hart, K. J., Guilmette, T. J., & Arkes, H. R. (1988). Neuropsychologists' capacity to detect adolescent malingerers. *Professional Psychology: Research and Practice, 19,* 508–515.

Fennig, S., Craig, T. J., Tanenberg-Karant, M., & Bromet, E. J. (1994). Comparison of facility and research diagnoses in first-admission psychotic patients. *American Journal of Psychiatry, 151,* 1423–1429.

Ferguson, R. J., Mittenberg, W., Barone, D. F., & Schneider, B. (1999). Postconcussion syndrome following sports-related head injury: Expectation as etiology. *Neuropsychology, 13,* 582–589.

Fernandez, A. L., & Marcopulos, B. A. (2008). A comparison of normative data for the Trail Making Test from several countries: Equivalence of norms and considerations for interpretation. *Scandinavian Journal of Psychology, 49,* 239–246.

Finn, S. E. (2007). *In our clients' shoes: Theory and techniques of therapeutic assessment.* Mahwah, NJ: Erlbaum.

Finn, S. E., & Tonsager, M. E. (1992). Therapeutic effects of providing MMPI-2 test feedback to college students awaiting therapy. *Psychological Assessment, 4,* 278–287.

Fishbain, D. A., Cole, B., Cutler, R. B., Lewis, J., Rosomoff, H. L., & Rosomoff, R. S. (2003). A structured evidence-based review on the meaning of nonorganic physical signs: Waddell signs. *Pain Medicine, 4,* 141–181.

Flanagan, D. P., Alfonso, V. C., & Ortiz, S. O. (2011). The cross-battery assessment approach: An overview, historical perspective, and current directions. In D. P. Flanagan & P. L. Harrison (Eds.), *Contemporary intellectual assessment; Theories, tests, and issues* (3rd ed., pp. 459–483). New York: Guilford Press.

Floyd, R. G., Shands, E. I., Rafael, F. A., Bergeron, R., & McGrew, K. S. (2009). The dependability of general-factor loadings: The effects of factor-extraction methods, test battery composition, test battery size, and their interactions. *Intelligence, 37,* 453–465.

Folstein, M. F., Folstein, S. E., & McHugh, P. R. (1975). Mini mental state: A practical method for grading the cognitive state of patients for the clinician. *Journal of Psychiatric Research, 12,* 189–198.

Forbey, J. D., Lee, T. T., & Handel, R. W. (2010). Correlates of the MMPI-2-RF in a college setting. *Psychological Assessment, 22,* 737–744.

Ford, M. R., & Widiger, T. A. (1989). Sex bias in the diagnosis of histrionic and antisocial personality disorders. *Journal of Consulting and Clinical Psychology, 57,* 301–305.

Förster, S., Teipel, S., Zach, C., Rominger, A., Cuming, P., La Fougere, C., et al. (2010). FDG-PET mapping the brain substrates of visuo-constructive processing in Alzheimer's disease. *Journal of Psychiatric Research, 44,* 462–469.

Fouad, N. A., Grus, C. L., Hatcher, R. L., Kaslow, N. J., Hutchings, P. S., Madison, M. B., et al. (2009). Competency benchmarks: A model for understanding and measuring competence in professional psychology across training levels. *Training and Education in Professional Psychology and Practice, 4,* S5–S26.

Frances, A. (2010, February 11). Opening Pandora's box: The 19 worst suggestions for DSM-5. *Psychiatric Times,* pp. 1–10.

Frances, A. (2013). *Saving normal: An insider's revolt against out-of-control psychiatric diagnosis, DSM-5, big pharma, and the medicalization of ordinary life.* New York: HarperCollins.

Francis-Rainer, E. L., Alloy, L. B., & Abramson, L. Y. (2006). Depressive personality styles and bipolar spectrum disorder: Prospective tests of the event congruency hypothesis. *Bipolar Disorders, 8,* 382–399.

Frank, J. D. (1974). Common features of psychotherapies and their patients. *Psychotherapy and Psychosomatics, 24,* 368–371.

Freeman, V. G., Rathore, S. S., Weinfurt, K. P., Schulman, K. A., & Sulmasy, D. P. (1999). Lying for patients: Physician deception of third party payers. *Archives of Internal Medicine, 159,* 2263–2270.

Freilich, B. M., & Hyer, L. A. (2007). Relation of the Repeatable Battery for Assessment of Neuropsychological Status to measures of daily functioning in dementia. *Psychological Reports, 10,* 119–129.

Frisch, M. B., Cornell, J., Villaneuva, M., & Retzlaff, P. J. (1991). Clinical validation of the Quality of Life Inventory: A measure of life satisfaction for use in treatment planning and outcome assessment. *Psychological Assessment, 4,* 92–101.

Frueh, B. C., Elhai, J. D., Grubaugh, A. L., Monnier, J., Kashdan, T. B., Sauvageot, J. A., et al. (2005). Documented combat exposure of US veterans seeking treatment for combat-related post-traumatic stress disorder. *British Journal of Psychiatry, 186,* 467–472.

Furnham, A., & Chamorro-Premuzic, T. (2010). Consensual beliefs about the fairness and accuracy of selection methods at university. *International Journal of Selection and Assessment, 18,* 417–424.

Gallagher, R. P. (2010). *National survey of counseling center directors.* Retrieved from *www.iacsinc.org/NSCCD%202010.pdf.*

Gambrill, E. (1990). *Critical thinking in clinical practice: Improving the quality of judgments and decisions.* San Francisco: Jossey-Bass.

Gambrill, E. (2005). *Critical thinking in clinical practice: Improving the quality of judgments and decisions* (2nd ed.). Hoboken, NJ: Wiley.

Garb, H. N. (1998a). Clinical judgment, clinical training, and professional experience. *Psychological Bulletin, 105,* 387–396.

Garb, H. N. (1998b). *Studying the clinician: Judgment research and psychological assessment.* Washington, DC: American Psychological Association.

Garb, H. N. (2007). Computer-administered interviews and rating scales. *Psychological Assessment, 19,* 4–13.

Garb, H. N., Lillienfeld, S. O., & Fowler, K. A. (2008). Psychological assessment and clinical judgment. In J. E. Maddux & B. A. Winstead (Eds.), *Psychopathology: Foundations for a contemporary understanding* (2nd ed., pp. 121–144). New York: Taylor & Francis.

Garcia, C., Leahy, B., Corradi, K., & Forchetti, C. (2008). Component structure of the Repeatable Battery for the Assessment of Neuropsychological Status in dementia. *Archives of Clinical Neuropsychology, 23,* 63–72.

Gasquoine, P. G. (2009). Race-norming of neuropsychological tests. *Neuropsychology Review, 19,* 250–262.

Gaultney, J. F. (2010). The prevalence of sleep disorders in college students: Impact on academic performance. *Journal of American College Health, 59,* 91–97.

Gervais, R. O., Ben-Porath, Y. S., Wygant, D. B., & Green, P. (2007). Development and validation of a Response Bias Scale (RBS) for the MMPI-2. *Assessment, 14,* 196–208.

Gervais, R. O., Russell, A. S., Green, P., Allen, L. M., Ferrari, R., & Pieschl, S. D. (2001). Effort testing in patients with fibromyalgia and disability incentives. *Journal of Rheumatology, 28,* 1892–1899.

Ghaemi, S. N. (2009). The rise and fall of the biopsychosocial model. *British Journal of Psychiatry, 195,* 3–4.

Gilbelman, M., & Mason, S. E. (2002). Treatment choices in a managed care environment: A multi-disciplinary exploration. *Clinical Social Work Journal, 30,* 199–214.

Glass, L. A., Ryan, J. J., & Charter, R. A. (2010). Discrepancy score reliabilities in the WAIS-IV standardization sample. *Journal of Psychoeducational Assessment, 28,* 201–208.

Glockner, A., & Witteman, C. (2010). Beyond dual-process models: A categorization of processes underlying intuitive judgment and decision making. *Thinking and Reasoning, 16,* 1–25.

Gogos, A., Joshua, N., & Rossell, S. L. (2010). Use of the Repeatable Battery for the Assessment of Neuropsychological Status (RBANS) to investigate group and gender differences in schizophrenia and bipolar disorder. *Australian and New Zealand Journal of Psychiatry, 44,* 220–229.

Gold, J. M., Queern, C., Iannone, V. N., & Buchanan, R. W. (1999). Repeatable Battery for the Assessment of Neuropsychological Status as a screening test in schizophrenia: I. Sensitivity, reliability, and validity. *American Journal of Psychiatry, 156,* 1944–1950.

Gontkovsky, S. T., Hillary, F. G., & Scott, J. G. (2002). Cross-validation and test sensitivity of the Repeatable Battery for the Assessment of Neuropsychological Status (RBANS). *Journal of Cognitive Rehabilitation, 20,* 26–31.

Goodwin, B. E., Sellbom, M., & Arbisi, P. A. (2013). Posttraumatic stress disorder in veterans: The utility of the MMPI-2-RF validity scales in detecting over-reported symptoms. *Psychological Assessment, 25,* 671–678.

Gottfredson, L. S. (1997). Mainstream science on intelligence: An editorial with 52 signatories, history, and bibliography. *Intelligence, 24,* 13–23.

Graber, M. L. (2009). Educational strategies to reduce diagnostic error: Can you teach this stuff? *Advances in Health Science Education, 14,* 63–69.

Graber, M. L., Franklin, N., & Gordon, R. R. (2005). Diagnostic error in internal medicine. *Archives of Internal Medicine, 165,* 1493–1499.

Green, A., Garrick, T., Sheedy, D., Blake, H., Shores, A., & Harper, C. (2008). Repeatable Battery for the Assessment of Neuropsychological Status (RBANS): Preliminary Australian normative data. *Australian Journal of Psychology, 60,* 72–90.

Green, A., Garrick, T., Sheedy, D., Blake, H., Shores, E. A., & Harper, C. (2010). The effect of moderate to heavy alcohol consumption on neuropsychological performance as measured by the Repeatable Battery for the Assessment of Neuropsychological Status. *Alcoholism: Clinical and Experimental Research, 34,* 443–450.

Green, P. (2005). *Green's Word Memory Test for Windows: User's manual.* Edmonton, Alberta, Canada: Author.

Green, P., Rohling, M. L., Lees-Haley, P. R., & Allen, L. M. (2001). Effort has a greater effect on test scores than severe brain injury in compensation claimants. *Brain Injury, 15,* 1045–1060.

Greene, J. P., & Foster, G. (2003). *Public high school graduation and college readiness rates in the United States.* New York: Manhattan Institute for Policy Research. Retrieved from *www.manhattan-institute.org/html/ewp_03.htm.*

Greiffenstein, M. F., Baker, W. J., & Johnson-Greene, D. (2002). Actual versus self-reported scholastic achievement of litigating postconcussion and severe closed head injury claimants. *Psychological Assessment, 14,* 202–208.

Greiffenstein, M. F., Gervais, R., Baker, W. J., Artiola, L., & Smith, H. (2013). Symptom validity testing in medically unexplained pain: A chronic regional pain syndrome type 1 case series. *The Clinical Neuropsychologist, 27,* 138–147.

Greve, K. W., Etherton, J. L., Ord, J., Bianchini, K. J., & Curtis, K. L. (2009). Detecting malingered pain-related disability: Classification accuracy of the Test of Memory Malingering. *The Clinical Neuropsychologist, 23,* 1250–1271.

Grothe, K. B., Dutton, G. R., Jones, G. N., Bodenlos, J., Ancona, M., & Brantley, P. J. (2005). Validation of the Beck Depression Inventory–II in a low-income African American sample of medical outpatients. *Psychological Assessment, 17,* 110–1114.

Groth-Marnat, G. (2009). *Handbook of psychological assessment* (5th ed.). Hoboken, NJ: Wiley.

Grove, W. M., Zald, D. H., Lebow, B. S., Snitz, B. E., & Nelson, C. (2000). Clinical versus mechanical prediction: A meta-analysis. *Psychological Assessment, 12,* 19–30.

Gunstad, J., & Suhr, J. A. (2001). "Expectation as Etiology" versus "The Good Old Days": Postconcussion syndrome symptom reporting in athletes, headache sufferers, and depressed individuals. *Journal of the International Neuropsychological Society, 7,* 323–333.

Gunstad, J., & Suhr, J. A. (2002). Perceptions of illness: Non-specificity of postconcussion syndrome symptom expectation. *Journal of the International Neuropsychological Society, 8*, 37–47.

Hagger, M. S., & Orbell, S. (2003). A meta-analytic review of the common-sense model of illness representations. *Psychology and Health, 18*, 141–184.

Hammen, C. (2006). Stress generation in depression: Reflections on originals, research, and future directions. *Journal of Clinical Psychology, 62*, 1065–1082.

Hammen, C., Kim, E. Y., Eberhart, N. K., & Brennan, P. A. (2009). Chronic and acute stress and the prediction of major depression in women. *Depression and Anxiety, 26*, 718–723.

Handler, L., & Smith, J. D. (2012). Education and training in psychological assessment. In J. R. Graham, J. A. Naglieri, & I. B. Weiner (Eds.), *Handbook of psychology: Vol. 10. Assessment psychology* (2nd ed., pp. 211–238). Hoboken, NJ: Wiley.

Harding, T. P. (2007). Clinical decision-making: How prepared are we? *Training and Education in Professional Psychology, 1*, 95–104.

Harkness, A. R., & McNulty, J. L. (1994). The Personality Psychopathology Five (PSY-5): Issues from the pages of a diagnostic manual instead of a dictionary. In S. Strack & M. Lorr (Eds.), *Differentiating normal and abnormal personality* (pp. 291–315). New York: Springer.

Harrison, A. G., Alexander, S. J., & Armstrong, I. T. (2013). Higher reported levels of depression, stress, and anxiety are associated with increased endorsement of ADHD symptoms by postsecondary students. *Canadian Journal of School Psychology, 28*, 243–260.

Harrison, A. G., & Edwards, M. J. (2010). Symptom exaggeration in post-secondary students: Preliminary base rates in a Canadian sample. *Applied Neuropsychology, 17*, 135–143.

Harrison, A. G., Green, P., & Flaro, L. (2012). The importance of symptom validity testing in adolescents and young adults undergoing assessments for learning or attention difficulties. *Canadian Journal of School Psychology, 27*, 98–113.

Hashem, A., Chi, M. T. H., & Friedman, C. P. (2003). Medical errors as a result of specialization. *Journal of Biomedical Informatics, 36*, 61–69.

Heaton, R. K., Chelune, G. J., Talley, J. L., Kay, G. G., & Curtiss, G. (1993). *Wisconsin Card Sorting Test manual: Revised and expanded*. Lutz, FL: Psychological Assessment Resources.

Heaton, R. K., Smith, H. H., Lehman, R. A. W., & Vogt, A. T. (1978). Prospects for faking believable deficits on neuropsychological testing. *Journal of Consulting and Clinical Psychology, 46*, 892–900.

Heilbronner, R. L., Sweet, J. J., Attix, D. K., Krull, K. R., Henry, G. K., & Hart, R. P. (2010). Official position of the American Academy of Clinical Neuropsychology on serial neuropsychological assessments: The utility and challenges of repeat test administrations in clinical and forensic contexts. *The Clinical Neuropsychologist, 24*, 1267–1278.

Heilbronner, R. L., Sweet, J. J., Morgan, J. E., Larrabee, G. J., Millis, S. R., & Conference Participants. (2009). American Academy of Clinical Neuropsychology Consensus Conference statement on the neuropsychological assessment of effort, response bias, and malingering. *The Clinical Neuropsychologist, 23*, 1093–1129.

Hendry, M. C., Douglas, K. S., Winter, E. A., & Edens, J. F. (2013). Construct measurement quality improves predictive accuracy in violence risk assessment:

An illustration using the Personality Assessment Inventory. *Behavioral Sciences and the Law, 31*, 477–493.

Henry, B., Moffit, T. E., Caspi, A., Langley, J., & Silva, P. A. (1994). On the "remembrance of things past": A longitudinal evaluation of the retrospective method. *Psychological Assessment, 6,* 92–101.

Hill, S. W., & Gale, S. D. (2011). Predicting psychogenic nonepileptic seizures with the Personality Assessment Inventory and seizure variables. *Epilepsy and Behavior, 22,* 505–510.

Hilsenroth, M. J., Peters, E. J., & Ackerman, S. J. (2004). The development of therapeutic alliance during psychological assessment: Patient and therapist perspectives across treatment. *Journal of Personality Assessment, 83,* 332–344.

Hobart, M. P., Goldberg, R., Bartko, J. J., & Gold, J. M. (1999). Repeatable Battery for the Assessment of Neuropsychological Status as a screening test in schizophrenia: II. Convergent/discriminant validity and diagnostic group comparisons. *American Journal of Psychiatry, 156,* 1951–1957.

Hobson, V. L., Hall, J. R., Humphreys-Clark, J. D., Schrimsher, G. W., & O'Bryant, S. E. (2010). Identifying functional impairment with scores from the Repeatable Battery for the Assessment of Neuropsychological Status (RBANS). *International Journal of Geriatric Psychiatry, 25,* 525–530.

Holzer, L., Chinet, L., Jaugey, L., Plancherel, B., Sofia, C., Halfon, O., et al. (2007). Detection of cognitive impairment with the Repeatable Battery for the Assessment of Neuropsychological Status (RBANS) in adolescents with psychotic symptomatology. *Schizophrenia Research, 95,* 48–53.

Hook, J. N., Marquine, M. J., & Hoelzle, J. B. (2009). Repeatable Battery for the Assessment of Neuropsychological Status Effort Index performance in a medically ill geriatric sample. *Archives of Clinical Neuropsychology, 24,* 231–235.

Hopwood, C. J., Orlando, M. J., & Clark, T. S. (2010). The detection of malingered pain-related disability with the Personality Assessment Inventory. *Rehabilitation Psychology, 55,* 307–310.

Hopwood, C. J., & Richard, D. C. (2005). Graduate student WAIS-III scoring accuracy is a function of Full Scale IQ and complexity of examiner tasks. *Assessment, 12,* 445–454.

Hunsley, J., & Mash, E. J. (2005). Introduction to the special section on developing guidelines for the evidence-based assessment (EBA) of adult disorders. *Psychological Assessment, 17,* 251–255.

Hunsley, J., & Mash, E. J. (2007). Evidence-based assessment. *Annual Review of Clinical Psychology, 3,* 57–79.

Hunsley, J., & Mash, E. J. (2008a). Developing criteria for evidence-based assessment: An introduction to assessments that work. In J. Hunsley & E. J. Mash (Eds.), *A guide to assessments that work* (pp. 3–14). New York: Oxford University Press.

Hunsley, J., & Mash, E. J. (Eds.). (2008b). *A guide to assessments that work.* New York: Oxford University Press.

Hunsley, J., & Mash, E. J. (2010). The role of assessment in evidence-based practice. In M. M. Antony & D. H. Barlow (Eds.), *Handbook of assessment and treatment planning for psychological disorders* (2nd ed., pp. 3–33). New York: Guilford Press.

Hunt, J., & Eisenberg, D. (2010). Mental health problems and help-seeking behavior among college students. *Journal of Adolescent Health, 46,* 3–10.

Individuals with Disabilities Education Act, 20 U. S. C. § 1400 (2004).

Ingram, P. B., Kelso, K. M., & McCord, D. M. (2011). Empirical correlates and expanded interpretation of the MMPI-2-RF Restructured Clinical Scale 3 (Cynicism). *Assessment, 18,* 95–101.

Insel, T., Cuthbert, B., Garvey, M., Heinssen, R., Pine, D. S., Quinn, K., et al. (2010). Research domain criteria (RDoC): Toward a new classification framework for research on mental disorders. *American Journal of Psychiatry, 167,* 748–751.

Iverson, G. L., Brooks, B. L., & Haley, G. M. T. (2009). Interpretation of the RBANS in inpatient psychiatry: Clinical normative data and prevalence of low scores for patients with schizophrenia. *Applied Neuropsychology, 16,* 31–41.

Jansen, C. E., Cooper, B. A., Dodd, M. J., & Miaskowski, C. A. (2011). A prospective longitudinal study of chemotherapy-induced cognitive changes in breast cancer patients. *Support Care Cancer, 19,* 1647–1656.

Jensen, A. R. (1980). *Bias in mental testing.* New York: Free Press.

Joe, S., Woolley, M. E., Brown, G. K., Ghahramanlou-Holloway, M., & Beck, A. T. (2008). Psychometric properties of the Beck Depression Inventory–II in low-income, African American suicide attempters. *Journal of Personality Assessment, 90,* 521–523.

Johnson, J. L., & Lesniak-Karpiak, K. (1997). The effect of warning on malingering on memory and motor tasks in college samples. *Archives of Clinical Neuropsychology, 12,* 231–238.

Johnson, L. A., Hobson, V., Jenkins, M., Dentino, A., Ragain, R. M., & O'Bryant, S. (2011). The influence of thyroid function on cognition in a sample of ethnically diverse, rural-dwelling women: A Project FRONTIER study. *Journal of Neuropsychiatry and Clinical Neurosciences, 23,* 219–222.

Jones, A., & Ingram, M. V. (2011). A comparison of selected MMPI-2 and MMPI-2-RF validity scales in assessing effort on cognitive tests in a military sample. *The Clinical Neuropsychologist, 25,* 1207–1227.

Jones, A., Ingram, M. V., & Ben-Porath, Y. S. (2012). Scores on the MMPI-2-RF scales as a function of increasing levels of failure on cognitive symptom validity tests in a military sample. *The Clinical Neuropsychologist, 26,* 790–815.

Jorge, R. E., Acion, L., Moser, D., Adams, H. P., & Robinson, R. G. (2010). Escitalopram and enhancement of cognitive recovery following stroke. *Archives of General Psychiatry, 67,* 187–196.

Kaiser, S. (1986). *Ability patterns of black and white adults on the WAIS-R independent of general intelligence and as a function of socioeconomic status.* Unpublished doctoral dissertation, Texas A&M University, College Station, TX.

Kamphuis, J. H., & Finn, S. E. (2002). Incorporating base rate information in daily clinical decision making. In J. N. Butcher (Ed.), *Clinical personality assessment: Practical approaches* (pp. 257–268). New York: Oxford University Press.

Kapci, E. G., & Cramer, D. (2000). The mediation component of the hopelessness depression in relation to negative life events. *Counseling Psychology Quarterly, 13,* 413–423.

Karantzoulis, S., Novitski, J., Gold, M., & Randolph, C. (2013). The Repeatable Battery for the Assessment of Neuropsychological Status (RBANS): Utility in detection and characterization of mild cognitive impairment due to Alzheimer's disease. *Archives of Clinical Neuropsychology, 28,* 837–844.

Kaufman, A. S. (1973). Comparison of the performance of matched groups of black children and white children on the Wechsler Preschool and Primary Scale of Intelligence. *Journal of Consulting and Clinical Psychology, 41,* 186–191.

Kaufman, A. S., & Kaufman, N. L. (1973). Black–white differences on the McCarthy Scales of Children's Abilities. *Journal of School Psychology, 11,* 196–206.

Kavale, K. A., & Spaulding, L. C. (2008). Is response to intervention good policy for specific learning disability? *Learning Disabilities Research and Practice, 23,* 169–179.

Kendler, K. S., & Gardner, C. O. (2010). Dependent stressful life events and prior depressive episodes in the prediction of major depression: The problem of causal inference in psychiatric epidemiology. *Archives of General Psychiatry, 67,* 1120–1127.

Keuntzel, J. G., Hetterscheidt, L. A., & Barnett, D. (2011). Testing intelligently includes double-checking Wechsler IQ scores. *Journal of Psychoeducational Assessment, 29,* 39–46.

Kielbasa, A. M., Pomerantz, A. M., Krohn, E. J., & Sullivan, B. F. (2004). How does clients' method of payment influence psychologists' diagnostic decisions? *Ethics and Behavior, 14,* 187–195.

King, L. C., Bailie, J. M., Kinney, D. I., & Nitch, S. R. (2012). Is the Repeatable Battery for the Assessment of Neuropsychological Status factor structure appropriate for inpatient psychiatry?: An exploratory and higher-order analysis. *Archives of Clinical Neuropsychology, 27,* 756–765.

Kojima, M., Furukawa, T. A., Takahashi, H., Kawai, M., Nagaya, T., & Tokudome, S. (2002). Cross-cultural validation of the Beck Depression Inventory–II in Japan. *Psychiatry Research, 110,* 291–299.

Larrabee, G. J. (Ed.). (2007). *Assessment of malingered neuropsychological deficits.* New York: Oxford University Press.

Larrabee, G. J. (2012). *Forensic neuropsychology: A scientific approach* (2nd ed.). New York: Oxford University Press.

Larson, E. B., Kirschner, K., Bode, R., Heinemann, A., & Goodman, R. (2005). Construct and predictive validity of the Repeatable Battery for the Assessment of Neuropsychological Status in the evaluation of stroke patients. *Journal of Clinical and Experimental Neuropsychology, 27,* 16–32.

Leventhal, H., Brissette, I., & Leventhal, E. A. (2003). The common-sense model of self-regulation of health and illness. In L. Cameron & H. Leventhal (Eds.), *The self regulation of health and illness behaviour* (pp. 42–65). New York: Routledge.

Lewandowski, L., Lovett, B. J., Codding, R. S., & Gordon, M. (2007). Symptoms of ADHD and academic concerns in college students with and without ADHD diagnoses. *Journal of Attention Disorders, 12,* 156–161.

Lezak, M. D., Howieson, D. B., Bigler, E. D., & Tranel, D. (2012). *Neuropsychological assessment* (5th ed.). New York: Oxford University Press.

Lichtenberger, E. O., & Kaufman, A. S. (2013). *Essentials of WAIS-IV assessment* (2nd ed.). Hoboken, NJ: Wiley.

Lilienfeld, S. O., Garb, H. N., & Wood, J. M. (2011). Unresolved questions concerning the effectiveness of psychological assessment as a therapeutic intervention: Comment on Poston and Hanson (2010). *Psychological Assessment, 23,* 1047–1055.

Lim, M., Collinson, S. L., Feng, L., & Ng, T. (2010). Cross-cultural application of the Repeatable Battery for the Assessment of Neuropsychological Status

(RBANS): Performances of elderly Chinese Singaporeans. *The Clinical Neuropsychologist, 24*, 811–826.

Lippa, S. M., Hawes, S., Jokic, E., & Caroselli, J. S. (2013). Sensitivity of the RBANS to acute traumatic brain injury and length of post-traumatic amnesia. *Brain Injury, 27*, 689–695.

Liu, R. T., & Alloy, L. B. (2010). Stress generation in depression: A systematic review of the empirical literature and recommendations for future study. *Clinical Psychology Review, 30*, 582–593.

Locke, D. E. C., Kirlin, K. A., Wershba, R., Osborne, D., Drazkowski, J. F., Sirven, J. I., et al. (2011). Randomized comparison of the Personality Assessment Inventory and the Minnesota Multiphasic Personality Inventory–2 in the epilepsy monitoring unit. *Epilepsy and Behavior, 21*, 397–401.

Lopez, S. R. (1989). Patient variable bases in clinical judgment: Conceptual overview and methodological considerations. *Psychological Bulletin, 106*, 184–203.

Lord, C., Petkova, E., Hus, V., Gan, W., Lu, F., Martin, D. M., et al. (2012). A multisite study of the clinical diagnosis of different autism spectrum disorders. *Archives of General Psychiatry, 69*, 306–313.

Lowe, J., Pomerantz, A. M., & Pettibone, J. C. (2007). The influence of payment method on psychologists' diagnostic decisions: Expanding the range of presenting problems. *Ethics and Behavior, 17*, 83–93.

Lowmaster, S. E., & Morey, L. C. (2012). Predicting law enforcement officer job performance with the personality assessment inventory. *Journal of Personality Assessment, 94*, 254–261.

Lucas, J. A., Ivnik, R. J., Willis, F. B., German, T. J., Smith, G. E., Parfitt, F. C., et al. (2005). Mayo's Older African Americans Normative Studies: Normative data for commonly used clinical neuropsychological measures. *The Clinical Neuropsychologist, 19*, 162–183.

Maddux, J. E., Gosselin, J. T., & Winstead, B. A. (2012). Conceptions of psychopathology: A social constructionist perspective. In J. E. Maddux & B. A. Winstead (Eds.), *Psychopathology: Foundations for a contemporary understanding* (3rd ed., pp. 3–22). New York: Routledge.

Magyar, M. S., Edens, J. F., Lilienfeld, S. O., Douglas, K. S., Poythress, N. G., & Skeem, J. L. (2012). Using the Personality Assessment Inventory to predict male offenders' conduct during and progression through substance abuse treatment. *Psychological Assessment, 24*, 216–225.

Manly, J. J. (2005). Advantages and disadvantages of separate norms for African Americans. *The Clinical Neuropsychologist, 19*, 270–275.

Manly, J. J., & Jacobs, D. M. (2002). Future directions in neuropsychological assessment with African Americans. In F. R. Ferraro (Ed.), *Minority and cross-cultural aspects of neuropsychological assessment* (pp. 79–96). Lisse, The Netherlands: Swets & Zeitlinger.

Marcotte, T. D., & Grant, I. (Eds.). (2010). *Neuropsychology of everyday functioning*. New York: Guilford Press.

Marcum, J. A. (2012). An integrated model of clinical reasoning: Dual-process theory of cognition and metacognition. *Journal of Evaluation in Clinical Practice, 18*, 954–961.

Marion, B. E., Sellbom, M., Salekin, R. T., Toomey, J. A., Kucharski, L. T., & Scott, D. (2013). An examination of the association between psychopathy and dissimulation using the MMPI-2-RF validity scales. *Law and Human Behavior, 37,* 219–230.

Marshall, P. S., Schroeder, R., O'Brien, J., Fisher, R., Ries, A., Blesi, B., et al. (2010). Effectiveness of symptom validity measures in identifying cognitive and behavioral symptom exaggeration in adult attention deficit hyperactivity disorder. *The Clinical Neuropsychologist, 24,* 1204–1237.

Mason, L. H., Shandera-Ochsner, A. L., Williamson, K. D., Harp, J. P., Edmundson, M., Berry, D. T. R., et al. (2013). Accuracy of MMPI-2-RF validity scales for identifying feigned PTSD symptoms, random responding, and genuine PTSD. *Journal of Personality Assessment, 95,* 585–593.

McCaffrey, R. J., Duff, K., & Westervelt, H. J. (Eds.). (2000). *Practitioner's guide to evaluating change with neuropsychological assessment instruments.* New York: Kluwer.

McCaffrey, R. J., Palav, A. A., O'Bryant, S. E., & Labarge, A. S. (Eds.). (2003). *Practitioner's guide to symptom base rates in clinical neuropsychology.* New York: Kluwer.

McDermott, A. T., & DeFilippis, N. A. (2010). Are the indices of the RBANS sufficient for differentiating Alzheimer's disease and subcortical vascular dementia? *Archives of Clinical Neuropsychology, 25,* 327–334.

McKay, C., Casey, J. E., Wertheimer, J., & Fichtenberg, N. L. (2007). Reliability and validity of the RBANS in a traumatic brain injured sample. *Archives of Clinical Neuropsychology, 22,* 91–98.

McKay, C., Wertheimer, J. C., Fichtenberg, N. L., & Casey, J. E. (2008). The Repeatable Battery for the Assessment of Neuropsychological Status (RBANS): Clinical utility in a traumatic brain injury sample. *The Clinical Neuropsychologist, 22,* 228–241.

McKeith, I. G., Dickson, D. W., Lowe, J., Emre, M., O'Brien, J. T., Feldman, H., et al. (2005). Diagnosis and management of dementia with Lewy bodies: Third report of the DLD Consortium. *Neurology, 65,* 1863–1872.

Messinis, L., Lyras, E., Andrian, V., Katsakiori, P., Panagis, G., Georgiou, V., et al. (2009). Neuropsychological functioning in buprenorphine maintained patients versus abstinent heroin abusers on naltrexone hydrochloride therapy. *Human Psychopharmacology: Clinical and Experimental, 24,* 524–531.

Meyer, G., Finn, S. E., Eyde, L. D., Kaye, G. G., Moreland, K. L., Dies, R. R., et al. (2001). Psychological testing and psychological assessment: A review of evidence and issues. *American Psychologist, 56,* 128–165.

Meyer, T. J., Miller, M. L., Metzgeer, R. L., & Borkovec, T. D. (1990). Development and validation of the Penn State Worry Questionnaire. *Behaviour Research and Therapy, 28,* 487–495.

Meyers, J. E., Millis, S. R., & Volkert, K. (2002). A validity index for the MMPI-2. *Archives of Clinical Neuropsychology, 17,* 157–169.

Michael, D. M. (2002). Psychological assessment as a therapeutic intervention in patients hospitalized with eating disorders. *Professional Psychology: Research and Practice, 33,* 470–477.

Miele, F. (1979). Cultural bias in the WISC. *Intelligence, 3,* 149–164.

Miller, E. (1983). A note on the interpretation of data derived from neuropsychological tests. *Cortex, 19,* 131–132.

Millis, S. R. (2009). What clinicians really need to know about symptom exaggeration, insufficient effort, and malingering: Statistical and measurement matters. In J. E. Morgan & J. J. Sweet (Eds.), *Neuropsychology of malingering casebook* (pp. 21–38). New York: Psychology Press.

Mitrushina, M. N., Boone, K. B., Razani, J., & D'Ella, L. F. (2005). *Handbook of normative data for neuropsychological assessment* (2nd ed). New York: Oxford University Press.

Mittenberg, W., DiGiulio, D. V., Perrin, S., & Bass, A. E. (1992). Symptoms following mild head injury: Expectation as etiology. *Journal of Neurology, Neurosurgery, and Psychiatry, 55*, 200–204.

Mittenberg, W., Patton, C., Canyock, E. M., & Condit, D. C. (2002). Base rates of malingering and symptom exaggeration. *Journal of Clinical and Experimental Neuropsychology, 24*, 1094–1102.

Moore, R. C., Davine, T., Harmell, A. L., Cardenas, V., Palmer, B. W., & Mausbach, B. T. (2013). Using the Repeatable Battery for the Assessment of Neuropsychological Status (RBANS) Effort Index to predict treatment group adherence in patients with schizophrenia. *Journal of the International Neuropsychological Society, 19*, 198–205.

Morey, L. C. (1991). *The Personality Assessment Inventory professional manual*. Odessa, FL: Psychological Assessment Resources.

Morey, L. C. (2003). *Essentials of PAI assessment*. Hoboken, NJ: Wiley.

Morey, L. C. (2007). *Personality Assessment Inventory professional manual* (2nd ed.). Lutz, FL: Psychological Assessment Resources.

Morgan, D. R., Linck, J., Scott, J., Adams, R., & Mold, J. (2010). Assessment of the RBANS visual and verbal indices in a sample of neurologically impaired elderly participants. *The Clinical Neuropsychologist, 24*, 1365–1378.

Mpofu, E., & Ortiz, S. O. (2009). Equitable assessment practices in diverse contexts. In E. L. Grigorenko (Ed.), *Multicultural psychoeducational assessment* (pp. 41–76). New York: Springer.

Mullins-Sweatt, S. N., & Widiger, T. A. (2009). Clinical utility and DSM-V. *Psychological Assessment, 21*, 302–312.

Mungas, D., Widaman, K. F., Reed, B. R., & Tomaszewski Farias, S. (2011). Measurement invariance of neuropsychological tests in diverse older persons. *Neuropsychology, 25*, 260–269.

Muntal Encinas, S., Gramunt-Fombuena, N., Badenes Guia, D., Casas Harnanz, L., & Aguilar Barbera, M. (2012). Spanish translation and adaptation of the Repeatable Battery for the Assessment of Neuropsychological Status (RBANS) Form A in a pilot sample. *Neurologia, 27*, 531–546.

Naglieri, J. A., & Graham, J. R. (2012). Current status and future directions of assessment psychology. In J. R. Graham, J. A. Naglieri, & I. B. Weiner (Eds.), *Handbook of psychology: Vol. 10. Assessment psychology* (2nd ed., pp. 645–658). Hoboken, NJ: Wiley.

Neisser, U., Boodoo, G., Bouchard, T. J., Jr., Boykin, A. W., Brody, N., Ceci, S. J. O., et al. (1996). Intelligence: Knowns and unknowns. *American Psychologist, 51*, 77–101.

Nelson, J. M., Canivez, G. L., & Watkins, M. W. (2013). Structural and incremental validity of the Wechsler Adult Intelligence Scale—Fourth Edition with a clinical sample. *Psychological Assessment, 25*, 618–630.

Nelson, N. W., Sweet, J. J., Berry, D. T. R., Bryant, F. B., & Granacher, R. P. (2007).

Response validity in forensic neuropsychology: Exploratory factor analytic evidence of distinct cognitive and psychological constructs. *Journal of the International Neuropsychological Society, 13,* 440–449.

Nelson, N. W., Sweet, J. J., & Demakis, G. J. (2006). Meta-analysis of the MMPI-2 Fake Bad Scale: Utility in forensic settings. *The Clinical Neuropsychologist, 20,* 39–58.

Newman, M. L. (2004). *Psychological assessment as brief psychotherapy: Therapeutic effects of providing MMPI-A test feedback to adolescents.* Unpublished doctoral dissertation, La Trobe University, Melbourne, Australia.

Newman, M. L., & Greenway, P. (1997). Therapeutic effects of providing MMPI-2 test feedback to clients at a university counseling service: A collaborative approach. *Psychological Assessment, 9,* 122–131.

Newman, T. B., & Kohn, M. A. (2009). *Evidence-based diagnosis.* New York: Cambridge University Press.

Nisbett, R. E. (2009). *Intelligence and how to get it: Why schools and cultures count.* New York: Norton.

Nisbett, R. E., Aronson, J., Blair, C., Dickens, W., Flynn, J., Halpern, D. F., et al. (2012). Intelligence: New findings and theoretical developments. *American Psychologist, 67,* 130–159.

Norman, G. R. (2009). Dual processing and diagnostic errors. *Advances in Health Sciences Education, 14,* 37–49.

Norman, G. R., Brooks, L. R., Colle, C. L., & Hatala, R. M. (2000). The benefit of diagnostic hypotheses in clinical reasoning: Experimental study of an instructional investigation for forward and backward reasoning. *Cognition and Instruction, 17,* 433–448.

Norman, G. R., & Eva, K. W. (2010). Diagnostic error and clinical reasoning. *Medical Education, 44,* 94–100.

Novitski, J., Steele, S., Karantzoulis, S., & Randolph, C. (2012). The Repeatable Battery for the Assessment of Neuropsychological Status effort scale. *Archives of Clinical Neuropsychology, 27,* 190–195.

O'Bryant, S. E., Falkowski, J., Hobson, V., Johnson, L., Hall, J., Schrimsher, G. W., et al. (2011). Executive functioning mediates the link between other neuropsychological domains and daily functioning: A Project FRONTIER study. *International Psychogeriatrics, 23,* 107–113.

O'Bryant, S. E., Hall, J. R., Cukrowicz, K. C., Edwards, M., Johnson, L. A., Lefforge, D., et al. (2011). The differential impact of depressive symptom clusters on cognition in a rural multi-ethnic cohort: A Project FRONTIER study. *International Journal of Geriatric Psychiatry, 26,* 199–205.

Odland, A., Martin, P., Perle, J., Simco, E. R., & Mittenberg, W. (2011). Rates of apparently abnormal MMPI-2 profiles in the normal population. *The Clinical Neuropsychologist, 25,* 1134–1144.

Osman, A., Kopper, B. A., Barrios, F., Gutierrez, P. M., & Bagge, C. L. (2004). Reliability and validity of the Beck Depression Inventory–II with adolescent psychiatric inpatients. *Psychological Assessment, 16,* 120–132.

Osmon, D. C., & Mano, Q. R. (2009). Malingered attention deficit hyperactivity disorder: Effort, depression, and dependence in the pursuit of academic accommodations. In J. E. Morgan & J. J. Sweet (Eds.), *Neuropsychology of malingering casebook* (pp. 386–398). New York: Psychology Press.

Ougrin, D., Ng, A. V., & Low, J. (2008). Therapeutic assessment based on cognitive-analytic therapy for young people presenting with self-harm: Pilot study. *Psychiatric Bulletin, 32,* 423–426.

Pachet, A. K. (2007). Construct validity of the Repeatable Battery for the Assessment of Neuropsychological Status (RBANS) with acquired brain injury patients. *The Clinical Neuropsychologist, 21,* 286–297.

Patton, D. E., Duff, K., Schoenberg, M. R., Mold, J. S., James, G., & Adams, R. L. (2003). Performance of cognitively normal African Americans on the RBANS in community-dwelling older adults. *The Clinical Neuropsychologist, 17,* 515–530.

Patton, D. E., Duff, K., Schoenberg, M. R., Mold, J., Scott, J. G., & Adams, R. L. (2006). RBANS index discrepancies: Base rates for older adults. *Archives of Clinical Neuropsychology, 21,* 151–160.

Patton, D. E., Duff, K., Schoenberg, M. R., Mold, J., Scott, J. G., & Adams, R. L. (2005). Base rates of longitudinal RBANS discrepancies at one- and two-year intervals in community-dwelling older adults. *The Clinical Neuropsychologist, 19,* 27–44.

Paulsen, J. S., & Mikos, A. (2008). Huntington's disease. In J. E. Morgan & J. H. Ricker (Eds.), *Textbook of clinical neuropsychology* (pp. 616–635). New York: Psychology Press.

Pearson. (2009a). *Advanced clinical solutions for WAIS-IV and WMS-IV.* San Antonio, TX: Author.

Pearson. (2009b). *Wechsler Individual Achievement Test—Third Edition technical manual.* San Antonio, TX: Author.

Pelham, W. E., Fabiano, G. A., & Massetti, G. M. (2005). Evidence-based assessment of attention deficit hyperactivity disorder in children and adolescents. *Journal of Clinical Child and Adolescent Psychology, 34,* 449–476.

Pella, R. D., Hill, B. D., Shelton, J. T., Elliott, E., & Gouvier, W. D. (2012). Evaluation of embedded malingering indices in a non-litigating clinical sample using control, clinical, and derived groups. *Archives of Clinical Neuropsychology, 27,* 45–57.

Penley, J. S., Wiebe, J. S., & Nwosu, A. (2003). Psychometric properties of the Spanish Beck Depression Inventory–II in a medical sample. *Psychological Assessment, 15,* 569–577.

Pennington, B. F. (2002). *The development of psychopathology: Nature and nurture.* New York: Guilford Press.

Percosky, A. B., Boccaccini, M. T., Bitting, B. S., & Hamilton, P. M. (2013). Personality Assessment Inventory scores as predictors of treatment compliance and misconduct among sex offenders participating in community-based treatment. *Journal of Forensic Psychology Practice, 13,* 192–203.

Perry, J. C. (1992). Problems and considerations in the valid assessment of personality disorders. *American Journal of Psychiatry, 149,* 1645–1653.

Persons, J. B., & Fresco, D. M. (2008). Adult depression. In J. Hunsley & E. J. Mash (Eds.), *A guide to assessments that work* (pp. 96–120). New York: Oxford University Press.

Phelps, R. P. (Ed.). (2009). *Correcting fallacies about educational and psychological testing.* Washington, DC: American Psychological Association.

Pilkonis, P. A., Heape, C. L., Prioetti, J. M., Clark, S. W., McDavid, J. D., & Pitts, T. E. (1995). The reliability and validity of two structured diagnostic interviews for personality disorders. *Archives of General Psychiatry, 52,* 1025–1033.

Poston, J. M., & Hanson, W. E. (2010). Meta-analysis of psychological assessment as a therapeutic intervention. *Psychological Assessment, 22,* 203–212.

Poston, J. M., & Hanson, W. E. (2011). Building confidence in psychological assessment as a therapeutic intervention: An empirically based replay to Lilienfeld, Gard, and Wood (2011). *Psychological Assessment, 23,* 1056–1062.

Proust, J. (2010). Metacognition. *Philosophy Compass, 5,* 989–998.

Rabin, L. A., Barr, W. B., & Burton, L. A. (2005). Assessment practices of clinical neuropsychologists in the United States and Canada: A survey of INS, NAN, and APA Division 40 members. *Archives of Clinical Psychology, 20,* 33–65.

Randolph, C. (1998). *Repeatable Battery for the Assessment of Neuropsychological Status (RBANS).* San Antonio, TX: Psychological Corporation.

Randolph, C. (2008). *RBANS update.* Bloomington, MN: Pearson.

Regier, D. A., & Narrow, W. E. (2002). Defining clinically significant psychopathology with epidemiologic data. In J. E. Helzer & J. J. Hudziak (Eds.), *Defining psychopathologies in the 21st century: DSM-V and beyond* (pp. 19–30). Arlington, VA: American Psychiatric Publishing.

Reitan, R. M., & Wolfson, D. (1997). *The Halstead–Reitan Neuropsychological Test Battery: Theory and clinical interpretation* (2nd ed.). Tucson, AZ: Neuropsychology Press.

Reschly, D. J. (2000). PASE v. Hannon. In C. R. Reynolds & E. Fletcher-Janzen (Eds.), *Encyclopedia of special education* (2nd ed., pp. 1156–1157). New York: Wiley.

Reynolds, C. R., & Gutkin, T. B. (1981). A multivariate comparison of the intellectual performance of blacks and whites matched on four demographic variables. *Personality and Individual Differences, 2,* 175–180.

Reynolds, C. R., Lowe, P. A., & Saenz, A. (1999). The problem of bias in psychological assessment. In T. B. Gutkin & C. R. Reynolds (Eds.), *The handbook of school psychology* (3rd ed.). New York: Wiley.

Reynolds, C. R., & Suzuki, L. A. (2013). Bias in psychological assessment: An empirical review and recommendations. In J. R. Graham, J. S. Naglieri, & I. B. Weiner (Eds.), *Handbook of psychology: Vol. 10. Assessment psychology* (2nd ed., pp. 82–113). Hoboken, NJ: Wiley.

Reynolds, M. R., Ingram, P. B., Seeley, J. S., & Newby, K. D. (2013). Investigating the structure and invariance of the Wechsler Adult Intelligence Scales, Fourth Edition in a sample of adults with intellectual disabilities. *Research in Developmental Disabilities, 34,* 3235–3245.

Rinehardt, E., Duff, K., Schoenberg, M., Mattingly, M., Bharucha, K., & Scott, J. (2010). Cognitive change on the Repeatable Battery for the Assessment of Neuropsychological Status (RBANS) in Parkinson's disease with and without bilateral subthalamic nucleus deep brain stimulation surgery. *The Clinical Neuropsychologist, 24,* 1339–1354.

Rios, J., & Morey, L. E. (2013). Detecting feigned ADHD in later adolescence: An examination of three PAI-A negative distortion indicators. *Journal of Personality Assessment, 95,* 594–599.

Rittel, H. W. J., & Webber, M. M. (1973). Dilemmas in a general theory of planning. *Policy Sciences, 4,* 155–169.

Rodolfa, E. R., Bent, R. J., Eisman, E., Nelson, P. D., Rehm, L., & Ritchie, P. (2005). A cube model for competency development: Implications for psychology educators and regulators. *Professional Psychology: Research and Practice, 36,* 347–354.

Rogers, R. (2003). Standardizing DSM-IV diagnoses: The clinical application of structured interviews. *Journal of Personality Assessment, 81*, 220–225.

Rogers, R. (Ed.). (2008a). *Clinical assessment of malingering and deception* (3rd ed.). New York: Guilford Press.

Rogers, R. (2008b). Structured interviews and dissimulation. In R. Rogers (Ed.), *Clinical assessment of malingering and deception* (3rd ed., pp. 301–322). New York: Guilford Press.

Rogers, R., Gillard, N. D., Berry, D. T. R., & Granacher, R. P. (2011). Effectiveness of the MMPI-2-RF validity scales for feigned mental disorders and cognitive impairment: A known-groups study. *Journal of Psychopathology and Behavioral Assessment, 33*, 355–367.

Rogers, R., Gillard, N. D., Wooley, C. N., & Kelsey, K. R. (2013). Cross-validation of the PAI Negative Distortion Scale for feigned mental disorders: A research report. *Assessment, 20*, 36–42.

Rohling, M. L., Binder, L., & Langhinrichen-Rohling, J. (1995). Money matters: A meta-analysis of the association between financial compensation and the experience and treatment of chronic pain. *Health Psychology, 14*, 537–547.

Rohling, M. L., & Boone, K. B. (2007). Future directions in effort assessment. In K. B. Boone (Ed.), *Assessment of feigned cognitive impairment: A neuropsychological perspective* (pp. 210–235). New York: Guilford Press.

Roid, G. H. (2003). *Stanford–Binet Intelligence Scales, Fifth Edition*. Austin, TX: PRO-ED.

Ruiz, M. A., Cox, J., Magyar, M. S., & Edens, J. F. (2014). Predictive validity of the Personality Assessment Inventory (PAI) for identifying criminal reoffending following completion of an in-jail addiction treatment program. *Psychological Assessment, 26*, 673–678.

Ryan, J. J., & Schnackenberger-Ott, S. D. (2003). Scoring reliability on the Wechsler Adult Intelligence Scale—Third Edition (WAIS-III). *Assessment, 10*, 151–159.

Salthouse, T. A. (2010). The paradox of cognitive change. *Journal of Clinical and Experimental Neuropsychology, 32*, 622–629.

Salthouse, T. A., & Saklofske, D. H. (2010). Do the WAIS-IV tests measure the same aspects of cognitive functioning in adults under and over age 65? In L. G. Weiss, D. H. Saklofske, D. L. Coalson, & S. E. Raiford (Eds.), *WAIS-IV clinical use and interpretation* (pp. 217–236). San Diego, CA: Academic Press.

Santor, D. A., Gregus, M., & Welch, A. (2006). Eight decades of measurement in depression. *Measurement, 4*, 135–155.

Sanz, J. C., Vargas, M. L., & Marin, J. J. (2009). Battery for assessment of neuropsychological status (RBANS) in schizophrenia: A pilot study in the Spanish population. *Acta Neuropsychiatrica, 21*, 18–25.

Sattler, J. M. (1988). *Assessment of children* (3rd ed.). San Diego, CA: Author.

Sattler, J. M., & Ryan, J. (2009). *Assessment with the WAIS-IV*. San Diego, CA: Authors.

Schmitt, A. L., Livingston, R. B., Smernoff, E. N., Reese, E. M., Hafer, D. G., & Harris, J. B. (2010). Factor analysis of the Repeatable Battery for the Assessment of Neuropsychological Status (RBANS) in a large sample of patients suspected of dementia. *Applied Neuropsychology, 17*, 8–17.

Schneider, W. J., & McGrew, K. S. (2012). The Cattel–Horn–Carroll model of intelligence. In D. P. Flanagan & P. L. Harrison (Eds.), *Contemporary intellectual assessment: Theories, tests, and issues* (3rd ed., pp. 99–144). New York: Guilford Press.

Schoenberg, M. R., Rinehardt, E., Duff, K., Mattingly, M., Bharucha, K. J., & Scott, J. G. (2012). Assessing reliable change using the Repeatable Battery for the Assessment of Neuropsychological Status (RBANS) for patents with Parkinson's disease undergoing deep brain stimulation surgery. *The Clinical Neuropsychologist, 26,* 255–270.

Schrank, F. A., & Wendling, B. J. (2012). The Woodcock–Johnson III Normative Update: Tests of Cognitive Abilities and Tests of Achievement. In D. P. Flanagan & P. L. Harrison (Eds.), *Contemporary intellectual assessment: Theories, tests, and issues* (3rd ed., pp. 297–335). New York: Guilford Press.

Schretlen, D. J., Munro, C. A., Anthony, J. C., & Pearlson, G. D. (2003). Examining the range of normal intraindividual variability in neuropsychological test performance. *Journal of the International Neuropsychological Society, 9,* 864–870.

Schrimsher, G. W., & Parker, J. D. (2008). Changes in cognitive function during substance use disorder treatment. *Journal of Psychopathology and Behavioral Assessment, 30,* 146–153.

Schroeder, R. W., Baade, L. E., Peck, C. P., VonDran, E. J., Brockman, C. J., Webster, B. K., et al. (2012). Validation of MMPI-2-RF Validity Scales in criterion group neuropsychological samples. *The Clinical Neuropsychologist, 26,* 129–146.

Segal, D. L., Mueller, A. E., & Coolidge, F. L. (2012). Structured and semistructured interviews for differential diagnosis: Fundamentals, applications, and essential features. In M. Hersen & D. C. Beidel (Eds.), *Adult psychopathology and diagnosis* (6th ed., pp. 91–116). Hoboken, NJ: Wiley.

Sellbom, M., Anderson, J. L., & Bagby, R. M. (2013). Assessing DSM-5 section III personality traits and disorders with the MMPI-2-RF. *Assessment, 20,* 709–722.

Sellbom, M., Marion, B. E., & Bagby, M. (2013). Psychological assessment in adult mental health settings. In J. R. Graham, J. A. Naglieri, & I. B. Weiner (Eds.), *Handbook of psychology: Vol. 10. Assessment psychology* (2nd ed., pp. 241–260). Hoboken, NJ: Wiley.

Sharland, M. J., & Gfeller, J. D. (2007). A survey of neuropsychologists' beliefs and practices with respect to the assessment of effort. *Archives of Clinical Neuropsychology, 22,* 213–223.

Sheehan, D. V., Lecrubier, Y., Harnett Sheehan, K., Amorim, P., Janavs, J., Weiller, E., et al. (1998). The Mini International Neuropsychiatric Interview (M.I.N.I): The development and validation of a structured diagnostic psychiatric interview for DSM-IV and ICD-10. *Journal of Clinical Psychiatry, 59*(Suppl. 20), 22–33.

Shemberg, K. M., & Doherty, M. E. (1999). Is diagnostic judgment influenced by a bias to see pathology? *Journal of Clinical Psychology, 55,* 513–518.

Sherrill-Pattison, S., Donders, J., & Thompson, E. (2000). Influence of demographic variables on neuropsychological test performance after traumatic brain injury. *The Clinical Neuropsychologist, 14,* 496–503.

Sideridis, G. D., Antoniou, F., & Padeliadu, S. (2008). Teacher biases in the identification of learning disabilities: An application of the logistic multilevel model. *Learning Disability Quarterly, 31,* 199–209.

Siedlecki, K. L., Manly, J. J., Brickman, A. M., Schupf, N., Tang, M., & Stern, Y.

(2010). Do neuropsychological tests have the same meaning in Spanish speakers as they do in English speakers? *Neuropsychology, 24,* 402–411.

Silverberg, N. D., & Millis, S. R. (2009). Impairment versus deficiency in neuropsychological assessment: Implications for ecological validity. *Journal of the
International Neuropsychological Society, 15,* 94–102.

Silverberg, N. D., Wertheimer, J. C., & Fichtenberg, N. L. (2007). An Effort Index
for the Repeatable Battery for the Assessment of Neuropsychological Status
(RBANS). *The Clinical Neuropsychologist, 21,* 841–854.

Sinclair, S. J., Bellow, I., Nyer, M., Slavin-Mulford, J., Stein, M. B., Renna, M., et
al. (2012). The Suicide (SPI) and Violence Potential Indices (VPI) from the
Personality Assessment Inventory: A preliminary exploration of validity in
an outpatient psychiatric sample. *Journal of Psychopathology and Behavioral
Assessment, 34,* 423–431.

Singh, H., & Weingart, S. N. (2009). Diagnostic errors in ambulatory care: Dimensions and preventive strategies. *Advances in Health Science Education Theory
and Practice, 14,* S27–S61.

Slavin-Mulford, J., Sinclair, S. J., Malone, J., Stein, M., Bello, I., & Blais, M. A.
(2013). External correlates of the Personality Assessment Inventory higher
order structures. *Journal of Personality Assessment, 95,* 432–434.

Slavin-Mulford, J., Sinclair, S. J., Stein, M., Malone, J., Bello, I., & Blais, M. (2012).
External validity of the Personality Assessment Inventory (PAI) in a clinical
sample. *Journal of Personality Assessment, 94,* 593–600.

Slick, D. J., Sherman, E. M., & Iverson, G. L. (1999). Diagnostic criteria for malingered neurocognitive dysfunction: Proposed standards for clinical practice
and research. *The Clinical Neuropsychologist, 13,* 545–561.

Slick, D. J., Tan, J. E., Strauss, E. H., & Hultsch, D. F. (2004). Detecting malingering: A survey of experts' practices. *Archives of Clinical Neuropsychology, 19,*
465–473.

Smith, G. E., Housen, P., Yaffe, K., Ruff, R., Kennison, R. F., Mahncke, H. W., et
al. (2009). A cognitive training program based on principles of brain plastic-
ity: Results from the Improvement in Memory with Plasticity-Based Cognitive Training (IMPACT) study. *Journal of the American Geriatrics Society, 57,*
594–603.

Smith, G. T. (2005). On construct validity: Issues of method and measurement.
Psychological Assessment, 17, 395–408.

Solanto, M. V., Etefia, K., & Marks, D. J. (2004). The utility of self-report measures
and the continuous performance test in the diagnosis of ADHD in adults. *CNS
Spectrums, 9,* 649–659.

Spengler, P. M. (2013). Clinical versus mechanical prediction. In J. R. Graham, J.
A. Naglieri, & I. B. Weiner (Eds.), *Handbook of psychology: Vol. 10. Assessment
psychology* (2nd ed., pp. 26–49). Hoboken, NJ: Wiley.

Spitzer, R. L. (1983). Psychiatric diagnosis: Are clinicians still necessary? *Comprehensive Psychiatry, 24,* 399–411.

Spitzer, R. L., Kroenke, K., Williams, J. B., & the Patient Health Questionnaire Primary Care Study Group. (1999). Validation and utility of a self-report version
of PRIME-MD. *Journal of the American Medical Association, 282,* 1737–1744.

Stanovich, K. E. (2011). *Rationality and the reflective mind.* New York: Oxford University Press.

Steer, R. A., Kumar, G., Ranieri, W. F., & Beck, A. T. (1998). Use of the Beck

Depression Inventory–II with adolescent depressed outpatients. *Journal of Psychopathology and Behavioral Assessment, 20*, 127–137.

Steer, R. A., Rissmiller, D. J., & Beck, A. T. (2000). Use of the Beck Depression Inventory–II with depressed geriatric inpatients. *Journal of Psychopathology and Behavioral Assessment, 20*, 127–137.

Stefan, J. S., Clopton, J. R., & Morgan, R. D. (2003). An MMPI-2 scale to detect malingered depression (Md scale). *Assessment, 10*, 382–392.

Stern, R. A., & White, T. (2003). *Neuropsychological Assessment Battery*. Lutz, FL: Psychological Assessment Resources.

Stone, J., & Moskowitz, G. B. (2011). Non-conscious bias in medical decision making: What can be done to reduce it? *Medical Education, 45*, 768–776.

Strauss, E., Sherman, E. M. S., & Spreen, O. (2006). *A compendium of neuropsychological tests* (3rd ed.). New York: Oxford University Press.

Stukenberg, K. W., Dura, J. R., & Kiecolt-Glaser, J. K. (1990). Depression screening scale validation in an elderly, community-dwelling population. *Psychological Assessment, 2*, 134–138.

Sue, D. W., & Sue, D. (2013). *Counseling the culturally diverse: Theory and practice* (6th ed.). Hoboken, NJ: Wiley.

Suhr, J. A., Buelow, M., & Riddle, T. (2011). Development of an infrequency index for the CAARS. *Journal of Psychoeducational Assessment, 29*, 160–170.

Suhr, J. A., & Gunstad, J. (2007). Coaching and malingering: A review. In G. Larrabee (Ed.), *Assessment of malingered neuropsychological deficits* (pp. 131–170). New York: Oxford University Press.

Suhr, J. A., Hammers, D., Dobbins-Buckland, K., Zimak, E., & Hughes, C. (2008). The relationship of malingering test failure to self-reported symptoms and neuropsychological findings in adults referred for ADHD evaluation. *Archives of Clinical Neuropsychology, 23*, 521–530.

Sullivan, B. K., May, K., & Galbally, L. (2007). Symptom exaggeration by college adults in attention-deficit hyperactivity disorder and learning disorder assessments. *Applied Neuropsychology, 14*, 189–207.

Summerfeldt, L. J., Kloosterman, P. H., & Antony, M. M. (2010). Structured and semistructured diagnostic interviews. In M. M. Antony & D. H. Barlow (Eds.), *Handbook of assessment and treatment planning for psychological disorders* (2nd ed., pp. 95–137). New York: Guilford Press.

Sweet, J. J., Moberg, P. J., & Suchy, Y. (2000). Ten-year follow-up survey of clinical neuropsychologists: Part 1. Practices and beliefs. *The Clinical Neuropsychologist, 14*, 18–37.

Sweet, J. J., Tovian, S. M., Guidotti Breting, L. M., & Suchy, Y. (2013). Psychological assessment in medical settings. In J. R. Graham, J. A. Naglieri, & I. B. Weiner (Eds.), *Handbook of psychology: Vol. 10. Assessment psychology* (2nd ed., pp. 315–346). Hoboken, NJ: Wiley.

Takaiwa, A., Hayashi, N., Kuwayama, N., Akioka, N., Kubo, M., & Endo, S. (2009). Changes in cognitive function during the 1-year period following endarterectomy and stenting of patients with high-grade carotid artery stenosis. *Acta Neurochirugica, 151*, 1593–1600.

Tarescavage, A. M., Wygant, D. B., Gervais, R. O., & Ben-Porath, Y. S. (2013). Association between the MMPI-2 Restructured Form (MMPI-2-RF) and malingered neurocognitive dysfunction among non-head injury disability claimants. *The Clinical Neuropsychologist, 27*, 313–335.

Tarter, R., & Kirisci, L. (1997). The Drug Use Screening Inventory for adults: Psychometric structure and discriminative sensitivity. *American Journal of Drug and Alcohol Abuse, 23*, 207–219.

Taub, G. E., & McGrew, K. S. (2004). A confirmatory factor analysis of Cattell–Horn–Carroll theory and cross-age invariance of the Woodcock–Johnson Tests of Cognitive Abilities III. *School Psychology Quarterly, 19*, 72–87.

Tellegen, A., & Ben-Porath, Y. S. (2011). *Minnesota Multiphasic Personality Inventory–2 Restructured Form technical manual.* Minneapolis: University of Minnesota Press.

Tellegen, A., Ben-Porath, Y. S., McNulty, J. L., Arbisi, P. A., Graham, J. R., & Kaemmer, B. (2003). *The MMPI-2 Restructured Clinical Scales: Development, validation, and interpretation.* Minneapolis: University of Minnesota Press.

Thomas, K. M., Hopwood, C. J., Orlando, M. J., Weathers, F. W., & McDevitt-Murphy, M. E. (2012). Detecting feigned PTSD using the Personality Assessment Inventory. *Psychological Injury and Law, 5*, 192–201.

Thomas, M. L., & Locke D. E. (2010). Psychometric properties of the MMPI-2-RF Somatic Complaints (RC1) Scale. *Psychological Assessment, 22*, 492–503.

Thompson, R., Bogner, H. R., Coyne, J. C., Gallo, J. J., & Eaton, W. W. (2004). Personal characteristics associated with consistency of recall of depressed or anhedonic mood in the 13-year follow-up of the Baltimore Epidemiologic Catchment Area Survey. *Acta Psychiatrica Scandinavica, 109*, 345–354.

Tubbs, P., & Pomerantz, A. M. (2001). Ethical behaviors of psychologists: Changes since 1987. *Journal of Clinical Psychology, 57*, 395–399.

Tverskey, A., & Kahneman, D. (1973). Availability: A heuristic for judging frequency and probability. *Cognitive Psychology, 5*, 207–232.

Tverskey, A., & Kahneman, D. (1974). Judgment under uncertainty: Heuristics and biases. *Science, 186*, 1124–1131.

Ursin, H. (2005). Press stop to start: The role of inhibition for choice and health. *Psychoneuroendocrinology, 30*, 1059–1065.

U.S. Department of Health and Human Services. (2013). *Results from the 2012 National Survey on Drug Use and Health: Summary of national findings.* Washington, DC: Author.

Valencia, R. A., Suzuki, L. A., & Salinas, M. (2001). Test bias. In R. R. Valencia & L. A. Suzuki (Eds.), *Intelligence testing with minority students: Foundations, performance factors and assessment issues* (pp. 111–181). Thousand Oaks, CA: Sage.

van der Heijden, P. T., Egger, J. I. M., Rossi, G. M. P., Grundel, G., & Derksen, J. J. L. (2013). The MMPI-2-Restructured Form and the Standard MMPI-2 clinical scales in relation to DSM-IV. *European Journal of Psychological Assessment, 29*, 182–188.

van der Heijden, P. T., Rossi, G. M. P., van der Velt, W. M., Derksen, J. J. L., & Egger, J. I. M. (2013). Personality and psychopathology: Higher-order relations between the five-factor model of personality and the MMPI-2 Restructured Form. *Journal of Research in Personality, 47*, 572–579.

van der Werf, S. P., Prins, J. D., Jongen, P. J. H., van der Meer, J. W. M., & Bleijenberg, G. (2000). Abnormal neuropsychological findings are not necessarily a sign of cerebral impairment: A matched comparison between chronic fatigue syndrome and multiple sclerosis. *Neuropsychiatry, Neuropsychology, and Behavioral Neurology, 13*, 199–203.

Van Vorhis, C. R. W., & Blumentritt, T. L. (2007). Psychometric properties of the Beck Depression Inventory–II in a clinically identified sample of Mexican American adolescents. *Journal of Child and Family Studies, 16*, 789–798.

Vervoort, T., Goubert, L., Eccleston, C., Bijttebier, P., & Crombez, G. (2006). Catastrophic thinking about pain is independently associated with pain severity, disability, and somatic complaints in school children and children with chronic pain. *Journal of Pediatric Psychology, 31*, 674–683.

Wagle, J., Farner, L., Flekkoy, K., Wyller, T. B., Sandvik, L. E., Eiklid, K. L., et al. (2009). Association between ApoE 4 and cognitive impairment after stroke. *Dementia and Geriatric Cognitive Disorders, 27*, 515–533.

Wagle, J., Farner, L., Flekkoy, K., Wyller, T. B., Sandvik, L. E., Eiklid, K. L., et al. (2010). Cognitive impairment and the role of the ApoE 4 allele after stroke—a 13 months follow-up study. *International Journal of Geriatric Psychiatry, 25*, 833–842.

Ward, L. C., Bergman, M. A., & Hebert, K. R. (2012). WAIS-IV subtest covariance structure: Conceptual and statistical considerations. *Psychological Assessment, 24*(2), 328–340.

Wasserman, J. D. (2013). Assessment of intellectual functioning. In J. R. Graham, J. A. Naglieri, & I. B. Weiner (Eds.), *Handbook of psychology: Vol. 10. Assessment psychology* (2nd ed., pp. 451–501). Hoboken, NJ: Wiley.

Wasserman, J. D., & Bracken, B. A. (2013). Fundamental psychometric considerations in assessment. In J. R. Graham, J. A. Naglieri, & I. B. Weiner (Eds.), *Handbook of psychology: Vol. 10. Assessment psychology* (pp. 50–81). Hoboken, NJ: Wiley.

Watson, D., & Pennebaker, J. W. (1989). Health complaints, stress, and distress: Exploring the central role of negative affectivity. *Psychological Review, 96*, 234–254.

Watson, D., & Tellegen, A. (1985). Toward a consensual structure of mood. *Psychological Bulletin, 98*, 219–235.

Wechsler, D. (1939). *Wechsler–Bellevue Intelligence Scale*. New York: Psychological Corporation.

Wechsler, D. (1997). *The Wechsler Memory Scale—Third Edition*. San Antonio, TX: Psychological Corporation.

Wechsler, D. (2001). *Wechsler Test of Adult Reading*. San Antonio, TX: Pearson.

Wechsler, D. (2003). *Wechsler Intelligence Scale for Children—Fourth Edition*. San Antonio, TX: Pearson.

Wechsler, D. (2008a). *WAIS-IV technical and interpretive manual*. San Antonio, TX: Pearson.

Wechsler, D. (2008b). *Wechsler Adult Intelligence Scale—Fourth Edition administration and scoring manual*. San Antonio, TX: Psychological Corporation.

Wechsler, D. (2011). *Wechsler Abbreviated Scale of Intelligence—Second Edition*. San Antonio, TX: Pearson.

Weiner, I. B. (2013). The assessment process. In J. R. Graham, J. A. Naglieri, & I. B. Weiner (Eds.), *Handbook of psychology: Vol. 10: Assessment psychology* (pp. 3–25). Hoboken, NJ: Wiley.

Weiss, L. G., Chen, H., Harris, J. G., Holdnack, J. A., & Saklofske, D. H. (2010). WAIS-IV use in a societal context. In L. G. Weiss, D. H., Saklofske, D. L. Coalson, & S. E. Raiford (Eds.), *WAIS-IV clinical use and interpretation* (pp. 97–140). San Diego, CA: Academic Press.

Weiss, L. G., Keith, T. X., Zhu, J. C., & Chen, H. (2013). WAIS-IV and clinical validation of the four- and five-factor interpretative approaches. *Journal of Psychoeducational Assessment, 31*, 94–113.

Weiss, L. G., Saklofske, D. H., Coalson, D., & Raiford, S. E. (Eds.). (2010). *WAIS-IV
clinical use and interpretation: Scientist-practitioner perspectives*. San Diego,
CA: Academic Press.

Whiteside, D. M., Clinton, C., Diamonti, C., Stroemel, J., White, C., Zimberoff, A.,
et al. (2010). Relationship between suboptimal cognitive effort and the clinical
scales of the Personality Assessment Inventory. *The Clinical Neuropsychologist, 24*, 315–325.

Whiteside, D. M., Galbreath, J., Brown, M., & Turnbull, J. (2012). Differential
response patterns on the Personality Assessment Inventory (PAI) in com-
pensation-seeking and non-compensation-seeking mild traumatic brain
injury patients. *Journal of Clinical and Experimental Neuropsychology, 34*,
172–182.

Widiger, T. A. (1998). Invited essay: Sex biases in the diagnoses of personality
disorders. *Journal of Personality Disorders, 12*, 95–118.

Widiger, T. A., & Edmundson, M. (2011). Diagnoses, dimensions, and DSM-5. In
D. H. Barlow (Ed.), *The Oxford handbook of clinical psychology* (pp. 254–278).
New York: Oxford University Press.

Wigdor, A. K., & Garner, W. R. (Eds.). (1982). *Ability testing: Uses, consequences,
and controversies*. Washington, DC: National Academy of Sciences.

Wiggins, C. W., Wygant, D. B., Hoelzle, J. B., & Gervais, R. O. (2012). The more
you say the less it means: Overreporting and attenuated criterion validity in a
forensic disability sample. *Psychological Injury and the Law, 5*, 162–173.

Wilde, M. C. (2006). The validity of the Repeatable Battery of Neuropsychological
Status in acute stroke. *The Clinical Neuropsychologist, 20*, 702–715.

Wilde, M. C. (2010). Lesion location and Repeatable Battery for the Assessment of
Neuropsychological Status performance in acute ischemic stroke. *The Clinical Neuropsychologist, 24*, 57–69.

Wilk, C. M., Gold, J. M., Humber, K., Dickerson, F., Fenton, W., & Buchanan, R. W.
(2004). Brief cognitive assessment in schizophrenia: Normative data for the
Repeatable Battery for the Assessment of Neuropsychological Status. *Schizophrenia Research, 70*, 175–186.

Wilkinson, G. S., & Robertson, G. J. (2006). *Wide Range Achievement Test–4*. Lutz,
FL: Psychological Assessment Resources.

Williams, T. H., McIntosh, D. E., Dixon, F., Newton, J. H., & Youman, E. (2010).
Confirmatory factor analysis of the Stanford–Binet Intelligence Scales, Fifth
Edition, with a high-achieving sample. *Psychology in the Schools, 47*, 1071–
1083.

Winstead, B. A., & Sanchez, J. (2012). The role of gender, race, and class in psychopathology. In J. E. Maddux & B. A. Winstead (Eds.), *Psychopathology: Foundations for a contemporary understanding* (3rd ed., pp. 69–100). New York:
Routledge.

Witteman, C. L. M., Harries, C., Bekker, H. L., & Van Aarle, E. J. M. (2007). Evaluating psychodiagnostic decisions. *Journal of Evaluation in Clinical Practice,
13*, 10–15.

Woodcock, R. W., McGrew, K. S., & Mather, N. (2007). *Woodcock–Johnson III Tests
of Achievement*. Rolling Meadows, IL: Riverside.

Woodcock, R. W., McGrew, K. S., Schrank, F. A., & Mather, N. (2007). *Woodcock–Johnson III normative update*. Rolling Meadows, IL: Riverside.

World Health Organization. (2012). *Measuring health and disability: Manual for WHO Disability Assessment Schedule (WHODAS 2.0)*. Geneva, Switzerland: Author.

Wynia, M. K., Cummins, D. S., VanGeest, J. B., & Wilson, I. B. (2000). Physician manipulation of reimbursement rules for patients: Between a rock and a hard place. *Journal of the American Medical Association, 283*, 1858–1865.

Young, J. C., Baughman, B. C., & Roper, B. L. (2012). Validation of the Repeatable Battery for the Assessment of Neuropsychological Status—Effort Index in a veteran sample. *The Clinical Neuropsychologist, 26*, 688–699.

Youngjohn, J. R., Lees-Haley, P. R., & Binder, L. M. (1999). Comment: Warning malingerers produces more sophisticated malingering. *Archives of Clinical Neuropsychology, 14*, 511–515.

Youngjohn, J. R., Wershba, R., Stevenson, M., Sturgeon, J., & Thomas, M. L. (2011). Independent validation of the MPI-2-RF somatic/cognitive and validity scales in TBI litigants tested for effort. *The Clinical Neuropsychologist, 25*, 463–476.

Zimmerman, M. D. (2003). What should the standard of care for psychiatric diagnostic evaluations be? *Journal of Nervous and Mental Disease, 191*, 281–286.

Zimmerman, M. D., & Mattia, J. I. (1999a). Differences between clinical and research practices in diagnosing borderline personality disorder. *American Journal of Psychiatry, 156*, 1570–1574.

Zimmerman, M. D., & Mattia, J. I. (1999b). Is posttraumatic stress disorder underdiagnosed in routine clinical practice? *Journal of Nervous and Mental Disorders, 187*, 420–428.

Zimmerman, M. D., & Mattia, J. I. (1999c). Psychiatric diagnosis in clinical psychiatry: Is comorbidity being missed? *Comprehensive Psychiatry, 40*, 182–191.

Index